Prostate Cancer from a Nuclear Oncology Perspective

Kalevi Kairemo

Prostate Cancer from a Nuclear Oncology Perspective

A Personal Journey

Springer

Kalevi Kairemo
Theranostics & Nuclear Medicine
Docrates Cancer Center
Helsinki, Finland

ISBN 978-3-031-90336-6 ISBN 978-3-031-90337-3 (eBook)
https://doi.org/10.1007/978-3-031-90337-3

This Springer imprint is published by the registered company Springer Nature Switzerland AG
The registered company address is: Gewerbestrasse 11, 6330 Cham, Switzerland

Preface

This book reviews diagnostic and therapeutic methods of prostate cancer (PCa) from a nuclear oncology point of view. The author has had a very special perspective on the development of PCa research, mainly through happy coincidences since 1980s. My academic dissertation dealt with radiolabeled monoclonal antibodies (MoAb) in clinical oncology; luckily there was also clinical grade MoAb production in Finland, against a target associated with PCa. I was extremely enthusiastic in participating in international scientific congresses and presenting tumor targeting work. I learned in Sydney in 1989 about the radiopharmaceutical ^{153}Sm-EDTMP for bone pain palliation; after being in another conference in New Zealand, I received from Australian researchers ten lyophilized kits, which I brought in my suitcase to Helsinki. In the same year I was about to start my fellowship at Memorial Sloan-Kettering Cancer Center in New York. At the same time, we in Finland managed to get enriched with ^{152}Sm from Kazakhstan and thus produce ^{153}Sm-EDTMP in Helsinki. Very soon we were running a clinical trial in Finland, which became the start of this kind of radionuclide therapy in PCa. Then, in New York I learned of scientists who worked in various fields of MoAb imaging. I became interested in targeted therapies and theranostics, and basically insisted on having a targetor for prostate cancer as well. Unfortunately, most of the attempts failed until 2010s. Some of this history has been described in this book, but again from a nuclear medicine point of view and the author's own history.

The diagnostics of PCa improved substantially since early 2000s, especially in the development of PET radiopharmaceuticals. I had the privilege to introduce many tracers into clinical routine practice in my home regions, including Na^{18}F, ^{18}F-FCH, ^{18}F-FACBC, ^{68}Ga-PSMA-11, ^{18}F-PSMA-1007, and ^{18}F-DCFPyL. Thus indications in various PCa subgroups have been discussed in detail as well the pros and cons in clinical practice. Surprisingly, during my affiliation at the Docrates Cancer Center in Helsinki there was tremendous interest in PCa, and a critical mass for supportive oncology and tumor biology research existed. In the author's practice, radiation therapy has been more important than surgery; therefore, e.g., PET-based dose planning for radiation therapy is presented in this book. The author has also followed the development of radiopharmaceutical treatments, bone pain palliation with several radiopharmaceuticals ($^{89}SrCl_2$, ^{186}ReHEDP, ^{153}SmEDTMP, ^{117m}SnDTPA, and $^{223}RaCl_2$), and targeted treatments (^{177}Lu-PSMSA-617, ^{177}Lu-PSMA-I&T, and ^{225}Ac-PSMA). Because we had production for clinical grade radiopharmaceuticals in Helsinki, I was able to start therapy tourism to Finland. This was very vivid, because patients were seeking for new effective radionuclide treatments in prostate cancer as well. Work periods in the pharmaceutical industry such as Advanced Accelerator Applications SA in France and a visiting professorship in the prestigious MD Anderson Cancer Center in Houston have contributed to my development and judgment. Because of this experience, I was asked to help other countries to set up new targeted treatments, first in Baltic and Nordic countries, then elsewhere in Europe, then in North America (e.g., Canada), and finally in Africa (e.g., Ghana).

My situation changed dramatically 3 years ago, when I was suspected of having PCa. The book includes my personal story as a prostate cancer survivor. Ironically, the ultimate diagnosis was made by the method that I had personally developed. Therefore, some sections of the book look at the developments from the patient's point of view.

This book is meant to be a comprehensive cross-section of history and the current situation of PCa theranostics, spiced up with my own experiences from both the doctor's and the patient's point of view. I wish you pleasant moments while reading the book.

Helsinki, Finland Kalevi Kairemo

Acknowledgments

Because the book describes the history of prostate cancer (PCa) since late 1980s, the key persons essential for the birth of this work are listed almost chronologically. I learned about prostate in early 1980s. My first contact with nuclear medicine took place as summer work in 1985 in the Nuclear Medicine Department of Helsinki University Hospital. Olof Alfthan, urology professor, taught me about basics of prostate cancer and Professor Kristian Liewendahl about basic elements of nuclear medicine. I learned very early in 1985 that nuclear medicine methods gave the best answer, e.g., in skeletal metastases of prostate cancer. In early 1987 I decided to focus on immunoscintigraphy (radioimmunodetection) in my dissertation. I traveled with my own money to the European Association of Nuclear Medicine (EANM) conference in Budapest, Hungary, in 1987. There I made multiple contacts with radiopharmaceutical companies. Ultimately, I had heard about Steven M. Larson's Georg de Hevesy lecture on radiolabeled monoclonal antibodies at the Budapest EANM 1987. I never could imagine that I would meet him personally at the 1988 Society of Nuclear Medicine and Molecular Imaging (SNMMI) conference in San Francisco (CA) and that I would present two clinical posters about immunoscintigraphy. After discussions, he offered a fellowship at Memorial Sloan-Kettering Cancer Center (MSKCC). One year after this meeting, I worked in Steve Larson's lab. At home, after the Budapest conference, I had conducted several clinical studies in hundreds of patients using multiple monoclonal antibodies. Additionally, I made contact with Professor Pirkko Vihko of University of Oulu in northern Finland where they had developed monoclonal antibodies against PCa. As a result of this collaboration we started clinical studies and trials in Helsinki with Prof. Alfthan using immunolymphoscintigraphy and intraprostatic injections.

Additionally, Prof. Alfthan came to see me in New York and introduced me to his urology professor colleague William H. Fair at MSKCC. Juha Ellmen from Farmos (Medipolar) came to see me in New York as well and provided some of their own antibodies to be studied in NYC. Prof. Fair's research fellow Craig Zippe had developed an animal model and we tested targeting with limited success. I also learned to know Warren "Skip" Heston and Carlos Cordon-Cardo who had worked on "PSMA" precursors, but not with in vivo targeting experiments. Steve Larson let me to also discuss with the North Carolina group who had developed monoclonal antibodies, i.e., "Prostascint® predecessors." To my disappointment, no greater interest was in the monoclonal antibody front at MSKCC. In 1989, before my MSKCC visit I went to Sydney, Australia, to a Radiopharmacology Congress. I learned there about bone pain palliation for PCa metastases using Sm-153-EDTMP. Australian Nuclear Science and Technology Organization (ANSTO) donated ten ethylenediamine tetramethylene phosphonic acid (EDTMP) kits, which I took in my suitcase to Finland. Under the leadership of Jukka Hiltunen from the Reactor Laboratory of the State Research Center (VTT, Otaniemi), I learned to label this compound with Sm-153. The original compound was developed by J. Harvey Turner whom I learned to know properly 10 years later. Jukka Hiltunen from MAP Medical Technologies (est. 1992) managed to get Sm-152 from Russia, and we started to produce Sm-153-EDTMP for clinical trials. Similarly, I introduced Re-186-HEDP for bone metastasis treatment in Finland 2 years later and presented my results at the EANM (European Association of Nuclear Medicine) conference in Lissabon, Portugal 1992. I never had time to publish these good results.

I went back to MSKCC and became next involved in the alpha therapy project. Prof. Sakari Rannikko, the new urology professor in Helsinki, contacted me and asked about the new tracers. This was the initiation of my estramustine project. My goal was to develop a "triple action" agent, i.e., a tumor targeting, cytotoxic (chemotherapy), radiotoxic (radionuclide therapy) agent, because I knew that estramustine targets prostate tissue. We wanted to develop labeled estramustine derivatives; this became Dr. Kaarlo Ståhlberg's academic dissertation project. Unfortunately, we could not develop such a compound for multiple reasons. The key person to help me in this was Per Björk at Astra in Lund, Sweden, and I got also their newest antibody for testing. We found interesting things that could be published in the scientific literature. In 1999 I was working in Norwegian University of Science and Technology (NTNU) in Norway when I heard about my father's PCa diagnosis. In 2001, I moved to the Uppsala University Hospital for almost 5 years; my task was to establish a new nuclear medicine clinic. There I learned from my predecessors that they were using Ra-223 for treating skeletal metastases. At the opening symposium of my clinic, Roy Larsen from Oslo gave a talk about treatment of skeletal metastases using alpha-emitters. Later I learned that that was the very first presentation in the whole world about the topic. Roy Larsen, Öyvind S. Bruland, and Sten Nilsson are Ra-223 patent holders, and their work resulted in marketing authorization in 2013 (first alpha emitter in clinical therapy). Uro-oncology professor Sten Nilsson at Karolinska Institute was my predecessor in Uppsala, Sweden. He also acted as an opponent for Kaarlo Ståhlberg's academic dissertation. Uppsala was a fruitful environment for my development in this field, because I was in charge of Experimental Nuclear Medicine, Per-Uno Malmström of Experimental Urology, Jörgen Carlsson of Radiobiology, and Hans Lundqvist of Radiation Physics. We built together the Medical Radiation Sciences. Our focus, however, was very little on prostate cancer. In the Nuclear Medicine Clinic, I learned from Jens Sörensen the role of ^{11}C-acetate-PET in PCa.

From Sweden I moved back to Finland because of family reasons and the increasing demand in our progress in the biotechnology industry.

Then the next milestone in my development in the field of prostate cancer was the work at Advanced Acceleration Applications SA (AAA) in France. The first compound for prostate cancer diagnosis was fluorocholine. I also learned about its production. From there I moved to Finland for the second time because of family reasons. At the same time, Docrates Cancer Center was about to start the radiotheranostics field. This was the first full service private oncology clinic in Northern Europe. The radiopharmaceutical Co. MAP had full service GMP production, and cyclotron for radiopharmaceuticals was located in the same building in the city center of Helsinki. The first new radiopharmaceuticals were introduced for routine clinics in 2010.

We started with GMP grade Na^{18}F-production. For this possibility I am very thankful to Jarmo Haukka (Chairman of the Board) and Mika Nyyssönen (CEO) at MAP. The Docrates Cancer Center turned out to be very friendly for prostate cancer diagnostics and therapeutics. Prof. Timo Joensuu was the local key opinion leader in prostate cancer supported by urology professor Martti Ala-Opas and radiology professor Kaarina Partanen. I learned a lot about prostate cancer MRI-imaging from Kaarina and from radiologist Merja Raade. The environment was very ideal to build a prostate theranostic facility. After Na^{18}F we introduced ^{18}F-choline, and to back up temporary problems in choline production, I introduced ^{18}F-fluciclovine, which was transported from my former institute, Uppsala University Hospital, by airplane. In mid-2010 we switched to PSMA-radiopharmaceuticals and we started with Ga-68-PSMA-11 production. Because of temporary problems in radiosynthesis and logistics, we switched to ^{18}F-PSMA-1007 production. At the same time we started to develop agents for PSMA therapy: for GMP production both ^{177}Lu-PSMA-617 and ^{177}Lu-PSMA-617-I&T.

A few years earlier we had done extensive therapy development with Ra-223. Together with Timo Joensuu and our physicists Aki Kangasmäki and Timo Kiljunen we developed dosimetry and response evaluation tools. In the practical therapy with ^{177}Lu-PSMA, I am very thankful for all the guidance from my European colleagues, Prof. Irene Virgolini from Innsbruck, Austria, and Prof. Richard P. Baum from Bad Berk, Germany. I am very thankful to Danish oncology professor colleague Finn Edler von Eyben. We shared the interest of prostate cancer research, and we could combine our forces by conducting systematic reviews of current situation. We made a meta-analysis about the characteristics of radiocholine imaging in prostate cancer diagnosis, the efficacy of ^{177}Lu-PSMA as third-line treatment (after radiotherapy/surgery and chemotherapy), and a network meta-analysis to be compared with the new therapies in similar patient populations of advanced disease. Additionally we analyzed the role of serum PSA (in the follow-up of prostate cancer) in very large population.

I was very fortunate to get a visiting professor position at The University of Texas MD Anderson Cancer Center (MDACC) in Houston, Texas, USA, in 2015. There I made acquaintance with very large patient populations, e.g., I was able to study thousands of cycles of Ra-223 in prostate cancer. In prostate cancer imaging I was able to analyze some tracers that I never used earlier in my studies, such as C-11-choline and F-18-DCFBC. The software for image analysis was very comprehensive and I was able develop new methods, e.g., for dual tracer imaging data from Finland. Additionally, I developed some new criteria for analyzing response. I am deeply thankful to Prof. Homer A. Macapinlac, the Chair of the Nuclear Medicine Department. I had multiple important collaborators at MDACC, but without the help of Vivek Subbiah (Investigative New Drugs and Phase One Department), S. Cheenu Kappadath (Physics Department), and Gregory Ravizzini (Center for ABI), I would not have been able to improve my own imaging modalities and develop new response criteria for radionuclide therapies. For practical matters in this book, I am thankful to Riku Parviainen, MSc, for drawing the chemical structures of the compounds, and to Timo Korkama, MSc, for practical assistance in computer problems.

I know that I have not been able to list all the names who should have been here. I have been very lucky to publish more than 50 prostate cancer-related publications, even the number of collaborators is a three-digit number. I am thankful to all these collaborations.

Finally I got my own prostate cancer diagnosis in 2022. I would not be writing this story without my own initiatives to challenge what conventional health care was providing. Actually the ultimate diagnosis was done with the method I established in Finland. Without this knowledge I would not have the treatments I got. Therefore, I am very thankful for the life path I had chosen. Without this experience I could not understand this disease from the patient's point view. Without this experience this book would never have been written.

Helsinki, Finland Kalevi Kairemo

Competing Interests The author has no competing interests to declare that are relevant to the content of this manuscript.

Contents

Introduction: Prostate Cancer from the Point of View of the Author and the History of Imaging

1

The book describes the history of prostate cancer diagnostics starting from prostate cancer specific or associated monoclonal antibodies and small molecules. The development includes introduction of multiple metabolic PET tracers, such as choline and acetate. Subsequently, amino acid targeting tracers were developed, and the discovery of PSMA changed the paradigm in the prostate cancer theragnostics. These PET tracers are discussed with various therapeutic applications. The therapy focus in this book lies on therapeutic radionuclide applications such as Ra-223-chloride, Lu-177-PSMA, and Ac-225-PSMA. Multicenter trials are presented as well as systematic reviews including meta-analyses and network meta-analyses.

The writer has worked almost 40 years in this field; thus, much of the presented work reflects own experience what comes to the nuclear oncology point of view. However, the writer is also a prostate cancer survivor so that he can look at the disease from a patient perspective. Therefore, general aspects of prostate cancer are reviewed in this chapter. Some of the facts have been controlled from two of my favorite textbooks of prostate cancer [1, 2].

Prostate Cancer in a Nutshell

The prostate gland produces seminal fluid and controls urine flow. Most common diseases are prostatitis, benign prostatic hyperplasia (BPH), and cancer, which have to be understood, e.g., in the differential diagnosis of imaging or clinical symptomatology. Very much is known of the nature of cancer; risk factors such as age, genetics, and diet; and the incidence of prostate cancer, especially among aging men. Diet and lifestyle changes could help reduce cancer risk, like increasing physical activity and consuming certain foods, but these are not discussed here. The diagnosis and detection methods are explained in detail, especially what comes to radionuclide imaging. Serum prostate-specific antigen (S-PSA) tests are discussed, because the author has laboratory medicine education (clinical chemistry specialist/professor). Some treatment options for prostate cancer are outlined, including radiation

K. Kairemo, *Prostate Cancer from a Nuclear Oncology Perspective*,
https://doi.org/10.1007/978-3-031-90337-3_1

therapy, hormone therapy, and new radionuclide therapies. Introduction of new effective radiopharmaceuticals has forced nuclear medicine physicians to become more treating clinicians, partly due to patient centered individual decision-making and partly due to balancing treatment effets with potential side effects.

This book discusses in a little extent life after treatment, focusing on recovery, managing side effects like urinary incontinence, and improving quality of life, but this information is mainly based on own experience as patient and what own patients have told. Most of the treated patients by the author have been more advanced cases, meaning that this book gives better guidance to metastatic prostate cancer treatments, bone pain management, and options for castration-resistant prostate cancer. The writer is aware of coping mechanisms for living with prostate cancer and maintaining a healthy lifestyle post-diagnosis, including stress management, diet, and exercise. But no recommendations to others will not be given. Own case is presented in a detail from the nuclear oncology point of view.

Some Specific Aspects of Prostate Cancer

Most common diseases, prostatitis, benign prostatic hyperplasia (BPH), and cancer, may all elevate S-PSA. Prostatitis can be acute or chronic. BPH is a noncancerous enlargement of the prostate, very common in older men, which may cause urinary symptoms. Prostate cancer is characterized by the uncontrolled growth of abnormal cells, which can spread beyond the prostate. It is the most common male cancer in the Western world and the second most common in the world, with 1.6 million new cases per year, with risk increasing with age.

There are no typical symptoms of prostate cancer, but they may include difficulty in urinating, frequent urination, or blood in the urine. Many cases are asymptomatic until the cancer has advanced, highlighting the importance of early detection through laboratory screening or imaging. The key idea is to identify high-risk cancers, because some prostate cancers do not need treatment besides active surveillance.

A blood test that measures serum PSA level may indicate prostate cancer, if elevated, but it is not specific and it may be elevated in other prostatic diseases. Thus, routine screening is controversial, unless combined with additional laboratory tests (including urine tests) or specific imaging. Additional imaging may also cause difficulties in the differential diagnosis. The focus in this book is in molecular imaging, because they turned out be powerful in high-risk cancers.

The diagnosis is based on biopsy which can be made, e.g., guided by transrectal ultrasound (TRUS) or magnetic resonance imaging (MRI) if a suspicious cite in the prostate is known. A biopsy involves removing tissue samples from the prostate to confirm cancer. If clear focus for biopsy cannot be identified, systemic sectoral prostate biopsies can be taken. After diagnosis, the stage will be determined (how far cancer has spread) and grade (how aggressive the cancer is) is crucial to know. The pathological classification is based on Gleason score (or now ISUP score).

The treatment options for localized and advanced prostate cancer include active surveillance, surgery (e.g., radical prostatectomy), radiation therapy, hormone therapy, chemotherapy, and immunotherapy. The selection of management depends based on the stage, grade, and other patient related factors.

Patients have to weigh their options by considering factors such as age, overall health, cancer stage, and personal preferences. The importance of informed patient centered decision-making and patient involvement in treatment plans is essential.

Different types of radiation therapy, external beam radiation therapy (EBRT) and brachytherapy, are discussed in this book, especially treatment planning, because molecular imaging can be applied there.

Surgery plays an essential role in the first line therapy, but not discussed in detail in this book. In brief, radical prostatectomy, a surgery that removes the entire prostate and surrounding tissues, which can be performed via laparoscopy and/or and by robotic techniques, is the most common procedure. Transurethral resection of the prostate (TURP) is a less invasive surgery used primarily to treat BPH by removing part of the prostate. Possible complications like urinary incontinence and erectile dysfunction may occur after surgery. These side effects may also occur after radiation therapy.

Prostate cancer is hormone dependent, and thus hormone therapy, also known as androgen deprivation therapy (ADT), reduces testosterone levels to slow cancer growth. Different approaches, including LHRH agonists and antiandrogens, and their potential side effects such as hot flashes and bone loss have to be taken into consideration.

When prostate cancer has metastasized, treatment focuses on controlling the spread and managing symptoms. Here ADT and radiation therapy have a certain role. Castration-resistant prostate cancer is a form of the disease that no longer responds to hormone therapy. Newer treatments like enzalutamide and abiraterone target cancer that continues to grow despite low testosterone levels. Staging is based on PSA tests and imaging, where especially PET methods have demonstrated their strength, in combination with morphology (CT or MRI).

Advanced diseases require systemic therapies, including chemotherapy and targeted therapies, for advanced stages. There are multiple new drugs which have been developed. Additionally, new radionuclide therapies have been developed. Multiple new technical innovations, such as high intensity focused ultrasound (HIFU), cryotherapy, and new forms of radiation therapy, have been introduced. This book describes also challenging cases, where these methods may provide a solution. Local symptoms, such as bone pain, may be treated with local approaches, e.g., with EBRT. In general, pain from bone metastases can be treated using radiation, pain medications, systemic radionuclide therapies, and treatments like bisphosphonates to strengthen bones and reduce pain.

In this book, estimates of the likely course of the disease based on the stage, grade, and other factors are given. Similarly, survival rates, including how early detection and less aggressive cancer types can lead to better outcomes, will be discussed.

About Own History

The writer knows how it feels to live with a diagnosis of prostate cancer. In the literature, there are multiple coping strategies for men diagnosed with prostate cancer, including emotional support, managing anxiety, and maintaining quality of life, but the writer can only speak from own experience. Therefore, the only real advice is to accept the situation and be in contact with real world specialists, i.e., with patient organizations and prostate cancer survivors.

I was personally aware of that certain risk factors (age, genetics, male sex); I was diagnosed at the age of 67, my father at age of 69, but he had a disease which only required active surveillance. But my lifestyle has been consisting of regular physical activity and a low-fat, high-fiber diet rich in fruits and vegetables, with no tobacco and no alcohol—in addition to a functional marriage of more than 42 years. With my own assumptions, I was convinced that with a marginally elevated PSA I could not have an aggressive prostate cancer that has to be treated. My history is discussed in detail in this book. I will discuss in detail the side effects of the treatment, such as urinary incontinence.

I hope that this book will help the prostate cancer community to interact with each other.

References

1. Roy Berger E, Lewis J Jr. Updated guidelines for surviving prostate cancer. 1st ed. Jericho: Health Education Literary Publisher; 2004. 464 p. ISBN 1-4107-9127-0
2. Larry Goldenberg S, Pickles T, Chi KN. Intelligent patient guide to prostate cancer. 4th ed. Granville Island Publishing Ltd.; 2014. 318 p. ISBN 978-0-9811599-2-8

Part I

Experimental

2 Integrated Summary of Research on Radioiodinated Estramustine Phosphate and Estramustine Binding Protein Antibody in Prostate Cancer Treatment

This chapter explores the therapeutic applications and mechanisms of estramustine phosphate (EMP) and radioiodinated estramustine binding protein antibody (EMBP-AB) in the treatment of prostate cancer [1, 2]. The studies reviewed provide insights into the use of these agents as radiosensitizers and targeted therapy options, respectively, highlighting both their potential and limitations in clinical settings.

Estramustine

Chemotherapeutic agents that targeted the nuclear matrix and microtubule function turned out to be particularly active in prostate cancer in late 1980s. Estramustine, a 17-β-estradiol phosphate derivative linked to a nor-nitrogen mustard molecule, was utilized in multiple chemotherapy regimens for prostate cancer. Its chemical structure is shown in Fig. 2.1.

Originally it was developed as an alkylating agent—estramustine had shown activity in prostate cancer possibly unrelated to its hormonal or alkylating effects. Estramustine binds to microtubule-associated proteins (MAPs) in the nuclear

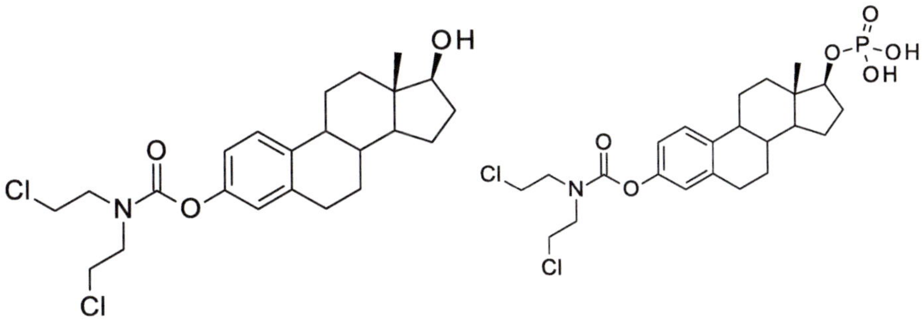

Fig. 2.1 Estramustine (left) and estramustine phosphate (right)

K. Kairemo, *Prostate Cancer from a Nuclear Oncology Perspective*,
https://doi.org/10.1007/978-3-031-90337-3_2

matrix and inhibits microtubule assembly and disassembly [3, 4]. The antimitotic effects of estramustine in prostate cancer have been shown in vivo in animals implanted with DU145 prostate tumor cell lines [5]. As a single agent, estramustine has shown an overall response rate of 14–48%, with subjective improvements in pain and performance status [6, 7]. Differing response criteria have resulted in the wide response rates. For example, in the Danish Prostatic Cancer Group (DAPROCA) 9002 trial, patients with a decline in prostate-specific antigen (PSA) of only 25% were classified as responders, while in other studies patients were classified as responders based on palliative endpoints [8]. The addition of estramustine to other chemotherapeutic agents that affect microtubule function improves response rates [9–13]. For example, Hudes et al. completed a phase III trial treating patients with either estramustine with vinblastine or vinblastine alone [13]. They demonstrated that patients receiving estramustine had an increased response rate and decreased time to progression. Overall survival was not significantly improved on the initial report but was significant on a later analysis with longer follow-up. Similarly, Berry et al. treated patients with HRPC with estramustine and paclitaxel or paclitaxel alone [14]. They found a similar result; estramustine improved PSA response rate but not overall survival. Studies with estramustine in combination with other antimicrotubule agents have also been completed, as described later in this chapter.

Radioiodinated Estramustine Phosphate

Estramustine phosphate, a chemotherapy agent with antimitotic properties, has been extensively used in the treatment of hormone-refractory prostate cancer since the early 1990s. Beyond its direct anticancer effects, EMP was investigated for its ability to enhance the effectiveness of radiotherapy. The primary mechanism by which EMP acts as a radiosensitizer is not through the induction of apoptosis, as might be expected, but rather through its impact on microtubule dynamics. The chemical structure of EMP is shown in Fig. 2.1.

EMP inhibits mitosis by binding to tubulin, leading to the depolymerization of microtubules, which are essential for cell division [3, 4]. This action arrests cells in the G2/M phase of the cell cycle, a stage where they are particularly susceptible to the effects of radiation. In studies involving human prostate cancer cells xenografted into mice, treatment with EMP alongside radiation led to significant tumor regression compared to radiation alone. Interestingly, this enhanced effect on tumor shrinkage was not accompanied by an increase in apoptotic cell death, suggesting that other cellular mechanisms might be at play [15].

Radioiodinated Estramustine Binding Protein Antibody

EMBP-AB targets estramustine binding proteins highly expressed in prostate tissue, making it a potential vehicle for delivering radioactive isotopes directly to cancer cells. Our studies assessed the distribution and efficacy of radioiodinated EMBP-AB in mice with prostate cancer xenografts [1, 2].

Although EMBP-AB effectively accumulates in prostate tissue, its rapid clearance from these sites and significant accumulation in nontarget organs pose major challenges. The studies demonstrated that while the prostate and tumor tissues initially take up the radioactive compound, the rapid decline in tumor-specific radioactivity limits the therapeutic usefulness of this approach [1, 2].

The findings indicate that the therapeutic potential of radioiodinated EMBP-AB is compromised by its biodistribution profile. High accumulation in nontarget tissues could lead to adverse effects if used in therapeutic doses, highlighting the need for carrier molecules with better selectivity and retention properties.

The methodologies employed in these investigations include experimental treatments of prostate cancer models in mice. These models were treated with EMP and/or subjected to radiotherapy to evaluate the radiosensitizing properties of EMP [1, 2]. Similarly, the distribution and therapeutic potential of EMBP-AB were assessed using biodistribution studies, where the compound's presence in various organs was meticulously tracked over time [1, 2]. The biodistribution data of radioiodinated EMBP-AB is shown in Fig. 2.2.

The use of EMP as a radiosensitizer should be optimized to leverage its cell cycle arrest capabilities without relying on apoptosis. This could involve combining EMP with other modalities that induce cell death or developing new EMP formulations that enhance its radiosensitizing efficiency.

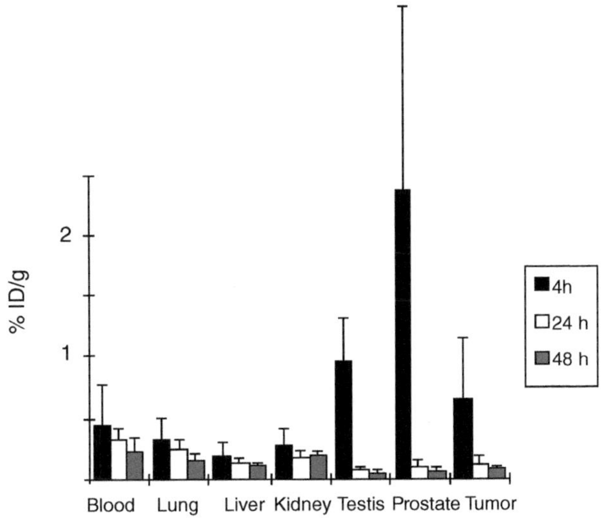

Fig. 2.2 Distribution of radioactivity 4–48 h after an injection of radioiodinated estramustine binding protein antibody in mice with DU-145 prostate cancer xenografts as percentage of the injected activity pre gram tissue (%ID/g); error bars indicate standard deviation [2]

Fig. 2.3 Organ-to-blood ratios of radioiodinated (I-125 or I-131) estramustine binding protein antibody in mice with DU-145 prostate cancer xenografts as a ratio of injected activity per tissue weight [2]

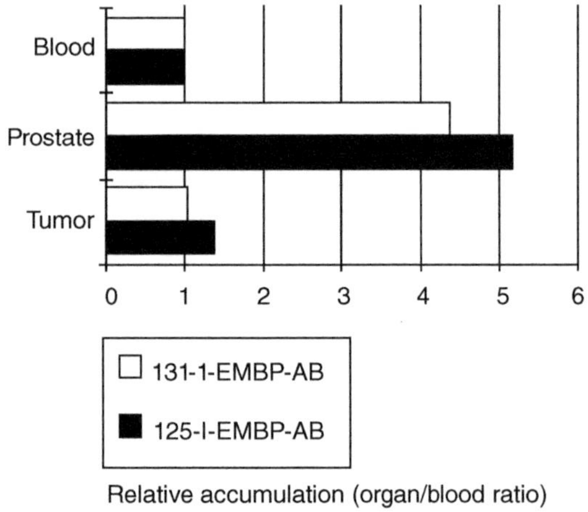

The application of radioiodinated EMBP-AB in prostate cancer treatment appears limited by its biodistribution characteristics [1, 2]. Figure 2.3 demonstrates that tumor-to-blood ratios are low as compared to prostate-to-blood ratios [2]. Therefore, we decided that our research should focus on improving the specificity and binding affinity of EMBP-AB or similar agents to ensure more targeted and effective radionuclide therapy.

The studies reviewed illustrate the complex interplay between drug mechanisms and therapeutic outcomes in the treatment of prostate cancer. While estramustine shows promise as a radiosensitizer, its clinical use must be carefully managed to maximize its benefits. Similarly, while radioiodinated EMBP-AB has potential as a targeted therapy, its current formulation does not meet the necessary criteria for effective and safe clinical application [1, 2]. Continued innovation and research are essential to overcome these challenges, with the ultimate goal of improving survival and quality of life for patients with prostate cancer.

Estramustine and Radiotherapy in Prostate Cancer

We analyzed the application of estramustine in the context of prostate cancer, particularly its use in conjunction with radiotherapy. Both works by Ståhlberg et al. [15, 16] explored different aspects of how estramustine, an antimitotic cytostatic drug, enhances the effects of radiotherapy by interacting with prostate cancer treatments.

Mechanism and Effects on Radiotherapy Enhancement

In the beginning, we delved into the role of estramustine as a radiosensitizer, which is not mediated through enhancing radiation-induced apoptosis [15]. The study involves DU-145 human prostate cancer cells xenografted into nude mice, treated

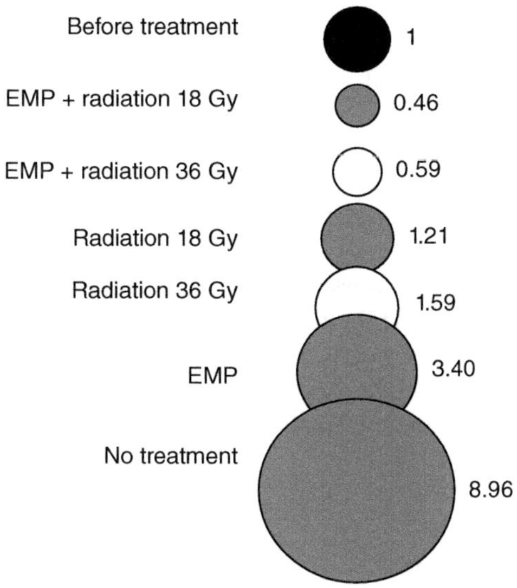

Fig. 2.4 Average change in tumor size in relation to the size before treatments. The area represents relative volume before treatments (black) and 4 weeks later after treatments (gray). The white circles are measured at 3 weeks with higher radiation dose (36 Gy), because of side effects. *EMP* estramustine phosphate [15]

with both estramustine and radiation. Results indicated that while tumor size regressed significantly in mice treated with both therapies, the expected increase in apoptosis was not observed, suggesting that radiosensitization by estramustine occurs through mechanisms other than apoptosis enhancement [15]. Figure 2.4 summarizes the results in mice treated with both estramustine and/or radiation in all combinations. It is obvious that EMP acts as a radiation sensitizer in combination with radiation in this experimental therapy and this combination has a clear therapeutic effect whereas estramustine or radiation alone are not effective [15]. Besides apoptosis, we discussed other potential mechanisms, such as mitotic arrest and microtubule interference, which could underpin the sensitization effect [15]. We analyzed tumor hypoxia in the same tumor model and found that EMP did not improve tumor oxygenation but enhanced the ability of radiotherapy to cause tumor necrosis [16]. The hypoxia was assessed by [^{18}F]FMISO uptake in experimental arrangement, where one group received only EMP, one only EBRT, one both EMP and EBRT, and one no treatment all [16].

Radioiodinated Estramustine Binding Protein Antibody in Treatment

After that, we investigated the distribution and potential therapeutic use of radioiodinated estramustine binding protein antibody (EMBP-AB) in mice with prostate cancer xenografts [2]. This study assessed whether EMBP-AB could effectively deliver radioactive iodine to prostate tumors. The findings revealed that while EMBP-AB accumulates in the prostate and tumor tissues, it does not offer significant therapeutic benefits over other organs which also accumulate the radioactive substance. Consequently, we learned the use of RI-EMBP-AB in radionuclide therapy for prostate cancer may not be beneficial due to its nonselective organ distribution and associated risks of high radioactivity in nontarget tissues.

Combining Estramustine with Other Treatments

Both these works [1, 2] underscored the complexity of using estramustine in cancer therapy. While it has a proven effect in enhancing the efficacy of radiotherapy, its mechanism does not involve simple augmentation of apoptosis. The exploration of EMBP-AB as a carrier for radioisotopes also brings to light the challenges of targeting treatment precisely at cancer cells without affecting surrounding healthy tissues [1, 2].

Therapeutic Implications and Future Directions

The research suggests a need for continued exploration of estramustine's radiosensitizing mechanisms and potential combination therapies that could better target tumor cells while minimizing side effects. Further studies could also explore the use of different isotopes or carrier molecules that might provide more effective and safer distribution patterns within the body.

Clinical Significance of Estramustine in Castration Resistant Prostate Cancer

A systematic review and meta-analysis by Qin et al. [17] investigates nine studies of a total of 956 patients treated between 1993 and 2010. The study aimed to assess the effectiveness and safety of adding estramustine to chemotherapy regimens for patients with CRPC, a condition where prostate cancer progresses despite androgen deprivation therapy. The primary endpoint was overall survival (OS), analyzed using hazard ratios (HRs). Secondary endpoints included PSA response rates and the incidence of grade 3 or 4 toxicities, both analyzed using odds ratios (ORs).

Key findings of the meta-analysis were as follows: Patients treated with chemotherapy plus estramustine had a significantly higher PSA response rate compared to those receiving chemotherapy alone (OR = 1.84, 95% CI = 1.20–2.80). There was no significant difference in OS between the two groups (HR = 0.90, 95% CI = 0.77–1.05), indicating that adding estramustine does not improve survival. No significant differences were observed in the incidence of grade 3 or 4 side effects between the groups, including serious conditions like anemia, neutropenia, and thromboembolic events [17].

The authors suggest that while estramustine improves PSA response, it does not confer a survival advantage or reduce the incidence of serious side effects [17]. The analysis highlights the need for careful consideration of estramustine's role in chemotherapy for CRPC, given its lack of impact on survival and manageable toxicity profile.

The authors suggest that while estramustine improves PSA response, it does not confer a survival advantage or reduce the incidence of serious side effects [17]. The analysis highlights the need for careful consideration of estramustine's role in chemotherapy for CRPC, given its lack of impact on survival and manageable toxicity profile [17]. Grade 3 and 4 toxicity data of chemotherapies with and without estramustine are shown in Table 2.1 [17].

The article by Goodin et al. [18] provides a detailed overview of the challenges and treatment strategies for CRPC, a condition where prostate cancer progresses despite hormone therapy.

Table 2.1 Outcomes of grade 3 or 4 toxicity comparing chemotherapy plus estramustine versus the same chemotherapy without estramustine

	Toxicity trials	Chemotherapy with estramustine	Chemotherapy without estramustine	OR[a] (95% CI[b])	P
Anemia	6	14/302	18/300	0.78 (0.38, 1.57)	0.481
Neutropenia	6	46/325	49/325	0.91 (0.59, 1.43)	0.694
Thrombocytopenia	4	2/247	4/250	0.68 (0.19, 2.42)	0.547
Nausea	5	10/280	3/278	2.34 (0.81, 6.72)	0.114
Vomiting	4	7/247	2/250	2.43 (0.69, 8.51)	0.166
Fatigue	5	11/292	18/297	0.67 (0.32, 1.41)	0.293
Neuropathy	3	6/199	12/204	0.54 (0.21, 1.44)	0.222
Allergic reaction	4	3/200	1/193	1.60 (0.37, 6.84)	0.529
Thromboembolic event	3	14/199	6/204	2.18 (0.86, 5.51)	0.101
Edema	2	2/154	2/157	1.02 (0.18, 5.95)	0.980

Modified from [17]

[a]*OR* odds ratio, [b]*CI* confidence interval

Table 2.2 Estramustine and taxane regimens studied in CRPC

	First patients reported	PSA response[a]	Measurable disease response	Final report
Estramustine 600 mg/m²/d po, paclitaxel 120 mg/m² continuous infusion over 96 h q 21 d	34	7/32 (53%)	4/9 (45%)	Hudes et al. [19]
Estramustine 280 mg bid d 0–2, paclitaxel 90 mg/m² q wk × 6 q 8 wk	63	36/62 (58.1%)	6/22 (27.3%)	Wong et al. [20]
Estramustine 280 mg bid d 1–3, 8–10, 15–17 and paclitaxel 100 mg/m² d 2, 9, 16 versus paclitaxel 100 mg/m² d 2, 9, 16	166	48%	n.a.	Berry et al. [21]
Estramustine 280 mg po tid d 1–5, docetaxel 40–80 mg/m² d 2 q 21 d	34	20/34 (63%)	5/18 (28%)	Petrylak et al. [22]

Updated from Goodin et al. [18]

[a]PSA response defined as a 50% or greater decrease in PSA from baseline

This work lists FDA-approved agents estramustine and mitoxantrone among the approved treatments for HRPC, noting that combinations of these drugs can induce a biochemical response in over 50% of patients, though the median response duration is typically 6 months.

The focus on estramustine in both reviews [17, 18] suggests its relevance in current treatment protocols but also highlights the need for therapies that can extend survival, not just manage symptoms or slow disease progression. The research dosing of estramustine and taxane regimens is shown in Table 2.2 [18]. As research evolves, the integration of new molecularly targeted therapies could provide breakthroughs necessary for significantly improving outcomes in HRPC treatment.

The management of CRPC by chemotherapy is complex and evolving, with a current focus on extending the duration of response and overall survival through combination therapies and novel agents targeting specific resistance mechanisms. The ongoing research aims to refine these strategies to improve outcomes for patients with this challenging form of cancer.

Conclusive Comments

Nonclinical

In conclusion, estramustine remains a valuable tool in the treatment of prostate cancer, particularly in its capacity to enhance the effects of radiotherapy. However, its exact mechanisms and optimal use protocols still require further research to fully harness its potential while ensuring patient safety. The ongoing exploration of molecular carriers like EMBP-AB also illustrates the potential for innovative approaches to cancer treatment, although with cautious consideration of their systemic effects. None of the radioligands of estramustine, estramustine phosphate, or

EMBP-AB did not fulfill the criteria required for a functional targeting chemoradiotherapy compound. Therefore, this field is not anymore active.

My own research contributed significantly to the understanding of estramustine's role in cancer therapy, providing insights into its benefits and limitations as a treatment enhancer. Further research and clinical trials will be crucial, if developing more effective and targeted therapeutic strategies using estramustine and related compounds.

Clinical

The synthesis of the findings in the reviews provides oncologists and researchers with a comprehensive view of the therapeutic challenges and innovations in treating advanced prostate cancer, guiding future strategies and research directions in oncology. It was found that adding estramustine to chemotherapy does not improve survival nor increase side effects. Therefore, new more potent agents have replaced it from current uro-oncology practice.

References

1. Ståhlberg K, Kairemo KJA, Karonen S-L, Jekunen AP, Taari K, Rannikko S. Biodistribution of radioiodinated estramustine phosphate and estramustine binding protein antibody in mice. Prostate. 1997;32:1–8.
2. Ståhlberg K, Kairemo K, Karonen SL, Taari K, Rannikko S. Distribution of radioiodinated estramustine binding protein antibody in mice with DU-145 prostate cancer xenograft. Anticancer Res. 2007;27:2275–8.
3. Hartley-Asp B, Kruse E. Nuclear protein matrix as a target for estramustine-induced cell death. Prostate. 1986;9:387–95.
4. Pienta KJ, Lehr JE. Inhibition of prostate cancer growth by estramustine and etoposide: evidence for interaction at the nuclear matrix. J Urol. 1993;149:1622–5.
5. Hartley-Asp B. Estramustine-induced mitotic arrest in two human prostatic carcinoma cell lines DU 145 and PC-3. Prostate. 1984;5:93–100.
6. Yagoda A, Smith JA, Soloway MS, et al. Phase II study of estramustine phosphate in advanced hormone refractory prostatic cancer with increasing prostate specific antigen levels. J Urol. 1991;145:384a.
7. Iversen P, Rasmussen F, Asmussen C, et al. Estramustine phosphate versus placebo as second line treatment after orchiectomy in patients with metastatic prostate cancer: DAPROCA study 9002. Danish Prostatic Cancer Group. J Urol. 1997;157:929–34.
8. Attivissimo LA, Fetten JV, Kreis W. Symptomatic improvement associated with combined estramustine and vinblastine chemotherapy for metastatic prostate cancer. Am J Clin Oncol. 1996;19:581–3.
9. Hudes GR, Greenberg R, Krigel RL, et al. Phase II study of estramustine and vinblastine, two microtubule inhibitors, in hormone-refractory prostate cancer. J Clin Oncol. 1992;10:1754–61.
10. Hudes GR, Nathan FE, Khater C, et al. Paclitaxel plus estramustine in metastatic hormone-refractory prostate cancer. Semin Oncol. 1995;22(suppl 12):41–5.
11. Petrylak DP, Shelton G, Judge T, et al. Phase I trial of docetaxel plus estramustine in androgen-insensitive prostate cancer. Proc Am Soc Clin Oncol. 1997;16:310a.

12. Mareel MM, Storme GA, Dragonetti CH, et al. Antiinvasive activity of estramustine on malignant MO4 mouse cells and on DU-145 human prostate carcinoma cells in vitro. Cancer Res. 1988;48:1842–9.
13. Hudes G, Einhorn L, Ross E, et al. Vinblastine versus vinblastine plus oral estramustine phosphate for patients with hormone-refractory prostate cancer: a Hoosier Oncology Group and Fox Chase Network phase III trial. J Clin Oncol. 1999;17:3160–6.
14. Berry W, Gregurish M, Dakhil S, et al. Phase II randomized trial of weekly paclitaxel (Taxol®) with or without estramustine phosphate in patients with symptomatic, hormone-refractory, metastatic prostate cancer. Proc Am Soc Clin Oncol. 2001;20:175a.
15. Ståhlberg K, Kairemo K, Erkkilä K, et al. Radiation sensitizing effect of estramustine is not dependent on apoptosis. Anticancer Res. 2005;25:2873–8.
16. Ståhlberg K, Kämäräinen E-L, Keyriläinen J, Virtanen I, Taari K, Kairemo K. Hypoxia in DU-145 prostate cancer xenografts after estramustine phosphate and radiotherapy. Curr Radiopharm. 2010;3:19–24.
17. Qin Z, Li X, Zhang J, et al. Chemotherapy with or without estramustine for treatment of castration-resistant prostate cancer: a systematic review and meta-analysis. Medicine (Baltimore). 2016;95(39):e4801.
18. Goodin S, Rao KV, DiPaola RS. State-of-the-art treatment of metastatic hormone-refractory prostate cancer. Oncologist. 2002;7:360–70.
19. Hudes GR, Nathan F, Khater C, et al. Phase II trial of 96-hour paclitaxel plus oral estramustine phosphate in metastatic hormone-refractory prostate cancer. J Clin Oncol. 1997;15:3156–63.
20. Wong YN, Manola J, Hudes GR, et al. Phase 2 study of weekly paclitaxel plus estramustine in metastatic hormone-refractory prostate carcinoma: ECOG-ACRIN Cancer Research Group (E1898) trial. Clin Genitourin Cancer. 2018;16:e315–22.
21. Berry WR, Hathorn JW, Dakhil SR, et al. Phase II randomized trial of weekly paclitaxel with or without estramustine phosphate in progressive, metastatic, hormone-refractory prostate cancer. Clin Prostate Cancer. 2004;3:104–11.
22. Petrylak DP, Macarthur RB, O'Connor J, et al. Phase I trial of docetaxel with estramustine in androgen-independent prostate cancer. J Clin Oncol. 1999;17:958–67.

Part II

Clinical Diagnostics

Summary of Diagnostic Accuracy of ^{18}F-Fluorocholine PET/CT in Prostate Cancer Staging

3

^{18}F-Fluorocholine (^{18}F-FCH) PET/CT

^{18}F-fluorocholine (^{18}F-FCH) PET/CT has been widely used in primary and recurrent prostate cancer (PCa) and has been shown to add valuable information. Although there is a correlation between the foci of activity and the areas of malignancy in the prostate gland, the clinical value of ^{18}F-FCH is still controversial for detection of the malignant focus in the prostate. For the T-staging of PCa at diagnosis, the value of ^{18}F-FCH is limited. This is probably due to limited resolution of PET system and positive findings in benign prostate diseases. Conversely, ^{18}F-FCH PET/CT is a promising imaging modality for the delineation of local and distant nodal recurrence and bone metastases and is poised to have an impact on therapy management. In this chapter, studies of ^{18}F-FCH PET/CT in PCa are summarized.

Choline acts as a precursor for the biosynthesis of phospholipids, e.g., phosphatidylcholine, the major component of the plasma membrane [1]. Carcinogenesis is characterized by enhanced cell proliferation and membrane synthesis with increased demand on phospholipids. Thus, as simplified, it reflects increased cellular membrane activity in prostate cancer. Figure 3.1 shows the chemical structures of most commonly used ^{11}C-choline or ^{18}F-choline.

Already the first studies in early 2010s indicated that ^{18}F-dluorocholine (^{18}F-FCH) PET/CT is superior in the diagnostic use in prostate cancer staging over traditional imaging techniques like CT or MRI. Several reviews emphasized the importance of precise lymph node staging for optimal treatment planning in prostate cancer patients [2, 3]. The systematic reviews [2, 3] collectively highlighted that ^{18}F-FCH PET/CT offers higher specificity but lower sensitivity when compared to

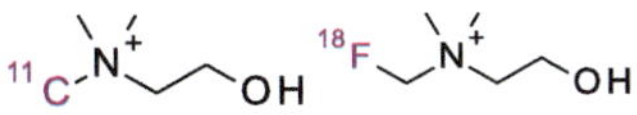

Fig. 3.1 The chemical structures of most commonly used ^{11}C-choline (left) or ^{18}F-choline (right)

K. Kairemo, *Prostate Cancer from a Nuclear Oncology Perspective*,
https://doi.org/10.1007/978-3-031-90337-3_3

conventional imaging techniques. This indicates that while ^{18}F-FCH PET/CT is excellent at confirming lymph node metastases when they are indeed present (high specificity), it struggles to detect all actual cases of lymph node metastases (low sensitivity).

Despite its high specificity, the relatively low sensitivity of ^{18}F-FCH PET/CT limits its utility as a stand-alone diagnostic tool. It is recommended for use in conjunction with other diagnostic modalities to improve accuracy in staging prostate cancer. Therefore, in the evolution, new tracers with higher sensitivity should be developed.

Lymph Node Staging

Seven studies involving a total of 627 patients were included in the analysis. The findings highlighted a pooled sensitivity of 57% and a specificity of 94% for ^{18}F-FCH PET/CT in lymph node staging [4]. The positive likelihood ratio was 10.2, suggesting that a positive test result is a strong indicator of lymph node metastases. Conversely, the negative likelihood ratio was 0.46, indicating moderate utility in ruling out lymph node metastases when the test result is negative. The diagnostic odds ratio was calculated to be 22, underscoring the method's overall diagnostic value [4].

^{18}F-FCH PET/CT shows high specificity but only moderate sensitivity for the detection of metastatic lymph nodes in newly diagnosed prostate cancer patients. It proves to be a valuable tool for confirming lymph node metastases when results are positive but has limitations as a stand-alone diagnostic tool for lymph node staging due to its moderate sensitivity. This study supports the use of ^{18}F-FCH PET/CT alongside traditional imaging methods to enhance the accuracy of preoperative lymph node staging in prostate cancer [4].

Bone Metastases

In the work by Guo et al. [5], the primary goal was to systematically review and meta-analyze the effectiveness of choline PET/CT, specifically using ^{11}C-choline or ^{18}F-choline, in detecting bone metastases in prostate cancer patients. This was prompted by the need for more reliable diagnostic tools beyond conventional imaging techniques like bone scans and MRI, which may lack sensitivity and specificity [5].

The methodological quality of included studies was evaluated using the Quality Assessment of Diagnostic Accuracy Studies-2 (QUADAS-2) tool, ensuring the robustness and reliability of the findings up to February 20, 2018. Fourteen studies consisting of 840 patients met the inclusion criteria and were deemed to have reasonable methodological quality [5].

In diagnostic performance metrics on a per-patient basis, the pooled results showed the following values: sensitivity of 0.89 (95% confidence interval [CI]

0.80–0.94), specificity of 0.98 (95% CI 0.95–0.99), positive likelihood ratio of 40.4 (95% CI 19.7–82.6), negative likelihood ratio of 0.12 (95% CI 0.07–0.20), and diagnostic odds ratio of 344 (95% CI 148–803) [5].

On a per-lesion basis, the pooled sensitivity was 0.91, and specificity was 0.97, further affirming the high diagnostic accuracy. Choline PET/CT demonstrated excellent sensitivity and specificity, making it a highly effective tool for detecting bone metastases in prostate cancer patients.

Despite its high accuracy, a negative choline PET/CT result could not conclusively rule out the presence of bone metastases, indicating the need for additional testing in some cases to ensure comprehensive diagnostic coverage [5].

Before the analysis by Guo et al. [5], MRI was studied in two Chinese meta-analyses [6, 7]. Concerning metastases detection, whole body MRI has been largely compared to choline PET/CT and to bone scintigraphy, reporting higher detection rates. Shen et al. [6] performed a meta-analysis comparing diagnostic performance for bone metastases in PCa patients of whole body MRI, ^{11}C-choline PET/CT, bone SPECT, and bone scintigraphy. The pooled sensitivities on a per-patient basis of MRI were 97% (95% CI 91–99%), compared to 91% with ^{11}C-choline PET/CT and 79% with bone scan [6]. Concerning specificity, the authors reported pooled specificities of 95% with whole body MRI and 99% with ^{11}C-choline PET/CT. These results should be interpreted with caution given the limitations of ^{11}C-choline PET/CT in PCa detection. Moreover, the utility of adding diffusion-weighted imaging to MRI was highlighted by a meta-analysis by Li et al. [7], in which 32 studies with 1507 patients were analyzed. On a per-patient based analysis, pooled sensitivity, specificity, and area under the curve for DWI were of 95% (95% CI 90–97%), 92% (95% CI 88–95%), and 0.98, respectively.

Own Meta-Analysis and Experience

We made 5 years earlier, before the last Chinese meta-analysis, a detailed meta-analysis evaluating the effectiveness of ^{11}C-choline or ^{18}F-choline PET/CT scans in managing prostate cancer. This analysis covered original studies from 1998 to September 2013, involving a total of 3167 patients reported in 47 articles [8].

Our meta-analysis highlights that choline PET/CT has a pooled sensitivity of 62% and a specificity of 92% for detecting pelvic lymph node metastases. This indicates a reliable performance in identifying metastatic nodes. We also found that choline PET/CT is more effective than bone scanning and [^{18}F]^{18}F-fluoro-2-deoxy-D-glucose (FDG) PET/CT in detecting prostate cancer recurrences, especially in patients with lower PSA levels who often show negative results with conventional imaging [8]. Additionally, in a significant portion of the study, 41% of patients with positive choline PET/CT findings experienced changes in their treatment plans based on imaging results [8]. These changes often led to a complete PSA response in 25% of cases, indicating that imaging findings directly contributed to effective management strategies [9]. We wrote an additional review where we included technical aspects related to the timing of acquisitions and other technical parameters [9],

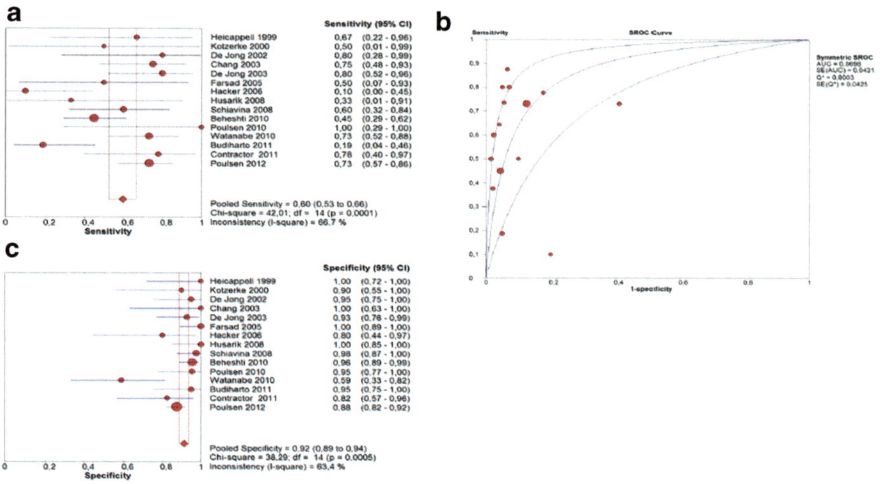

Fig. 3.2 Sensitivity (**a**), specificity (**b**), and SROC curve (**c**) for detection of pelvic lymph node metastases according to PET/CT and pelvic node dissection for patients with biochemical recurrence [8]

and additionally we presented data up to 6000 patients in 2 conferences in November 2013: in the first Indian Cancer Congress in New Delhi and in the eighth ICRT World Congress in Radiopharmaceutical Therapy in Manila in the Philippines. These larger population numbers were never published, because the characteristics remained almost identical, and we were about to introduce new radiopharmaceuticals with higher sensitivity. Figure 3.2 from our data demonstrates the performance characteristics of the analysis by von Eyben and Kairemo [8]—sensitivity (A), specificity (B), and SROC curve (C)—for detection of pelvic lymph node metastases according to PET/CT and pelvic node dissection for patients with biochemical recurrence [8].

Already more than 10 years ago, choline PET/CT was presented as a preferable first-line imaging option for restaging prostate cancer in patients with biochemical recurrence, specifically those with PSA levels between 1.0 and 50 ng/ml [8].

It is especially valuable for identifying the locations of recurrence and guiding subsequent treatment modifications, which may range from intensified localized treatment to adjustments in systemic therapy [8].

A strange meta-analysis with the QUADAS-2 tool was performed a short time after our meta-analysis was published [10]. It compared ^{18}F-FDG, ^{11}C-choline, ^{18}F-choline, and ^{11}C-acetate in a total of 56 studies containing 3586 patients. ^{18}F-FCH-PET/CT was considered as a superior diagnostic tool over the other three radiotracers [10]. Area under ROC curve (AUC) of SROC was 0.94, 95% CI 0.92–0.96, for ^{18}F-choline and 0.73, 95% CI 0.69–0.77, for ^{18}F-FDG [10].

Patient Image Examples of Using Choline PET

Biochemical Recurrence

Figures 3.3, 3.4 and 3.5 demonstrate three patient cases imaged with biochemical recurrence and with low PSA values using ^{11}C-choline. Figure 3.3 demonstrates a lymph node metastasis in the left internal iliac region (PSA = 2.9 μg/l). Figure 3.4 demonstrates a local recurrence in the prostate bed (PSA = 2.2 μg/l). Figure 3.5 shows a recurrence in the skeleton (PSA = 4.4 μg/l). All images are from the pelvic region. In general, the short 20-min half-life of ^{11}C limits the imaging possibilities besides the radiopharmacokinetics of choline.

At the beginning, imaging with ^{18}F-choline often included imaging at different time points, because the uptake increased in metastases as a function of time. The introduction of ^{18}F-choline allowed imaging at 1–3 h and increased specificity in findings.

Figure 3.6 shows a patient with biochemical recurrence after radical prostatectomy and with a rather low PSA value (S-PSA = 6.3 μg/l) using ^{18}F-choline. His case was presented in a Russian journal because of a rather intense therapy tourism from Central Asia to Western Europe [11].

Figure 3.7 shows how with multiple time points the diagnostic accuracy of ^{18}F-choline imaging can be increased. With lipophilic tracers, such as ^{18}F-choline, the assessment of liver metastases can be cumbersome because of high physiologic uptake in the liver and in the reticuloendothelial system. This patient had multiple liver metastases at the time of show up. With the knowledge of limitations of ^{18}F-choline in the assessment of liver metastases, multiple time points were applied [12]. The SUVmax values with ^{18}F-choline varied from 9.3 to 12.6 in early images (at 15 min) and from 9.4 to 13.0 in late images (at 60 min). This showed that the normal is physiologic uptake in the liver decreased substantially to late images, whereas the uptake in the liver metastases still increased slightly. This helped the visualization and most importantly we confirmed the findings with a liver biopsy [12].

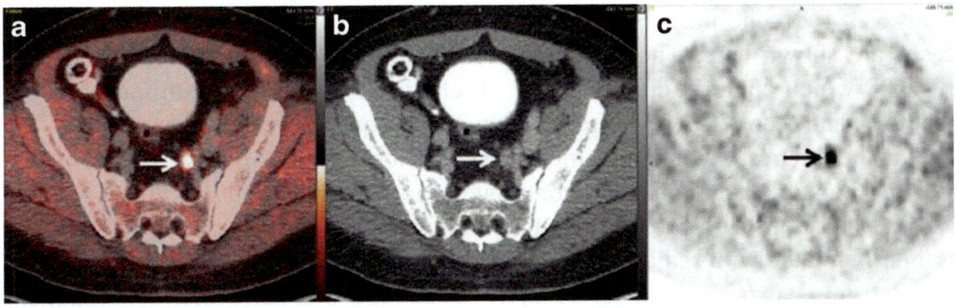

Fig. 3.3 A 58-year old man with prostate adenocarcinoma with biochemical recurrence (S-PSA = 2.9 μg/l) after radiation therapy. Axial ^{11}C-choline PET/CT fusions (**a**), CT (**b**), and PET (**c**) demonstrate a lymph node metastasis in the left internal iliac region; size 2.1 cm × 1.1 cm

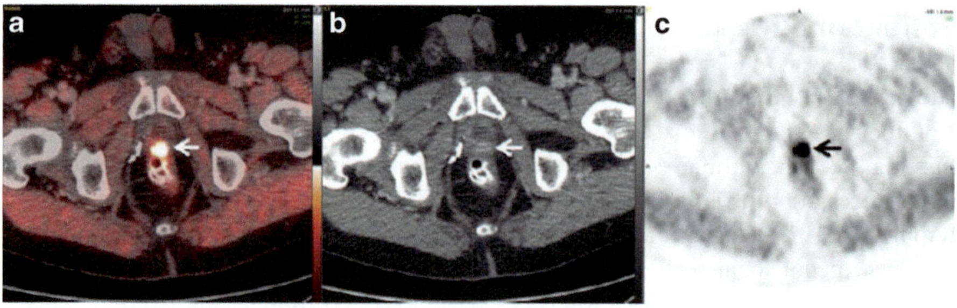

Fig. 3.4 A 71-year-old man with prostate adenocarcinoma with biochemical recurrence (S-PSA = 2.2 μg/l) after radical prostatectomy. Axial PET/CT fusions (**a**), CT (**b**), and PET (**c**) demonstrate a local recurrence in the prostate bed. SUVmax of 5.0 with ^{11}C-choline

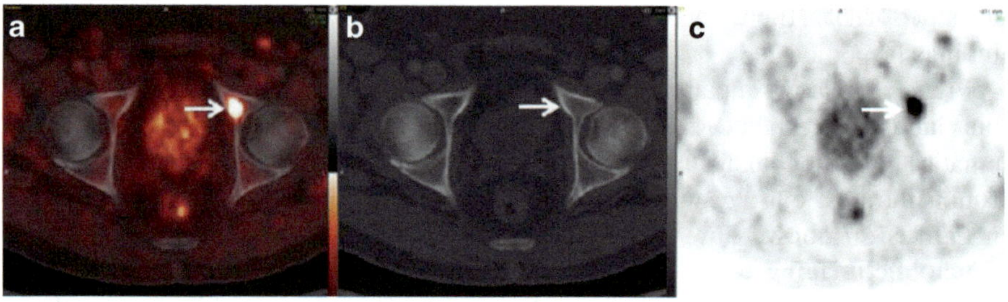

Fig. 3.5 A 68-year-old man with prostate adenocarcinoma with biochemical recurrence (S-PSA = 4.4 μg/l) after radical prostatectomy. Axial PET/CT fusions (**a**), CT (**b**), and PET (**c**) demonstrate a local skeletal metastasis in the left acetabulum. SUVmax of 6.1 with ^{11}C-choline

Response Evaluation

Molecular imaging in the differential diagnosis of prostate has been powerful from the very beginning, and it has increased our knowledge about the metastatic disease. Extremely peculiar cases have been shown in the literature, and these molecular imaging methods have help to identify new exotic locations of recurrence and guided subsequent treatment modifications, as we already concluded in our meta-analysis [8]. ^{18}F-choline can be used for assessing therapy response. Two additional cases are shown here. The first case is unusual and rare perineural invasion in Fig. 3.8 which could be identified by ^{18}F-choline PET but not with morphologic methods, and there was a clear response to a subsequent new treatment.

Another interesting patient demonstrated left locoregional disease (lymph nodes, soft tissues, and skeleton) and a contralateral testicular metastasis (Fig. 3.9). This 71-year-old male with prostate adenocarcinoma (Gleason score 8, T3N0M0) was primarily treated with radiation therapy and adjuvant hormone therapy. The S-PSA elevated in 3 years to the level 29 ug/l. ^{18}F-choline was performed for treatment planning. A large (max size 10 cm) parailiac soft-tissue uptake and another soft-tissue (max size 5 cm) uptake were seen in the funicle of the right testis. A skeletal

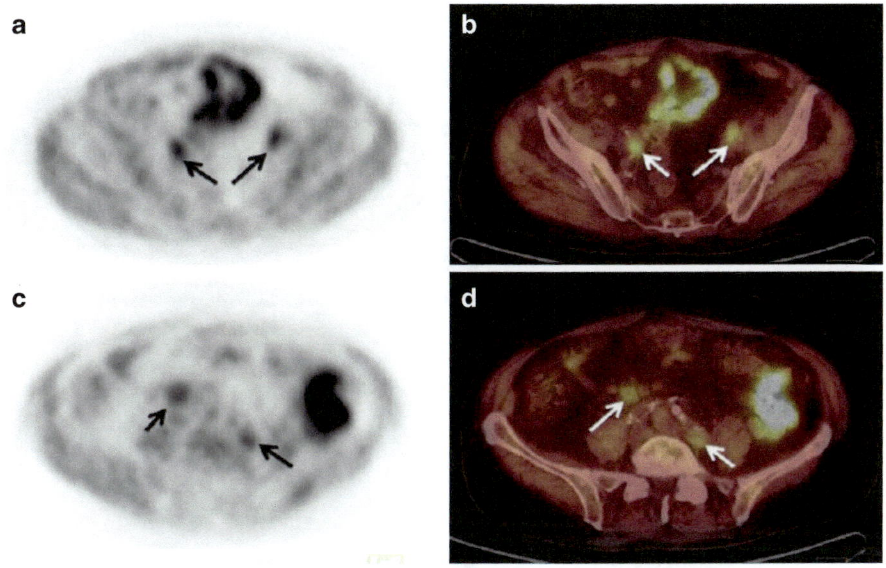

Fig. 3.6 An 83-year-old man with prostate adenocarcinoma and biochemical recurrence (S-PSA = 6.3 μg/l) after radical prostatectomy. Axial ^{18}F-choline PET images (**a**, **c**) and PET/CT fusions (**b**, **d**) demonstrate uptakes bilaterally in internal iliac regions (**a**, **b**) and in enlarged lymph nodes retroperitoneally (**c**, **d**). SUVmax values varied from 4.5 to 5.4 in these lymph nodes compatible with lymph node metastases. There is physiologic uptake in the bowel due to enterohepatic clearance [9]

lesion was found in the left pelvic region including the sacrum, acetabulum, and os ilium, which was also seen on Na^{18}F-PET. These pelvic lesions were treated with radiation therapy using PET guidance, and the testicular lesion was operated. Histology of the 30-g testis showed extensive metastatic lesions in the testicle, rete testis and epididymis, metastatic prostate adenocarcinoma, a poorly differentiated adeno-PCa (upper right), and positive staining with PSA (lower right) (Fig. 3.9).

Interestingly, in this patient, the contralateral testicular metastasis might be due to hematogenic spread, but in an extreme unusual location for prostatic adenocarcinoma. After orchiectomy and radiotherapy, PSA decreased down to 1.1 ug/l.

Interestingly, I managed to report a patient with no findings in the literature [13]. A 57-year-old man was administered with 326 MBq (8.81 mCi) ^{18}F-choline at 12:50 p.m. for a PET study. The next morning at 7:00 a.m. when he entered his workplace at a nuclear power plant, all alarms sounded. His radioactivity level was measured to be 0.35 MBq (9.5 μCi), i.e., approximately of 1/930 original activity corresponding physical decay of fluorine-18 which has 110 min half-life.

Already these practical examples show how much complementary and sometimes crucial information can be obtained by prostate PET imaging. All this development led to prostate PET becoming part of everyday practice—already ^{18}F-choline fulfilled the required criteria.

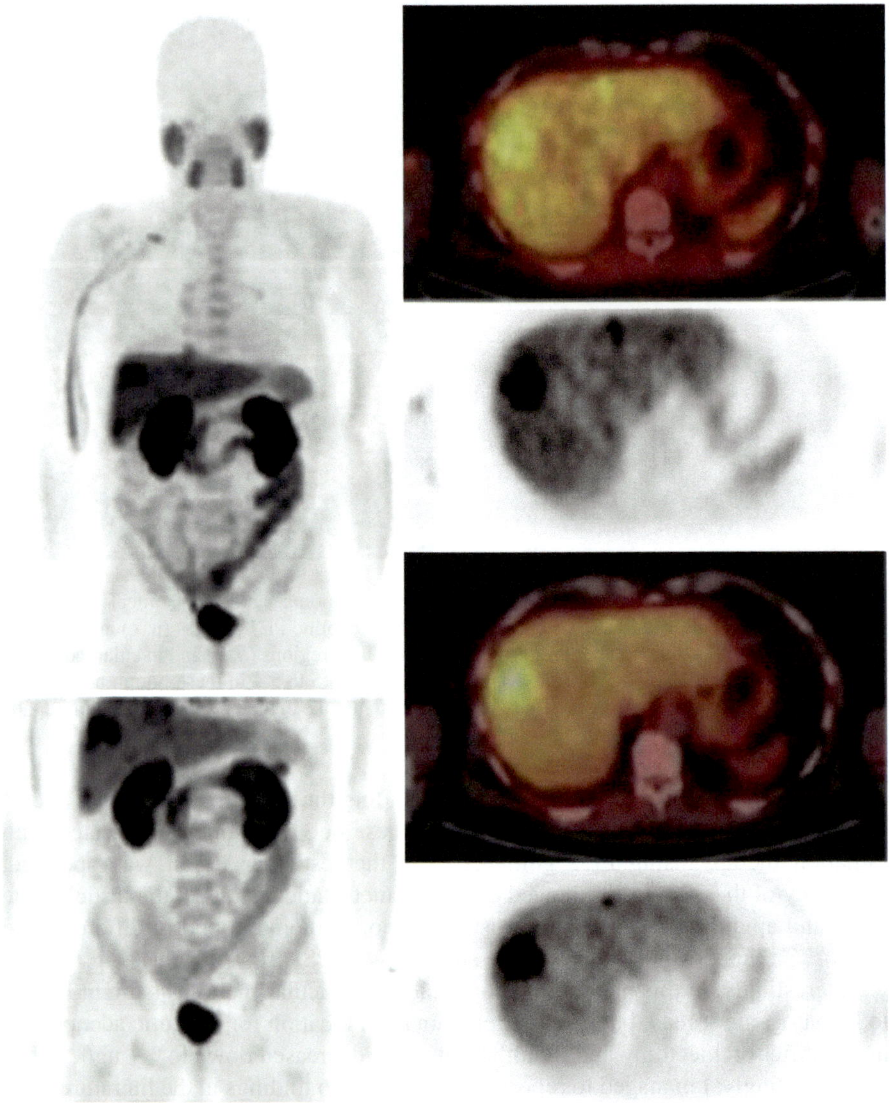

Fig. 3.7 A 62-year-old man with prostate adenocarcinoma and biochemical recurrence (S-PSA = 6.7 μg/l) after radical prostatectomy. Whole body MIP images on the left, early time point at 15 min (upper panel) and late at 60 min (lower panel). On the right, corresponding axial ^{18}F-choline PET/CT fusions and PET images at early and late time points are shown. Early images (upper panel) demonstrate one large uptake, whereas late images demonstrate clearly multiple (four) lesions (lower panel). The SUVmax values varied from 9.3 to 12.6 in early images and from 9.4 to 13.0 in late images. This means that the normal is physiologic uptake in the liver decreases to late images, whereas the uptake in the liver metastases slightly increases. The histology (HE staining) from the liver biopsy including PSA staining showed that the findings were consistent with prostate cancer liver metastases [12]

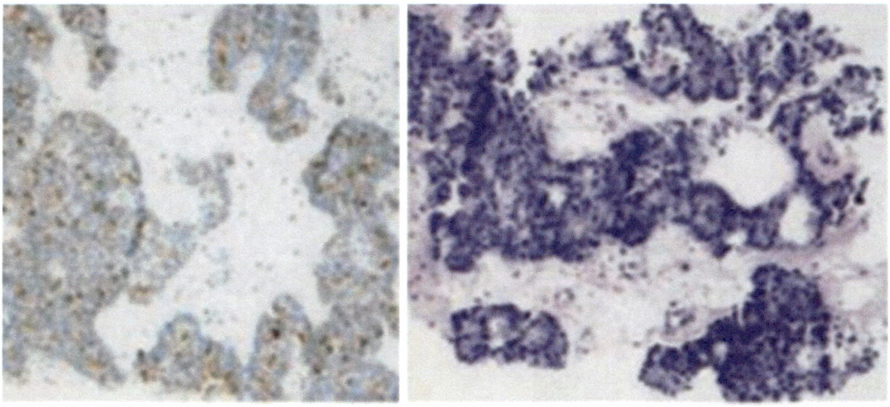

Fig. 3.7 (continued)

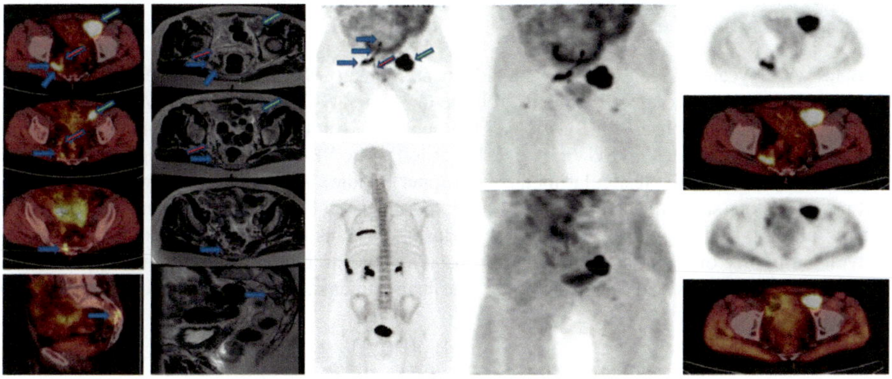

Fig. 3.8 A 67-year-old man with prostate adenocarcinoma (GS 10, ISUP 5) and biochemical recurrence after prostatectomy developed immediately skeletal metastases which could be controlled with zolendronic acid (S-PSA = 0.2 μg/l), but now a new relapse (S-PSA = 18.5 μg/l). On the left, ^{18}F-choline PET/CT fusions and corresponding MRI images (three axial, one sagittal) and ^{18}F-choline PET MIP image from the pelvic region and whole body Na^{18}F image. Na^{18}F PET shows lesions in the left VII and VIII ribs. Arrows indicate lesion sites in PET/CT fusion, MRI, and pelvic images to better understand the anatomic locations. On the right, whole body MIP images in the left panels, baseline before chemotherapy (upper panel) and 5 weeks later (lower panel). In the panels most right corresponding axial ^{18}F-choline PET images and PET/CT fusions at the time of relapse and 5 weeks later after chemotherapy (docetaxel). Baseline images (upper panel) demonstrate one large uptake in the left iliac lymph node and a longitudinal uptake in sacral canal (perineural invasion) and in mesorectal fascia. In later images (lower panel), the the uptakes in sacral and mesorectal fascia have disappeared, and the uptake in the large left iliac lymph node has decreased. There is thus a clear response to the chemotherapy

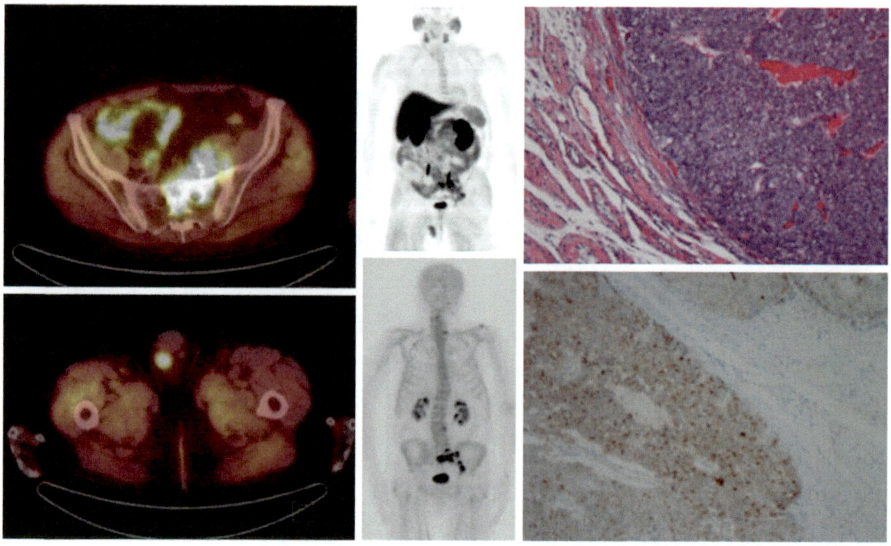

Fig. 3.9 A 71-year-old man with prostate adenocarcinoma (GS 8, ISUP 4) treated with radiation therapy and hormone therapy developed a relapse in 3 years (S-PSA = 29.1 μg/l). A left parailiacic soft-tissue uptake was observed (SUVmax 7.0; upper left). Another soft-tissue uptake was seen in the funicle of the right testis (SUVmax 6.7; lower left). The ^{18}F-choline MIP image demonstrates the pelvic lesions and the testicular metastasis (upper middle). A skeletal lesion was found in the left pelvic region (sacrum, acetabulum, os ilium; SUVmax 11.4) and was also seen on Na^{18}F-PET [lower middle]. Histology showed extensive metastatic lesions in the testicle, rete testis, and epididymis, a poorly differentiated metastatic prostate adenocarcinoma (HE staining; upper right), and positive staining with PSA (lower right). After treatments, the S-PSA is decreased down to 1.1 μg/l

Conclusive Comment

The reviewed material in this chapter and own wide experience underline the role of ^{18}F-choline PET/CT in the staging of prostate cancer, particularly in assessing lymph node metastasis. While it offers a high degree of specificity, its application is limited by lower sensitivity. Therefore, it should not be used as the sole diagnostic tool but rather as part of a multimodal diagnostic approach. This combination can help in making more informed decisions regarding the management and treatment planning of prostate cancer patients.

For further reading and deeper insights into the research discussed, accessing the original studies and systematic reviews can provide additional details on the methodologies and patient outcomes associated with this diagnostic technology.

The meta-analyses solidify the role of ^{11}C-choline and ^{18}F-choline PET/CT in enhancing the diagnostic pathway for prostate cancer, particularly in cases of biochemical recurrence. By providing detailed information on metastatic locations and the likelihood of recurrence, choline PET/CT assists in optimizing treatment strategies and potentially improving patient outcomes. This review supports broader use of choline PET/CT in clinical practice, underlining its superior diagnostic capabilities compared to traditional methods. Nowadays, ^{18}F-choline PET has been widely replaced with more sensitive PET tracers which are discussed in other chapters.

References

1. Zeisel SH. Dietary choline: biochemistry, physiology, and pharmacology. Annu Rev Nutr. 1981;1:95–121.
2. Bauman G, Belhocine T, Kovacs M, Ward A, Beheshti M, Rachinsky I. 18F-fluorocholine for prostate cancer imaging: a systematic review of the literature. Prostate Cancer Prostatic Dis. 2012;15:45–55.
3. Evangelista L, Zattoni F, Guttilla A, et al. Choline PET or PET/CT and biochemical relapse of prostate cancer: a systematic review and meta-analysis. Clin Nucl Med. 2013;38:305–14.
4. Kim SJ, Lee SW. Diagnostic accuracy of ^{F}18 flucholine PET/CT for preoperative lymph node staging in newly diagnosed prostate cancer patients; a systematic review and meta-analysis. Br J Radiol. 2019;92:20190193.
5. Guo Y, Wang L, Hu J, Feng D, Xu L. Diagnostic performance of choline PET/CT for the detection of bone metastasis in prostate cancer: a systematic review and meta-analysis. PLoS One. 2018;13:e0203400.
6. Li B, Li Q, Nie W, Liu S. Diagnostic value of whole-body diffusion-weighted magnetic resonance imaging for detection of primary and metastatic malignancies: a meta-analysis. Eur J Radiol. 2014;83:338–44.
7. Shen G, Deng H, Hu S, Jia Z. Comparison of choline- PET/CT, MRI, SPECT, and bone scintigraphy in the diagnosis of bone metastases in patients with prostate cancer: a meta-analysis. Skeletal Radiol. 2014;43:1503–13.
8. von Eyben FE, Kairemo K. Meta-analysis of (^{11})C-choline and (^{18})F-choline PET/CT for management of patients with prostate cancer. Nucl Med Commun. 2014;35:221–30.
9. von Eyben FE, Kairemo K. Acquisition with (^{11})C-choline and (^{18})F-fluorocholine PET/CT for patients with biochemical recurrence of prostate cancer: a systematic review and meta-analysis. Ann Nucl Med. 2016;30:385–92.
10. Liu J, Chen Z, Wang T, et al. Influence of four radiotracers in PET/CT on diagnostic accuracy for prostate cancer: a bivariate random-effects meta-analysis. Cell Physiol Biochem. 2016;39:467–80.
11. Kairemo K. Приложение к статье с объяснением находок на ПЭТ/КТ с 18-F холином у больных раком простаты (F-18 choline imaging in prostate cancer). Consilium. 2014;3-4:73–4.
12. Kairemo K, Partanen K, Bützow A, Valle T, Ala-Opas M, Joensuu T. Personalized imaging approach in the clinical diagnosis of prostate cancer with suspicion of liver metastases. Medical case reports. iMedJournals. 2015;10:1. http://medical-case-reports.imedpub.com/personalized-imaging-approach-in-the-clinicaldiagnosis-of-prostate-cancer-with-suspicion-ofliver-metastases.php?aid=8000—A4
13. Kairemo K. Radiation safety matters. Letters to the Editor. Radiat Prot Dosim. 2017;174:291.

Overview of ^{18}F-NaF PET/CT Imaging

4

^{18}F-sodium fluoride (^{18}F-NaF) PET/CT has established its place in the oncologic clinical routine. It has essential role in initial staging, detection of suspected first osseous metastasis, suspected progression of osseous metastasis, or treatment monitoring in many types of cancer, such as prostate, lung, and breast cancer.

Bone uptake of ^{18}F-NaF reflects bone remodeling, and the uptake of ^{18}F-NaF is part of the mineralization of bone matrix. $^{18}F^-$ (fluoride-ion) is exchanged for OH^- (oxonium ion), so hydroxyapatite bone matrix is transformed into fluorapatite, indicating that high uptake of ^{18}F-NaF reflects bone reactions to bone metastases, not to cancer itself. Therefore, positive findings with ^{18}F-NaF PET/CT may be due to both benign and malignant bone disorders. Figure 4.1 illustrates how hydroxyapatite bone matrix is transformed into fluoroapatite. In this chapter, the use of ^{18}F-NaF PET/CT in prostate has been reviewed.

K. Kairemo, *Prostate Cancer from a Nuclear Oncology Perspective*,
https://doi.org/10.1007/978-3-031-90337-3_4

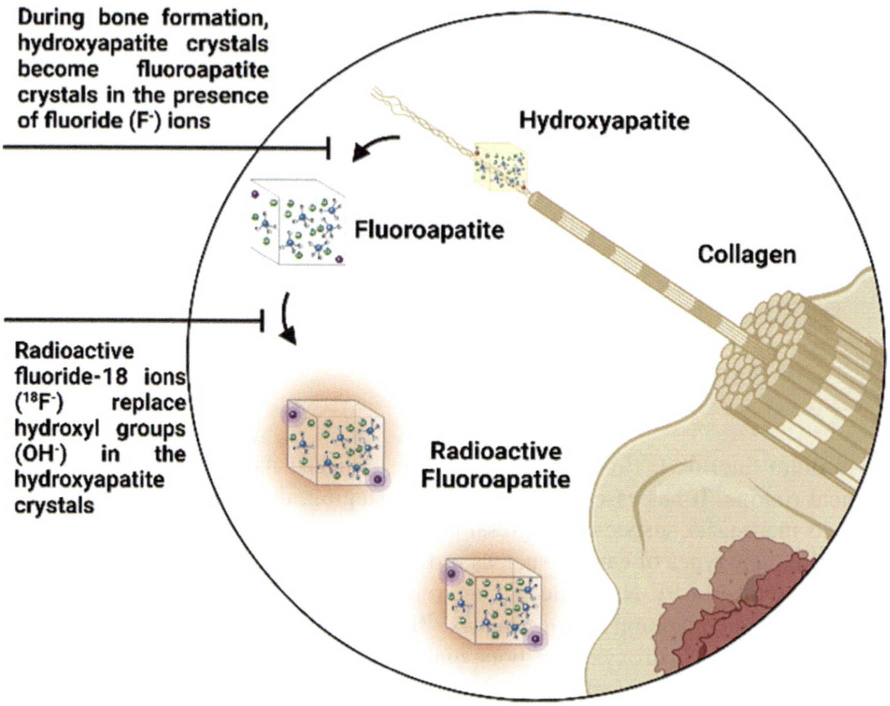

Fig. 4.1 Mechanism of $^{18}F^-$ (fluoride-ion) uptake in the reactive bone tissue, e.g., in a metastasis. During bone formation, hydroxyapatite crystals become fluoroapatite crystals in the presence of $^{18}F^-$ radioactive $^{18}F^-$ (fluoride-ion) replace hydroxyl group OH^- of the hydroxyapatite crystal. (Part of the figure from Kairemo et al. [27])

Historical Context and Development

^{18}F-NaF is an old tracer, initially utilized in the 1960s and 1970s. ^{18}F-NaF's use in bone scanning waned due to technological limitations of gamma cameras at the time [1]. With the advent of hybrid PET/CT cameras in the late 1990s, there has been a resurgence in its use due to enhanced imaging capabilities; the hybrid PET/CT technology combines the high-resolution and sensitive PET scan with the anatomical detail provided by CT, offering superior diagnostic accuracy over older methods like SPECT and planar bone scintigraphy [2, 3]. This superior imaging quality is crucial for the initial staging of prostate cancer, the detection of new or suspected skeletal metastases, monitoring disease progression, and assessing responses to treatment [4–6].

Prostate cancer frequently metastasizes to the bones, necessitating precise imaging to guide treatment. ^{18}F-sodium fluoride PET/CT has emerged as a superior modality for identifying skeletal metastases due to its high sensitivity and specificity compared to traditional bone scintigraphy [7, 8]. This imaging technique is particularly adept at detecting osteoblastic lesions, which are common in prostate cancer. Approximately 80% of the skeletal metastases are osteoblastic in prostate cancer. Studies underscore its utility in initial staging and monitoring treatment response, especially in metastatic contexts where early detection significantly impacts therapeutic outcomes.

It is especially useful in assessing the skeletal burden of metastatic disease and in planning treatment strategies. The ^{18}F-NaF fluoride PET/CT methodology allows for the simultaneous characterization of the alterations of metastatic bone density and the tracer uptake, which both are well-established markers of lesion severity and may be essential in judging the necessity of early implementation of radionuclide therapies for bone pain palliation and treatment. For instance, most lytic lesions are not detectable at bone scintigraphy. It has been reported that in cancer patients with multiple skeletal metastases, an increased ^{18}F-NaF fluoride uptake may be detected both in lesions with sclerotic characteristics on CT and in mixed sclerotic and lytic metastases [9].

Diagnostic Performance and Clinical Utility

Comparison with other imaging modalities (CT, MRI) is necessary when ^{18}F-NaF used in the diagnosis of skeletal metastases of prostate cancer. In spite of the fact that ^{18}F-NaF PET/CT demonstrates higher sensitivity and specificity in detecting bone metastases compared to traditional bone scintigraphy and SPECT, it must be compared with morphological imaging. It is particularly effective in identifying osteoblastic metastases, which are common in prostate cancer. Figure 4.2 illustrates how osteoblastic changes may be traumatic or degenerative. It may be challenging to detect the presence of malignant disorders as Fig. 4.2 shows.

The accuracy of ^{18}F-NaF PET/CT aids in upstaging or downstaging cancer, impacting decisions between curative and palliative care. It also helps in monitoring response to therapies like chemotherapy or radionuclide treatments, guiding adjustments in treatment plans. It is especially useful in assessing the skeletal burden of metastatic disease and in planning treatment strategies. There are even certain quantitative response criteria for ^{18}F-NaF PET imaging and methods of how to calculate tumor burden [10–12]. These are discussed in Chap. 16 in detail which discusses bone targeted therapies.

Studies have shown that the whole-body skeletal tumor burden assessed by ^{18}F-NaF PET/CT at baseline can serve as a potent prognostic biomarker in prostate cancer, influencing survival outcomes and treatment choices [12]. Beyond detecting metastases, ^{18}F-NaF PET/CT provides prognostic value by assessing tumor burden and response to therapies like radium-223. This capability enables personalized treatment plans and predicts patient outcomes, enhancing both the strategic approach to care and its efficacy. The quantitative analysis of skeletal tumor burden, facilitated by ^{18}F-NaF PET/CT, offers a robust framework for evaluating progression or regression of bone metastases.

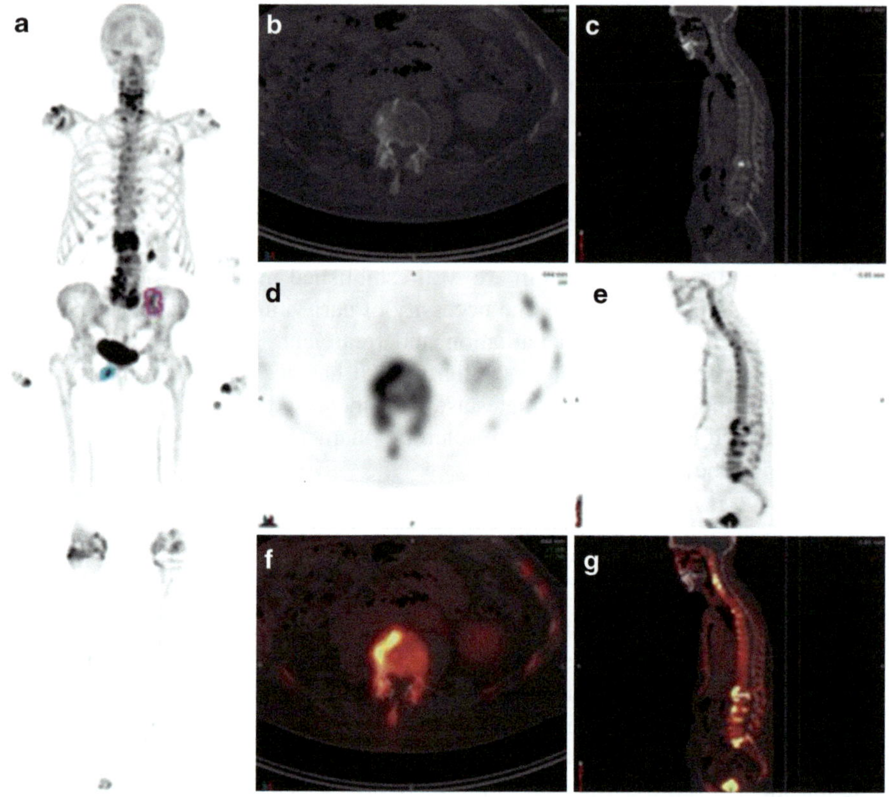

Fig. 4.2 An 81-year-old male with skeletal metastases imaged with Na^{18}F. MIP image (**a**) demonstrates increased uptakes of the left iliac bone (purple contour) and right inferior pubic ramus (light blue contour) which were metastatic. All other uptakes were of benign nature. Transaxial CT (**b**), PET (**c**), and PET/CT fusion (**d**) images show degenerative changes in the lumbar spine, and sagittal CT (**e**), PET (**f**), and PET/CT fusion (**g**) images demonstrate focal degenerations in the spine. Additionally, there was an anamnestic vertebroplasty at the level of L1. This case illustrates how important the anamestic trauma/surgery information, correlative morphologic imaging, and case history for correct diagnosis and how difficult it will be to distinguish malignant lesions from trauma or degenerative changes

^{18}F-NaF PET/CT has been used clinically to enhance the detection of skeletal metastases with greater accuracy than other radiotracers like ^{18}F-choline; this was already discussed in Chap. 3 discussing the characteristics of choline PET. While both tracers are effective at staging prostate cancer, ^{18}F-choline tends to have higher specificity at restaging for recurrent disease. Figure 4.3 presents an example of a patient who was imaged quantitatively with ^{18}F-choline and ^{18}F-NaF on consecutive days [13].

It is shown clearly in Fig. 4.3 that ^{18}F-choline, ^{18}F-NaF, and CT measure different entities, and this is shown at the voxel level. The ^{18}F-choline and ^{18}F-NaF studies are aligned on each other with the help of 3D skeleton. Figure 4.4 summarizes how the

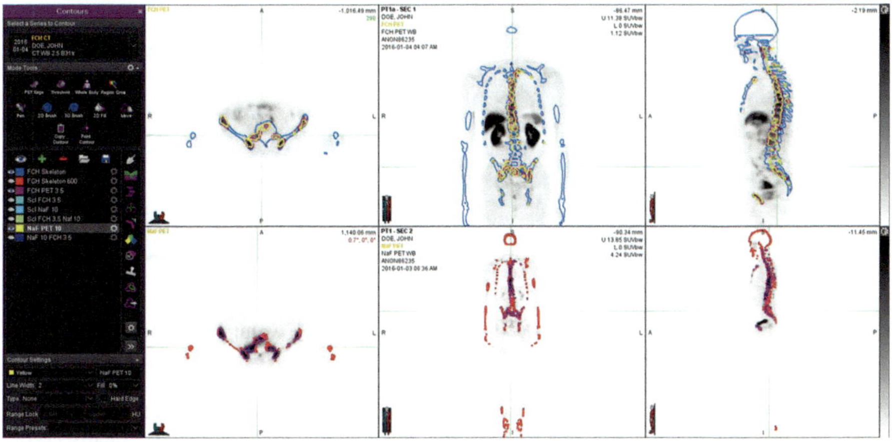

Fig. 4.3 Example of a 67-year-old patient who had an aggressive prostate cancer, T4N1M1, when initially diagnosed with Gleason score of 9. S-PSA was 40. The upper row shows FCH PET study one transaxial, coronaand sagittal section. The lower row illustrates the same sections in the NaF PET study. Here, normal skeleton (HU > 150 as measured from simultaneous CT) is shown in red on NaF PET (lower row) and blue on FCH PET (upper row). Pathologic NaF (SUV > 10) is shown in yellow on FCH PET (upper row) and pathologic FCH (SUV > 3.5) in purple on NaF PET (lower row). This demonstrates clearly that volume regions differ significantly from each other, and PET tracers show different distributions, i.e., NaF is targeting cortical bone and FCH bone marrow [13]

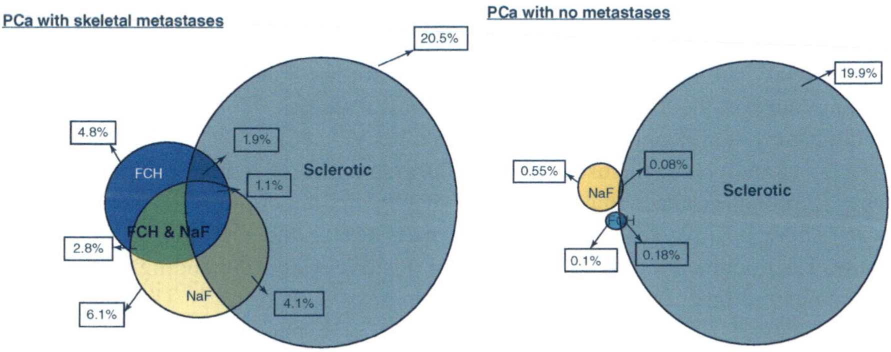

Fig. 4.4 Fluorocholine vs. sodium fluoride. Pathologic PET/CT volumes as percentages of the skeletal volumes (when HU > 150 on CT) are presented as spheres. Pathologic volumes for FCH (SUV > 3.5) are in blue and NaF (SUV > 10) in yellow. Sclerosis is measured from CT (HU > 600) volume (gray). The volumes are shown for patients with bone metastases (M) and for control prostate cancer patients with no skeletal metastases (N). The amount of sclerosis (gray spheres) does not statistically differ in these patient groups. All pathological volumes, including overlapping regions, differ statistically significantly from each other between M and N group [13]

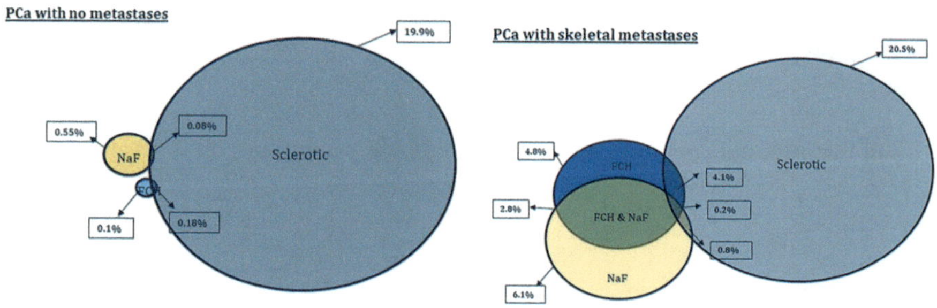

Fig. 4.5 Fluorocholine vs. Ga-68-PSMA-11. Pathologic PET/CT volumes as percentages of the skeletal volumes (when HU > 150 on CT) are presented as spheres. Pathologic volumes for ^{68}Ga-PSMA-11 (SUV > 3.0) are in blue and NaF (SUV > 10) in yellow. Sclerosis is measured from CT (HU > 600) volume (gray). The volumes are shown for patients with bone metastases (M) and for control prostate cancer patients with no skeletal metastases (N). The amount of sclerosis (gray spheres) does not statistically differ in these patient groups. All pathological volumes, including overlapping regions, differ statistically significantly from each other between M and N group [14]

volumes of ^{18}F-choline, ^{18}F-NaF, and CT overlap percentually in patients with skeletal metastases and in prostate cancer patients who do not have skeletal metastases but have same amount of sclerosis in the skeleton. Roughly, ^{18}F-NaF is targeting cortical bone and ^{18}F-FCH bone marrow [13].

We performed similar study with ^{68}Ga-PSMA, ^{18}F-NaF, and CT [14]. Summary data is shown in Fig. 4.5. The findings were very similar to those of ^{18}F-choline, ^{18}F-NaF, and CT [13] in that sense that all these modalities measure different things. It seems that ^{68}Ga-PSMA and ^{18}F-NaF overlap less with each other than ^{18}F-choline and ^{18}F-NaF, but the numbers are too small for further conclusions [13, 14]. These findings support the findings seen in other clinical studies. ^{18}F-Choline and ^{18}F-NaF findings may significantly differ from each other [15, 16].

A meta-analysis of the use of sodium fluoride in the detection of skeletal metastases in prostate cancer that about 33% of patients undergoing ^{18}F-NaF PET/CT scans show positive results for skeletal metastases, underscoring its diagnostic value. The document notes varying rates of positive results depending on the clinical context—higher in cases suspected of progressive metastases. The small meta-analysis about ^{18}F-NaF PET/CT consisted of 3918 patients, with 1289 having positive scans [17]. In the US National Oncologic PET Registry (NOPR) [18, 19], the indication for the PET/CT was reflected in the PET/CT findings: 14% of patients had a positive ^{18}F-NaF PET/CT at staging; 29% of the patients had positive ^{18}F-NaF PET/CT if the examination was an initial test for bone metastases; 76% of the patients had positive ^{18}F-NaFPET/CT if the examination was requested as a test for progressive bone metastases. ^{18}F-NaF and ^{18}F-choline PET/CT had similar diagnostic accuracy at staging for patients with prostate cancer, but ^{18}F-choline has higher specificity at restaging for recurrence [15, 16]. Patients with positive ^{18}F-NaF PET/CT scans have a high risk of having dissemination of prostate cancer to the bones. Bone metastases occur in nearly all patients with castration resistant prostate cancer and are the primary cause of disability, impaired quality of life, and death, due to an increased risk of pathologic fractures, spinal cord or nerve root compression, and hypercalcemia of malignancy [20]. In this context, the skeletal involvement from prostate cancer can be assessed using ^{18}F-NaF fluoride PET/CT. This imaging modality allows the identification and quantification of bone metastatic lesions [1]. The NOPR Registry has collected Na^{18}F PET results linked to Medicare claims (federal insurance) by imaging initial staging, detection of new suspected skeletal metastases, suspected progression of skeletal disease, or assessing treatment response in prostate, lung, or breast cancer. In an analysis from NOPR of 21,167 ^{18}F-NaF PET/CT studies [19], the results were associated with subsequent hospice claims and with patient survival. ^{18}F-NaF-PET provides important information on the presence of osseous metastasis and prognosis to assist patients and their physicians when making decisions on whether to select palliative care and transition to hospice or whether to continue treatment [19]. The Society for Nuclear Medicine has published guidelines for ^{18}F-NaF PET/CT [21]. Some international recommendations already include ^{18}F-NaF as a radiotracer for skeletal imaging [22].

Current drugs for the treatment of bone metastases also include ADT and systemic chemotherapy, but monoclonal antibodies, analgesics, EBRT, radiopharmaceuticals, and bisphosphonates specifically target osseous disease alone or in combination. However, ^{18}F-NaF fluoride PET/CT is best in the evaluation of bone targeted therapies and in bone dominant metastatic prostate cancer. This ^{18}F-fluoride PET/CT methodology can be used for assessing the final outcome of many treatments [23]. Despite benefits, challenges occur in using interim ^{18}F-fluoride PET/CT scans to predict outcomes after ^{223}Ra therapy, as changes in uptake may not distinguish between progression and response [24]. This complicates its use in monitoring the effectiveness of various treatments, including chemotherapeutic and hormonal agents. However, the Na^{18}F burden data is convincing, because serum markers, such as alkaline phosphatase (AFOS) or prostate-specific antigen (PSA), seldom reflect small changes in the overall cancer burden. ^{18}F-NaF fluoride PET/CT may also be used for radiation therapy treatment planning [25, 26].

Conclusive Remarks

The chapter compares ^{18}F-fluoride PET/CT with other imaging modalities, establishing it as superior in detecting osteoblastic metastases in prostate cancer. The use of ^{18}F-fluoride PET/CT as a prognostic tool is emphasized, especially for assessing the skeletal tumor burden in prostate cancer. It helps in quantifying osteoblastic metastases, which is pivotal for tailoring individual treatment plans and predicting responses to therapies like ^{223}Ra, a bone-seeking radionuclide.

The review underscores the critical role of ^{18}F-NaF PET/CT in modern oncological practice, particularly for bone metastasis management. As technology and access improve, its integration into clinical pathways is likely to expand, enhancing cancer diagnosis, staging, and treatment planning.

This synthesis from multiple sources highlights the evolution, applications, and significant impact of ^{18}F-NaF PET/CT, suggesting its continued importance in medical imaging and patient care strategies in uro-oncology. However, challenges remain, particularly regarding the widespread adoption of advanced imaging and radionuclide therapies due to cost and availability constraints.

Prostate cancer management is poised at a transformative juncture, with advanced imaging and targeted therapies offering new avenues for effective treatment. The integration of ^{18}F-NaF PET/CT in clinical practice exemplifies this shift, providing a more nuanced understanding of disease progression and treatment response. As research continues to advance, these tools are expected to become central components of prostate cancer care, leading to better patient outcomes and more personalized therapeutic approaches. The synergy between innovative diagnostic tools and targeted treatment regimens heralds a new era in oncology, where precision medicine becomes the standard of care in battling prostate cancer.

Overall, the importance of ^{18}F-fluoride PET/CT in the advanced diagnostic imaging landscape, particularly for managing prostate cancer through precise detection and evaluation of skeletal metastases, aids in better clinical decision-making and improved patient outcomes.

References

1. Kairemo K, Macapinlac HA, editors. Sodium fluoride PET/CT in clinical use, Clinicians' guides to radionuclide hybrid imaging. Cham: Springer; 2020. Available at: https://link.springer.com/book/10.1007/978-3-030-23577-2#bibliographic-information
2. Even-Sapir E, Metser U, Mishani E, et al. The detection of bone metastases in patients with high-risk prostate cancer: 99mTc-MDP Planar bone scintigraphy; single- and multi-field-of-view SPECT; ^{18}F-fluoride PET; and ^{18}Ffluoride PET/CT. J Nucl Med. 2006;47:287–97.
3. Löfgren J, Mortensen J, Rasmussen SH, et al. A prospective study comparing ^{99m}Tc-hydroxyethylene-diphosphonate planar bone scintigraphy and whole-body SPECT/CT with ^{18}F-fluoride PET/CT and ^{18}F-fluoride PET/MRI for diagnosing bone metastases. J Nucl Med. 2017;58:1778–85.
4. Fox JJ, Schöder H, Larson SM. Molecular imaging of prostate cancer. Curr Opin Urol. 2012;22:320–7.
5. Cho SY, Szabo Z. Molecular imaging of urogenital diseases. Semin Nucl Med. 2014;44:93–109.
6. Kulshrestha RK, Vinjamuri S, England A, Nightingale J, Hogg P. The role of ^{18}F-sodium fluoride PET/CT bone scans in the diagnosis of metastatic bone disease from breast and prostate cancer. J Nucl Med Technol. 2016;44:217–22.
7. Bagheri MH, Ahlman MA, Lindenberg L, et al. Advances in medical imaging for the diagnosis and management of common genitourinary cancers. Urol Oncol. 2017;35:473–91.
8. Fraum TJ, Ludwig DR, Kim EH, Schroeder P, Hope TA, Ippolito JE. Prostate cancer PET tracers: essentials for the urologist. Can J Urol. 2018;25:9371–83.
9. Capitanio S, Bongioanni F, Piccardo A, et al. Comparisons between glucose analogue 2-deoxy-2-((^{18})F)fluoro-D-glucose and (^{18})F-sodium fluoride positron emission tomography/computed tomography in breast cancer patients with bone lesions. World J Radiol. 2016;8:200.
10. Kairemo K, Joensuu T. Radium-223-dichloride in castration resistant metastatic prostate cancer-preliminary results of the response evaluation using F-18-fluoride PET/CT. Diagnostics (Basel). 2015;5:413–27.

11. Etchebehere E, Brito AE, Rezaee A, et al. Therapy assessment of bone metastatic disease in the era of 223 radium. Eur J Nucl Med Mol Imaging. 2017;44(Suppl 1):84–96.
12. Etchebehere EC, Araujo JC, Fox PS, Swanston NM, Macapinlac HA, Rohren EM. Prognostic factors in patients treated with ^{223}Ra: the role of skeletal tumor turden on baseline ^{18}Ffluoride PET/CT in predicting overall survival. J Nucl Med. 2015;56:1177–84.
13. Kairemo K, Kappadath SC, Joensuu T, Macapinlac HA. A retrospective comparative study of sodium fluoride (NaF-18)-PET/CT and fluorocholine (F-18-CH) PET/CT in the evaluation of skeletal metastases in metastatic prostate cancer using a volumetric 3-D radiomics analysis. Diagnostics (Basel). 2020;11(1):17.
14. Kairemo K, Kangasmäki A, Kappadath SC, Joensuu T, Macapinlac HA. A retrospective comparative study of sodium fluoride Na^{18}F-PET/CT and ^{68}Ga-PSMA-11 PET/CT in the bone metastases of prostate cancer using a volumetric 3-D radiomic analysis. Life (Basel). 2022;12:1977.
15. Beheshti M, Rezaee A, Geinitz H, Loidl W, Pirich C, Langsteger W. Evaluation of prostate cancer bone metastases with ^{18}F-NaF and ^{18}F-fluorocholine PET/CT. J Nucl Med. 2016;57:55S–60S.
16. Langsteger W, Balogova S, Huchet V, et al. Fluorocholine (^{18}F) and sodium fluoride (^{18}F) PET/CT in the detection of prostate cancer: prospective comparison of diagnostic performance determined by masked reading. Q J Nucl Med Mol Imaging. 2011;55:448–57.
17. von Eyben FE, Kairemo K, Kiljunen T, Joensuu T. Planning of external beam radiotherapy for prostate cancer guided by PET/CT. Curr Radiopharm. 2015;8:19–31.
18. Hillner BE, Siegel BA, Hanna L, Duan F, Shields AF, Coleman RE. Impact of ^{18}F-fluoride PET in patients with known prostate cancer: initial results from the national oncologic PET registry. J Nucl Med. 2014;55:574–81.
19. Gareen IF, Hillner BE, Hanna L, et al. Hospice admission and survival after ^{18}F-fluoride PET performed for evaluation of osseous metastatic disease in the national oncologic PET registry. J Nucl Med. 2018;59:427–33.
20. Scher HI, Sawyers CL. Biology of progressive, castration resistant prostate cancer: directed therapies targeting the androgen receptor signaling axis. J Clin Oncol. 2005;23:8253–61.
21. Segall G, Delbeke D, Stabin MG, et al. SNM practice guideline for sodium ^{18}F-fluoride PET/CT bone scans 1.0. J Nucl Med. 2010;51:1813–20.
22. Oyen W, Sundram F, Haug AR, et al. Radium-223 dichloride (Ra-223) for the treatment of metastatic castration-resistant prostate cancer: optimizing clinical practice in nuclear medicine centers. J Oncopathol. 2015;3:1–25.
23. Kairemo K, Milton DR, Etchebehere E, et al. Final outcome of ^{223}Ra-therapy and the role of ^{18}F-fluoride-PET in response evaluation in metastatic castration-resistant prostate cancer—a single institution experience. Curr Radiopharm. 2018;11:152–7.
24. Etchebehere E, Brito AE, Kairemo K, Rohren E, Araujo J, Macapinlac H. Is interim ^{18}F-fluoride PET/CT a predictor of outcomes after radium-223 therapy? Radiol Bras. 2019;52:33–40.
25. Kairemo KJA. PET/computed tomography for radiation therapy planning of prostate cancer. PET Clin. 2017;12:257–67.
26. Kairemo K, Rasulova N, Kiljunen T, Partanen K, Kangasmäki A, Joensuu T. PET/CT dose planning for volumetric modulated arc radiation therapy (VMAT)—comparison with conventional approach in advanced prostate cancer patients. Curr Radiopharm. 2015;8:2–8.
27. Kairemo K, Gouda MA, Buschhorn L, et al. Sodium fluoride (Na^{18}F) PET response criteria in solid tumors (NAFCIST): a framework for response assessment in bone tumors. ESMO Open. 2023;8:101575.

^{18}F-Fluciclovine (^{18}F-FACBC) Positron Emission Tomography in Prostate Cancer

5

Fluciclovine (^{18}F), also known as anti-1-amino-3-18F-fluorocyclobutane-1-carboxylic acid (anti-3[^{18}F] FACBC), is a diagnostic agent used for positron emission tomography (PET) imaging in men with suspected prostate cancer (PCa) recurrence based on elevated prostate-specific antigen (PSA) levels [1–4].

Fluciclovine is a [^{18}F]-tagged synthetic analogue of the amino acid L-leucine [1, 4]. Its chemical structure is shown in Fig. 5.1. FACBC uptake by the tumor is related to functional activity of two amino acid transporters [1, 2], specifically sodium-dependent system ASCT-2, with a lesser contribution by sodium-independent system LAT-1 [1, 2]. Although it is handled by the amino acid transporter system, it does not undergo terminally incorporative metabolism within the body [1, 2].

In the literature, there are two rather new systematic reviews of the use of ^{18}F-fluciclovine positron emission tomography in the diagnosis of prostate cancer [5, 6]. Its effectiveness has been assessed in multiple clinical settings—initial staging, lymph node (LN) staging before surgery, and recurrence detection. Prostate cancer is the second most common cancer in men, and accurate detection of its recurrence is crucial for effective treatment. ^{18}F-fluciclovine (Axumin®) has been approved by both by the US and EU authorities, the FDA and EMA, for its use in detecting biochemical recurrence in prostate cancer patients when PSMA (prostate-specific membrane antigen) PET imaging is not available. The newer systematic review and meta-analysis in compliance with PRISMA guidelines [5] selected 15 studies out of 283 studies published between 2011 and 2020. These studies had to

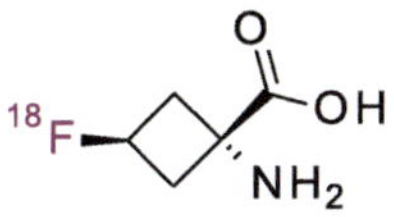

Fig. 5.1 The chemical structure of fluciclovine a.k.a. anti-1-amino-3-18F-fluorocyclobutane-1-carboxylic acid (anti-3[^{18}F] FACBC)

K. Kairemo, *Prostate Cancer from a Nuclear Oncology Perspective*,
https://doi.org/10.1007/978-3-031-90337-3_5

report diagnostic accuracy data: true positives, false positives, true negatives, and false negatives for ^{18}F-fluciclovine in diagnosing primary cancer, staging lymph nodes, and detecting recurrent prostate cancer. The final analysis accounted 697 patients.

The pooled sensitivity for ^{18}F-fluciclovine PET/CT for diagnosis of primary PCa was 0.83 (95% CI 0.80–0.86) and specificity of 0.77 (95% CI 0.74–0.80). The meta-analysis suggested that ^{18}F-fluciclovine PET/CT is effective in detecting primary prostate cancer, with a reasonable balance between sensitivity (= ability to correctly detect disease) and specificity (= ability to correctly rule out disease). The pooled sensitivity for preoperative lymph node staging was 0.57 (95% CI 0.39–0.73) and specificity of 0.99 (95% CI 0.94–1.00). The test showed high specificity in detecting lymph node metastases (close to 100%), but sensitivity was relatively low, indicating that while it can reliably confirm lymph node involvement when detected, it may miss some positive cases. The pooled sensitivity for the overall detection of recurrence in relapsed patients was 0.68 (95% CI 0.63–0.73) and specificity of 0.68 (95% CI 0.60–0.75). In the detection of recurrence, ^{18}F-fluciclovine PET/CT demonstrated moderate sensitivity and specificity. The authors note that this imaging modality is useful in identifying sites of prostate cancer relapse, particularly when conventional imaging (like CT or MRI) fails to provide conclusive result [5].

There was insufficient data to perform a comprehensive meta-analysis for bone metastases, as only one relevant study was identified. The article highlights the need for further research in this area, particularly regarding the physiological uptake of ^{18}F-fluciclovine in bones, which can complicate its interpretation [5]. The data from the meta-analysis had several overall limitations, because there was significant variability in the study designs, patient cohorts, and imaging protocols across the included studies, which might affect the consistency of the findings. Certain analyses, such as lymph node staging, were based on only a few studies, reducing the statistical power of the conclusions. In many cases, validation of PET/CT findings is challenging, particularly in the recurrent setting, where histological confirmation is not always feasible. The authors emphasize the need for further studies that include biopsy validation [5].

The former large systematic review and meta-analysis included also 15 studies for the detection of primary and 9 studies for recurrent prostate cancer [6]. Table 5.1 summarizes the selected studies for this meta-analysis. At patient-based analysis, the pooled sensitivity and specificity of ^{18}F-fluciclovine PET/CT for the assessment of PCa were 86.3% and 75.9%, respectively [6]. The pooled diagnostic odds ratio value was 16.45, with heterogeneity of 30%. At the regional-based analysis, the pooled sensitivity of ^{18}F-fluciclovine PET/CT for the evaluation of primary/recurrent disease in the prostatic bed was higher than in the extra-prostatic regions (90.4% vs. 76.5%, respectively); conversely, the pooled specificity was higher for the evaluation of extra-prostatic region than the prostatic bed (89% vs. 45%, respectively) [6]. Our own study [4] was included into those 15 studies in both meta-analyses [5, 6]. We found that the PSA doubling time (PDT) in patients with positive findings was significantly shorter than PDT in patients with negative findings: 3.25 ± 2.09 months (0.3–6 months) versus 31.2 ± 22.0 months

Table 5.1 Selected studies for detecting primary/recurrent prostate cancer using ^{18}F-FACBC

First author, year, ref number, country	Study design	*N.* pts	Mean age (range)	Gleason score (*n*)	Type of treatment (*n*)	Mean PSA (range)	Mean PSA doubling time (range)
Schuster 2007 [7] USA	Prospective staging (*n* = 9) Restaging (*n* = 6)	15	62 years (45–76)	6–10	Misc.	15µg/l (1.9–71)	NA
Schuster 2011 [8] USA	Prospective restaging	50	68.3 years (50–90)	NA	Misc.	6.62µg/l (0.11–44.74)	NA
Turkbey 2014 [9] USA	Prospective staging	21	62 years (44–73)	6–9	RARP + LND (21)	13.5µg/l (3.55–37.3)	NA
Kairemo 2014 [4] Finland	Retrospective restaging	26	68.1 years (56–77)	5–9	Misc.	7.9µg/l (0.11–69)	Positive FACBC 3.2mo (0.3–6) Negative FACBC 31.2mo (8–84)
Nanni 2014 [10] Italy	Prospective restaging	28	67 years (55–78)	6–10	RP (28), RT (11), ADT (14)	2.9µg/l (0.2–14.6)	NA
Nanni 2015 [11] Italy	Prospective restaging	50	67 years (55–78)	6–10	RP (50), RT (23), ADT (21)	3.2µg/l (0.24–15.6)	NA
Odewole 2016 [12] USA	Retrospective staging	53	67.57 years (49–90)	7 (49) NA (4)	Misc.	7.2µg/l (0.11–44.8)	18.6mo (−31.6–357.8)
Bach-Gansmo 2017 [13] Norway Italy USA	Retrospective restaging	596	67 years (42–90)	6.7 (110) 7.4 (355)	Misc.	5.43µg/l (0.05–82.0)	NA
Akin-Akintayo 2017 [14] USA	Prospective restaging	42	62 years (42–75)	7 (42)	RP (42)	2.1µg/l (0.07–11.15)	NA

(continued)

Table 5.1 (continued)

First author, year, ref number, country	Study design	*N.* pts	Mean age (range)	Gleason score (*n*)	Type of treatment (*n*)	Mean PSA (range)	Mean PSA doubling time (range)
Selnaes 2018 [15] Norway	Prospective staging	26	66.2 years (55–71.9)	7–9	RARP + LND (26)	14.6μg/l (3.7–56.9)	NA
Jambor 2018 [16]. Finland	Prospective staging	26	65 years (49–76)	6–9	RARP + LND (26)	12μg/l (4.1–35)	NA
Akin-Akintayo 2018 [17] USA	Prospective staging	24	70.8 years (60–83)	7 (24)	Misc.	8.5μg/l (2.2–29.3)	NA
Andriole 2019 [18] USA	Prospective restaging	213	66.4 years (46–90)	5–10	Misc.	4.24μg/l (0.2–93.5)	NA
England 2019 [19] USA	Retrospective restaging	28	67.1 years (53–77)	7–9	Misc.	0.44μg/l (0.1–1.0)	6.38mo (1.6–16.8)
Suzuki 2019 [20] Japan	Prospective staging	28	67.9 years (57–77)	6–9	RARP + LND (28)	17.94μg/l (1.20–82.38)	NA

Modified from Ref. [6]

(8–84 months), $P < 0.0001$ [4]. Additionally, there was a strong positive correlation between PSA value and number of metabolically active lesions ($R = 0.74$) and a negative correlation between PDT and number of metabolically active lesions ($R = -0.56$). There was only a weak negative correlation between PDT and SUVmax ($R = -0.30$) [4].

After these two meta-analyses, two larger studies have been reported: in 165 patients [21] and 81 patients [22] with detection rates of 66.7% and 76.9%, respectively. In the former study, the detection rate was 15.4% with PSA values <0.5 and 93.7% with PSA values >5.0 [21], whereas in the latter study, the detection rate was 66.7% with PSA values <0.57 and 90.0% with PSA values >1.5 [22]. This demonstrates that the patient cohort plays essential role, but the trend is clear and this data confirms the findings of the meta-analyses. In a study investigating biochemical recurrence, in patients with very low PSA levels (<0.3μg/l), the detection rate was 43.8% for patients with PSA level below 0.1μg/l, increasing up to 65.2% for patients with PSA between 0.2 and 0.3μg/l [23]. There are multiple comparisons between two tracers in the literature. In an early prospective study that compared the accuracy of ^{18}F-FACBC and ^{11}C-choline in the detection of PCa relapse, the detection rate was 32% for ^{11}C-choline versus 38% for ^{18}F-FACBC [24]. The diagnostic performance of ^{18}F-FACBC was compared to that of ^{11}C-choline PET/CT for the primary staging of PCa. The respective sensitivity, specificity, and accuracy were 50%, 70%, and 65% for ^{11}C-choline and 50%, 81%, and 74% for ^{18}F-FACBC [25].

In patients with recurrent PCa, an ^{18}F-FACBC PET/CT scan led to mainly major changes in clinical management for 40% of patients [25]. However, its low sensitivity in preoperative PCa patients means that not all lymph node metastases (LNM) could be detected even in patients with a positive ^{18}F-FACBC PET scan. The detection rate when using ^{18}F-FACBC correlates with the tumor size: detection rates of 23.7% and 83.3% for metastases with the respective diameters of 3 mm and 9 mm have been reported [26].

Patient Image Examples of Using ^{18}F-FACBC PET

Biochemical Recurrence and Response Evaluation

Figures 5.2 and 5.3 demonstrate two patient cases imaged with biochemical recurrence and with low PSA values using ^{18}F-FACBC-PET. Figure 5.2 demonstrates a patient with a small lymph node, <1 cm, and with a low SUVmax value of 3.4, when S-PSA = 7.70μg/l. Figure 5.3 demonstrates a patient with two S-PSA values within 3 months. The ^{18}F-FACBC-PET was negative with the S-PSA value of 0.54 but turned positive with the S-PSA value of 1.50; this lymph node was smaller than 1 cm. Figure 5.4 shows a biochemical recurrence with a rather large tumors and multiple lymph nodes in the pelvic, retroperitoneal, and supraclavicular regions, with SUVmax values up to 11.9. The follow-up ^{18}F-FACBC-PET 3 months later showed that all lymph node uptakes had disappeared indicating a major response to the therapy.

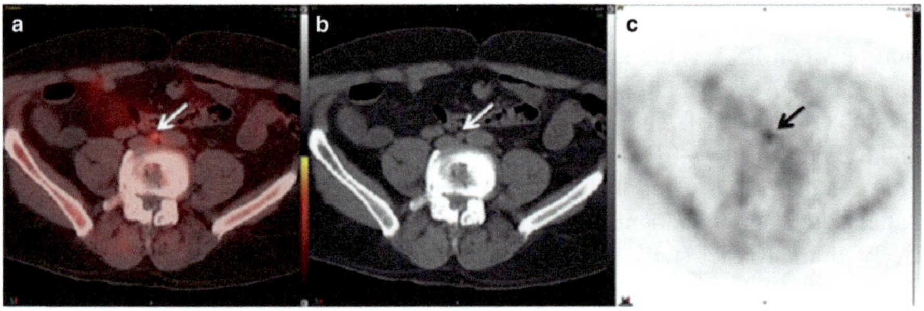

Fig. 5.2 A 65-year-old man with prostate adenocarcinoma (GS 9) treated originally with radical prostatectomy developed a biochemical recurrence (S-PSA = 7.70μg/l). Axial ^{18}F-fluciclovine PET/CT fusions (**a**), CT (**b**), and PET (**c**) demonstrate a lymph node metastasis in the aortocaval region. SUVmax 3.4; max size 1.0 cm

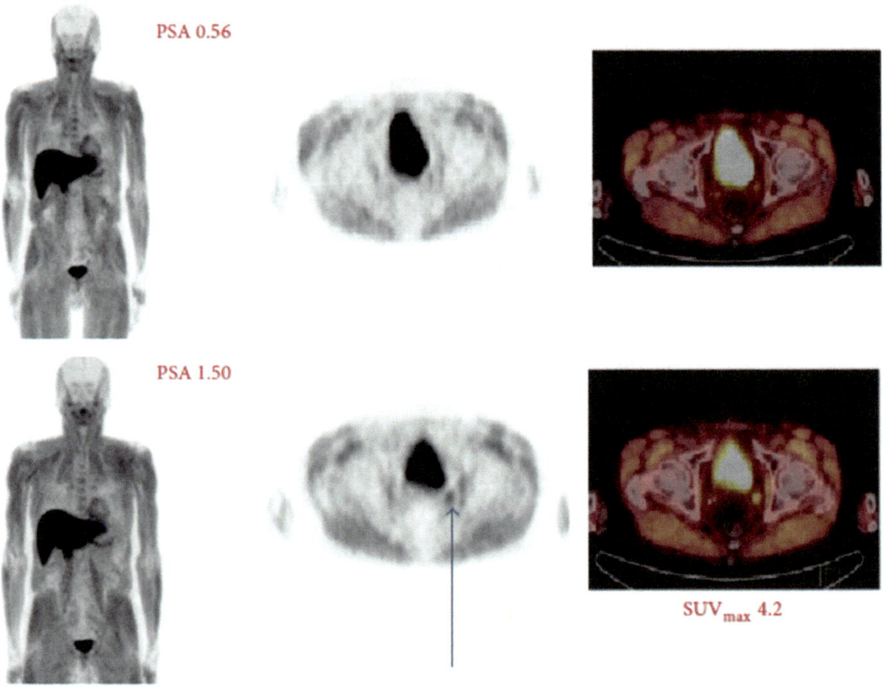

Fig. 5.3 A 70-year-old man with prostate adenocarcinoma (GS 9) with a suspicion of biochemical recurrence (S-PSA = 0.56μg/l) after radical prostatectomy (upper panel). This examination was negative, but the second examination (S-PSA = 1.50μg/l) 3 months later became positive (lower panel, arrow). MIP images (left), axial PET images (middle), and axial PET/CT fusions (right) demonstrate a local recurrence in an obturator lymph node. SUVmax 4.2 with ^{18}F-fluciclovine, whereas it was 1.7 in the first study [4]

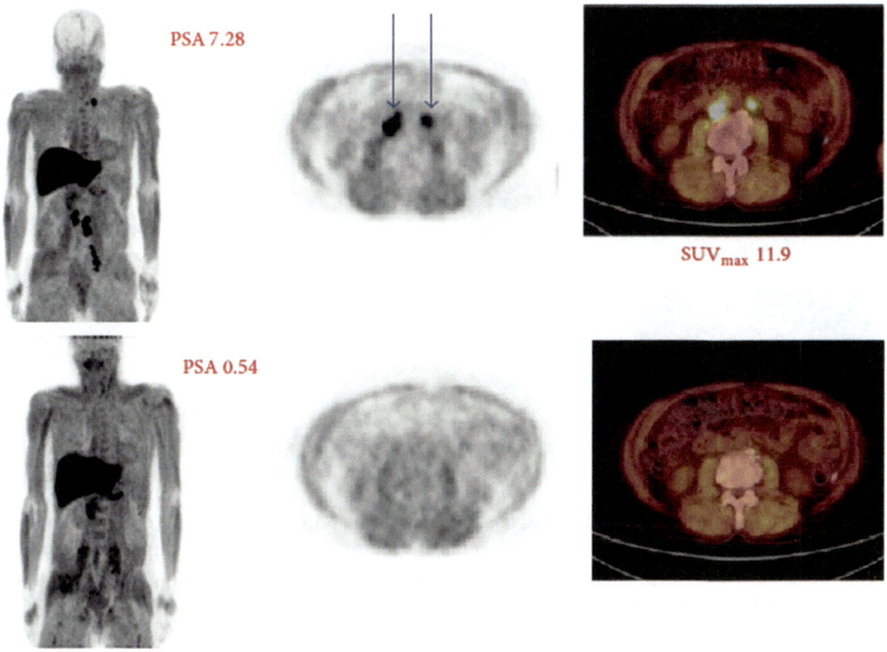

Fig. 5.4 A 67-year-old man with prostate adenocarcinoma (GS 9) treated with radiation therapy 4 years earlier combined with ADT but developed a biochemical recurrence (S-PSA = 7.28µg/l). The first examination demonstrates a large tumor burden in the left parailiac, para-aortic, aortocaval, and left supraclavicular lymph nodes (upper panel), but in the second examination (S-PSA = 0.55µg/l) 3 months later (lower panel), all these lymph node uptakes that have disappeared. MIP images (left), axial PET images (middle), and axial PET/CT fusions (right) demonstrate a major response in all lymph node regions. SUVmax levels were up to 11.9 with ^{18}F-fluciclovine in the first study [4]

Differential Diagnosis and Biochemical Recurrence

Figure 5.5 demonstrates a patient case with low PSA value imaged for biochemical recurrence of both ^{18}F-FACBC-PET and Na^{18}PET. These studies were performed on consecutive days. The Na^{18}F-PET-study shows multiple uptakes (seen in the MIP image; Fig. 5.5) in the skeleton (e.g., cervical spine, multiple ribs, pelvic bones, and right femur); some of these were considered to be trauma related, such as the femur, pelvic bones, ribs (anamnestic car accident), and some degenerative changes, such as cervical spine due to spondylarthrosis. From this study, it is almost impossible to diagnose possible skeletal metastases. Fortunately, ^{18}F-FACBC-PET revealed only one single pathologic tiny uptake, seen in the MIP image dorsocranially from the urinary bladder and clearly in the axial PET image and PET/CT fusion image. This sacral was also seen in the Na^{18}F-PET, but the uptake was actually lower than in the known healing fractures. This finding dramatically gave the diagnosis, even though the role of ^{18}F-FACBC-PET in the detection of skeletal metastases is unclear as discussed earlier in this chapter.

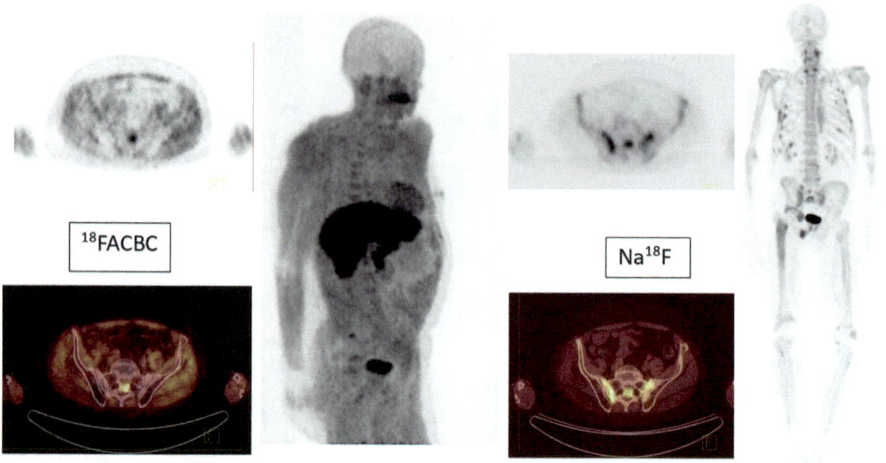

Fig. 5.5 A 75-year-old man with prostate adenocarcinoma (GS 8) treated with radiation therapy combined with ADT but developed a biochemical recurrence (S-PSA = 4.20µg/l). On the left, ^{18}F-fluciclovine-PET images and, on the right, Na^{18}F-PET images are shown; whole body MIP images (right panel), axial PET images (upper panels), and axial PET/CT fusions (lower panels) are shown at the same level on consecutive days. Na^{18}F-PET images show three separate uptakes in the pelvic bones, whereas ^{18}F-FACBC-PET demonstrates only one uptake in the middle of sacral bone. This example demonstrates the nonspecific nature of Na^{18}F-PET in skeletal disease, whereas ^{18}F-FACBC-PET finding was associated with the prostate cancer. This patient had been earlier in a car accident, and the larger uptakes were associated with healing bone fractures. In the follow-up with local treatment, the uptake disappeared and S-PSA normalized

Conclusive Remarks

The chapter summarizes that ^{18}F-fluciclovine PET/CT is a valuable tool, especially for detecting recurrent prostate cancer when other old imaging methods (e.g., choline PET or conventional CT/MRI) fail. The high specificity in preoperative lymph node staging highlights its reliability in confirming positive cases, though the lower sensitivity suggests that it might not detect all metastatic nodes. The European Association of Urology (EAU) recommends its use when PSMA-PET is not available, especially in patients with biochemical recurrence and PSA levels >1µg/l.^{18}F-FACBC-PET/CT seems to be promising in recurrent PCa, particularly for the evaluation of the prostatic bed.

FDA and EMA approved 2022 ^{18}F-fluciclovine only for recurrent PCa, but emerging data supports its potential use in high-risk primary cases.

The meta-analyses show that ^{18}F-fluciclovine PET/CT demonstrates promising diagnostic accuracy in various clinical settings, particularly in detecting recurrent prostate cancer and staging lymph nodes. However, these results should be interpreted carefully due to the heterogeneity of the included studies. More research is needed to confirm its role in bone metastasis and improve sensitivity in preoperative lymph node staging. Despite of the presented limitations ^{18}F-fluciclovine remains an important tool in managing prostate cancer, especially in the context of biochemical recurrence.

References

1. Oka S, Okudaira H, Yoshida Y, Schuster DM, Goodman MM, Shirakami Y. Transport mechanisms of trans-1-amino-3-fluoro[1-(14)C]cyclobutanecarboxylic acid in prostate cancer cells. Nucl Med Biol. 2012;39:109–19.
2. Schuster DM, Nanni C, Fanti S, et al. Anti-1-amino-3-18F-fluorocyclobutane-1-carboxylic acid: physiologic uptake patterns, incidental findings, and variants that may simulate disease. J Nucl Med. 2014;55(12):1986–92.
3. Schiavina R, Brunocilla E, Martorana G. The new promise of FACBC position emission tomography/computed tomography in the localization of disease relapse after radical treatment for prostate cancer: are we turning to the right radiotracer? Eur Urol. 2014;65(1):255–6.
4. Kairemo K, Rasulova N, Partanen K, Joensuu T. Preliminary clinical experience of trans-1-Amino-3-(^{18})F-fluorocyclobutanecarboxylic acid (anti-(^{18})F-FACBC) PET/CT imaging in prostate cancer patients. Biomed Res Int. 2014;2014:305182.
5. Biscontini G, Romagnolo C, Cottignoli C, et al. ^{18}F-fluciclovine positron emission tomography in prostate cancer: a systematic review and diagnostic meta-analysis. Diagnostics. 2021;11:304. https://doi.org/10.3390/diagnostics11020304.
6. Laudicella R, Albano D, Alongi P, et al. ^{18}F-FACBC in prostate cancer: a systematic review and meta-analysis. Cancers (Basel). 2019;11(9):1348.
7. Schuster DM, Votaw JR, Nieh PT, et al. Initial experience with the radiotracer anti-1-amino-3-18F-fluorocyclobutane-1-carboxylic acid with PET/CT in prostate carcinoma. J Nucl Med. 2007;48(1):56–63.
8. Schuster DM, Savir-Baruch B, Nieh PT, et al. Detection of recurrent prostate carcinoma with anti-1-amino-3-18F-fluorocyclobutane-1-carboxylic acid PET/CT and 111In-capromab pendetide SPECT/CT. Radiology. 2011;259(3):852–61.
9. Turkbey B, Mena E, Shih J, et al. Localized prostate cancer detection with 18F FACBC PET/CT: comparison with MR imaging and histopathologic analysis. Radiology. 2014;270(3):849–56.
10. Nanni C, Schiavina R, Brunocilla E, et al. ^{18}F-FACBC compared with 11C-choline PET/CT in patients with biochemical relapse after radical prostatectomy: a prospective study in 28 patients. Clin Genitourin Cancer. 2014;12(2):106–10.
11. Nanni C, Schiavina R, Brunocilla E, et al. ^{18}F-fluciclovine PET/CT for the detection of prostate cancer relapse: a comparison to ^{11}C-choline PET/CT. Clin Nucl Med. 2015;40:e386–91.
12. Odewole OA, Tade FI, Nieh PT, et al. Recurrent prostate cancer detection with anti-3-[(^{18})F]FACBC PET/CT: comparison with CT. Eur J Nucl Med Mol Imaging. 2016;43:1773–83.
13. Bach-GansmoBach-Gansmo T, Nanni C, Nieh PT, et al. Multisite experience of the safety, detection rate and diagnostic performance of fluciclovine (^{18}F) positron emission tomography/computerized tomography imaging in the staging of biochemically recurrent prostate cancer. J Urol. 2017;197:676–83.
14. Akin-Akintayo OO, Jani AB, Odewole O, et al. Change in salvage radiotherapy management based on guidance with FACBC (fluciclovine) PET/CT in postprostatectomy recurrent prostate cancer. Clin Nucl Med. 2017;42(1):e22–8.
15. Selnæs KM, Krüger-Stokke B, Elschot M, et al. ^{18}F-fluciclovine PET/MRI for preoperative lymph node staging in high-risk prostate cancer patients. Eur Radiol. 2018;28:3151–9.
16. Jambor I, Kuisma A, Kähkönen E, et al. Prospective evaluation of ^{18}F-FACBC PET/CT and PET/MRI versus multiparametric MRI in intermediate- to high-risk prostate cancer patients (FLUCIPRO trial). Eur J Nucl Med Mol Imaging. 2018;45(3):355–64.

17. Akin-Akintayo O, Tade F, Mittal P, et al. Prospective evaluation of fluciclovine (^{18}F) PET-CT and MRI in detection of recurrent prostate cancer in non-prostatectomy patients. Eur J Radiol. 2018;102:1–8.
18. Andriole GL, Kostakoglu L, Chau A, et al. The impact of positron emission tomography with ^{18}F-fluciclovine on the treatment of biochemical recurrence of prostate cancer: results from the LOCATE trial. J Urol. 2019;201(2):322–31.
19. England JR, Paluch J, Ballas LK, Jadvar H. ^{18}F-fluciclovine PET/CT detection of recurrent prostate carcinoma in patients with serum PSA $\leq$ 1 ng/mL after definitive primary treatment. Clin Nucl Med. 2019;44:e128–32.
20. Suzuki H, Jinnouchi S, Kaji Y, et al. Diagnostic performance of ^{18}F-fluciclovine PET/CT for regional lymph node metastases in patients with primary prostate cancer: a multicenter phase II clinical trial. Jpn J Clin Oncol. 2019;49(9):803–11.
21. Nakamoto R, Harrison C, Song H, et al. The clinical utility of ^{18}F-fluciclovine PET/CT in biochemically recurrent prostate cancer: an academic center experience post FDA approval. Mol Imaging Biol. 2021;23:614–23.
22. Filippi L, Bagni O, Crisafulli C, et al. Detection rate and clinical impact of PET/CT with ^{18}F-FACBC in patients with biochemical recurrence of prostate cancer: a retrospective bicentric study. Biomedicine. 2022;10:177.
23. Marcus C, Abiodun-Ojo OA, Jani AB, Schuster MD. Clinical utility of ^{18}F-fluciclovine PET/CT in recurrent prostate cancer with very low (_0.3 ng/mL) prostate-specific antigen levels. Am J Nucl Med Mol Imaging. 2021;11:406–14.
24. Nanni C, Zanoni L, Pultrone C, et al. (^{18})F-FACBC (anti1-amino-3-(^{18})F-fluorocyclobutane-1-carboxylic acid) versus (^{11})C-choline PET/CT in prostate cancer relapse: results of a prospective trial. Eur J Nucl Med Mol Imaging. 2016;43:1601–10.
25. Zanoni L, Bianchi L, Nanni C, et al. [^{18}F]-fluciclovine PET/CT for preoperative nodal staging in high-risk primary prostate cancer: final results of a prospective trial. Eur J Nucl Med Mol Imaging. 2021;49:390–409.
26. Seierstad T, Hole KH, Tulipan AJ, et al. ^{18}F-fluciclovine PET for assessment of prostate cancer with histopathology as reference standard. PET Clin. 2021;16:167–76.

PSMA-PET in Prostate Cancer

6

^{68}Ga-PSMA-PET/CT detects metastases in prostate cancer (PCa) better than conventional imaging [1], so some countries already recommend that patients initially are staged with PSMA PET. The Food and Drug Administration (FDA) of the United States approved three PSMA PET/CTs: ^{68}Ga-PSMA-11 [1], ^{18}F-DCFPyL [2], and ^{18}F-rh-PSMA-7.3 [3]. Today, half of high-risk (HRPCa) patients are staged with PSMA PET [4], and its use increases. The structures of ^{68}Ga-PSMA-11 and ^{18}F-DCFPyL are shown in Fig. 6.1.

The literature on staging with PSMA PET is extensive [5], but there is no consensus on whether and how PCa metastases at diagnosis indicated only on PSMA PET should be treated [6–9]. We undertook a systematic review and meta-analysis (SR and MA) of PCa. This chapter summarizes the role of PSMA PET for delineation of metastases and its impact on staging and initial diagnosis.

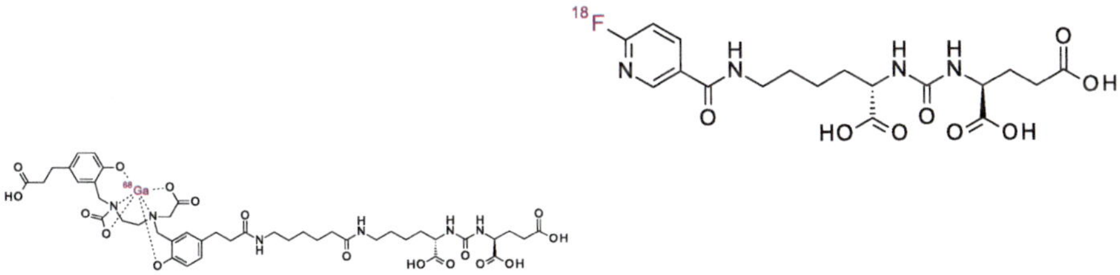

Fig. 6.1 The structures of ^{68}Ga-PSMA-11 (left) and ^{18}F-DCFPyL (right)

K. Kairemo, *Prostate Cancer from a Nuclear Oncology Perspective*,
https://doi.org/10.1007/978-3-031-90337-3_6

^{68}Ga-PSMA PET

This section focuses on how ^{68}Ga-PSMA PET imaging helps in the initial diagnosis of prostate cancer, particularly in patients with ambiguous MRI results. It discusses the strengths of ^{68}Ga-PSMA PET compared to traditional imaging, showing higher sensitivity and specificity in detecting prostate cancer and its metastases.

Initial Diagnosis Integration of ^{68}Ga-PSMA-PET with MRI-targeted biopsy enhances the initial diagnosis of clinically significant prostate cancer, particularly in ambiguous lesions like PIRADS 3 (scale 1–5), offering added value beyond MRI alone [10]. A comprehensive review by Evangelista et al. [11] highlighted that integrated PET/MRI proved to be of greater diagnostic value in locating PCa than either mpMRI or PET imaging alone. This conclusion was supported by several primary studies cited within the review.

The literature review by Satapathy et al. [12] noted that the ^{68}Ga-PSMA-PET has a high sensitivity (0.97) in the initial detection of prostate cancer. A major drawback is its moderate specificity (0.66). Other studies in the literature review reported specificities ranging from 44.6% to 81.8%—with only one reporting 100% specificity. A possible explanation for this might be the use of normal metabolic activity found in the prostate gland as the threshold for determining pet-positive lesions and also interobserver variability in the way the imaging is performed and reported [12, 13].

In cases with equivocal MRI findings or suspicion of clinically significant disease, ^{68}Ga-PSMA PET/CT demonstrates promise as a noninvasive imaging modality for the initial diagnosis of prostate cancer, complementing MRI [14]. Prospective trials have underscored the importance of ^{68}Ga-PSMA PET in primary prostate cancer diagnosis. However, a systematic review noted notable variability in imaging protocols and reporting methods, necessitating standardized reporting practices to enhance the broader applicability of trial results [13].

^{68}Ga-PSMA PET accuracy in detecting primary PCa lesions and its potential to aid in recurrence detection and staging make it a promising screening method, particularly when combined with other modalities like MRI [9]. ^{68}Ga-PSMA PET demonstrates high diagnostic accuracy for primary prostatic lesions, with comparable sensitivity, specificity, and diagnostic odds ratios, supporting ^{68}Ga-PSMA PET's incorporation into the initial workup of high-risk prostate cancer patients [15]. Table 6.1 shows the summary of the main findings of the articles in this indication. These reviews highlight the strong association between ^{68}Ga-PSMA PET readings, PSA levels, and Gleason scores, helping to stratify risk and guide treatment for patients. PSMA, a type 2 transmembrane glycoprotein, is overexpressed in prostate tumors—it correlates with elevated serum levels of prostate-specific antigen (PSA) and a higher Gleason score, indicating its potential as a biomarker for prostate cancer severity and progression [16, 17]. There is a significant association between the intensity of ^{68}Ga-PSMA uptake and Gleason score in confirmed lesions suggesting that parameters such as SUV_{max} and SUV_{ratio} of the primary tumor could serve as predictors of clinically significant prostate cancer [14].

Table 6.1 Systematic reviews and meta-analyses in the initial diagnosis of prostate cancer

Author and reference	Sample size	Sensitivity	Specificity	Conclusion
Kawada et al. [10]	497	0.89 (CI 0.85–0.93)	0.56 (CI 0.29–0.80)	^{68}Ga-PSMA-PET shows promise but needs more validation in diagnosis
Evangelista et al. [11]	2104	0.949 (CI 0.875–0.986)	0.909 (CI 0.437–0.789)	^{68}Ga-PSMA-PET shows promising accuracy in diagnosing primary prostate cancer
Satapathy et al. [12]	389	0.97 (CI 0.90–0.99)	0.66 (95% CI 0.52–0.78)	^{68}Ga-PSMA PET/CT is highly sensitive for initial diagnosis but with moderate specificity
Caracciolo et al. [14]	1379	NR	NR	^{68}Ga PSMA PET/CT is highly sensitive for initial prostate cancer diagnosis

The use of ^{68}Ga-PSMA PET demonstrates promising potential as a noninvasive diagnostic tool for prostate cancer, closely correlating with Gleason score and PSA levels for risk assessment and treatment planning [18–20]. The uptake of ^{68}Ga-PSMA on PET/CT is notably higher in individuals with PCa having a Gleason score of ≥8 or a PSA level of ≥10 ng/mL compared to those with GS ≤ 7 or PSA ≤ 10 ng/ml. This shows the potential of PET findings to reflect the aggressiveness and severity of prostate cancer, as assessed by Gleason score and PSA levels [9]. Review by Jiao et al. [21] has also shown that SUV_{max} values are significantly higher in patients with GS > 7 or PSA > 10 ng/ml compared to those with GS ≤ 7 or PSA ≤ 10 ng/ml.

TNM Staging PSMA PET imaging, particularly ^{68}Ga-PSMA PET/CT, has emerged as a superior method for N and M staging in high-risk prostate cancer patients, showing increased sensitivity and accuracy in detecting lymph nodes and distant metastases. Additionally, ^{68}Ga-PSMA PET demonstrates remarkable sensitivity in the early detection of prostate cancer, surpassing conventional imaging techniques. The integration of ^{68}Ga-PSMA PET/CT with clinical nomograms enhances the prediction of lymph node metastasis, potentially reducing unnecessary surgeries and improving nodal staging accuracy [22–24]. ^{68}Ga-PSMA-PET exhibits moderate sensitivity and outstanding specificity in detecting seminal vesicle invasion and extraprostatic extension in newly diagnosed prostate cancer patients undergoing radical prostatectomy. Studies comparing PET/MRI to PET/CT suggest PET/MRI's superior sensitivity in detecting seminal vesicle invasion, potentially attributed to its multiparametric approach, while variability in imaging protocols underscores the need for standardized assessment criteria to enhance ^{68}Ga-PSMA-PET's accuracy in local staging [22, 23]. However, the analysis revealed comparable diagnostic accuracy for extraprostatic extension detection between ^{68}Ga-PSMA PET/MRI and ^{68}Ga-PSMA PET/CT, with overlapping ranges [22]. ^{68}Ga-PSMA PET/CT, while capable of detecting smaller lesions, is less accurate than mpMRI in T staging, particularly in identifying extraprostatic extension and seminal vesicle invasion. SUV_{max} cutoff values ranging from 3.0 to 4.0 aid in differentiating prostate cancer lesions, with ^{68}Ga-PSMA PET showing greater correspondence with histopathology in detecting gross tumor volume compared to mpMRI [24]. For T staging, ^{68}Ga-PSMA PET/MRI offers superior accuracy in identifying T3 prostate cancer, particularly discerning extraprostatic extension and seminal vesicle invasion [21].

For the identification of lymph node metastases, analysis of diagnostic accuracy and detection rate indicated potentially better performance with ^{68}Ga-PSMA PET/MRI compared to ^{68}Ga-PSMA PET/CT [11, 20]. In a comprehensive review of 18 diagnostic test accuracy trials evaluating ^{68}Ga-PSMA PET for primary lymph node staging in prostate cancer, it was found to exhibit superior sensitivity (59%) and specificity (93%) compared to conventional CT and MRI. Despite variations in diagnostic accuracy attributed to factors like research design and technical aspects, these findings underscore the potential of ^{68}Ga-PSMA PET as a valuable imaging tool for primary staging [25]. ^{68}Ga-PSMA PET imaging, especially ^{68}Ga-PSMA PET/CT, exhibits heightened sensitivity and specificity in detecting lymph node metastases compared to conventional methods, highlighting its potential utility in primary staging [21, 26].

^{68}Ga-PSMA PET imaging outperforms conventional imaging in N and M staging for high-risk prostate cancer patients, offering superior sensitivity and accuracy in detecting lymph nodes and distant metastases [24]. ^{68}Ga-PSMA PET imaging demonstrates superior sensitivity and specificity compared to conventional imaging techniques such as bone scans, detecting more metastases, including those missed by bone scans, with an additional 17.6% involvement of bone regions. In intermediate to high-risk prostate cancer patients, ^{68}Ga-PSMA PET reveals lymph node metastases in extrapelvic sites (M1a) in up to 36.0% of cases, highlighting its efficacy in identifying distant metastases, particularly in high-risk populations.[26] In a review by Jiao et al. [21], it was noted that ^{68}Ga-PSMA PET/CT also demonstrates the same result stated above when compared to conventional imaging in detecting metastasis with sensitivity of 96.2% and specificity of 99.1%. ^{68}Ga-PSMA PET/CT can detect more undetected metastases, especially extrapelvic lesions, highlighting its utility in the M staging of prostate cancer [21].

In general, the lack of standardized SUVmax cutoff values is still a challenge, which may lead to variability in results of multiple reviews from the literature discussed here. Therefore, further research after the establishment of standardized protocols will improve reporting and outcome for ^{68}Ga-PSMA PET imaging.

It is obvious that ^{68}Ga-PSMA PET imaging is providing more accurate diagnostic and staging capabilities compared to traditional methods, but improved protocols are needed to maximize its clinical benefits and comparable results.

^{18}F-PSMA-PET

While wading through literature about PSMA-PET including meta-analyses, I came to a conclusion that approximately three-fourths of literature is dealing with ^{68}Ga-PSMA-PET and more than 95% of these reports concern ^{68}Ga-PSMA-11 (Illuccix®, Locametz®). Thus, less than one-fourth of literature is dealing with ^{18}F-PSMA-PET. More than ten different ^{18}F-PSMA-PET tracers have been introduced into clinical practice [27], these include ^{18}F-PSMA-1007 and ^{18}F-DCFPyL [2] with the tradenames Pylarify® and Pylclari®, and ^{18}F-rh-PSMA-7.3 [3] with the tradename Posluma®. Still, the most reported ^{18}F-PSMA-PET tracer is ^{18}F-PSMA-1007. This is a lipophilic tracer and its structure is shown in Fig. 6.2. ^{68}Ga PSMA PET and ^{18}F-PSMA-1007 have been compared in two studies where the tracers turned out to be equally effective to indicate positive sites [28, 29].

^{68}Ga-PSMA PET/CT is extensively documented and it has lower costs than ^{18}F-PSMA PET, and the effective radiation dose is lower, because lower activities are used. A factor not favoring ^{68}Ga-PSMA PET/CT is that it is excreted in the urine and can disturb the interpretation in the region of the urinary bladder [30]. ^{18}F-PSMA-1007 PET/CT is lipophilic and not excreted in the urine, but enterohepatic clearance may hamper differential diagnosis of liver metastases. A recent study reports that patients with oligometastatic prostate have a higher progression-free survival after staging with ^{68}Ga PSMA PET than after staging with ^{18}F-PSMA [31], but the numbers are small ($n = 44$). However, the data with ^{18}F PSMA is not that extensive, and there are no head-to-head comparisons between ^{18}F-PSMA tracers. Personally, I have not found any major difference by using three different ^{18}F-PSMA tracers for patient diagnosis (as a consulting physician). For my own diagnosis, I studied two ^{18}F-PSMA tracers, pictures shown in that chapter, and the minor difference is discussed which changed therapy planning. There are no reported adverse effects from PSMA PET.

In the following, some cases are shown which deal with metastatic detection, biochemical recurrence, and response to radionuclide therapy.

Figure 6.3 shows a ^{68}Ga-PSMA-11-PET study of a 62-year-old male with a castrate resistant metastatic prostate cancer. His original diagnosis was T4N1M1 Gleason score 8 cancer 2 years earlier—first he developed relapse with skeletal

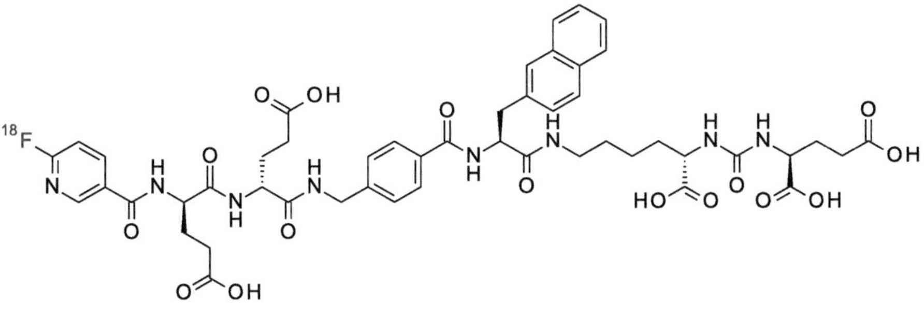

Fig. 6.2 The structure of ^{18}F-PSMA-1007

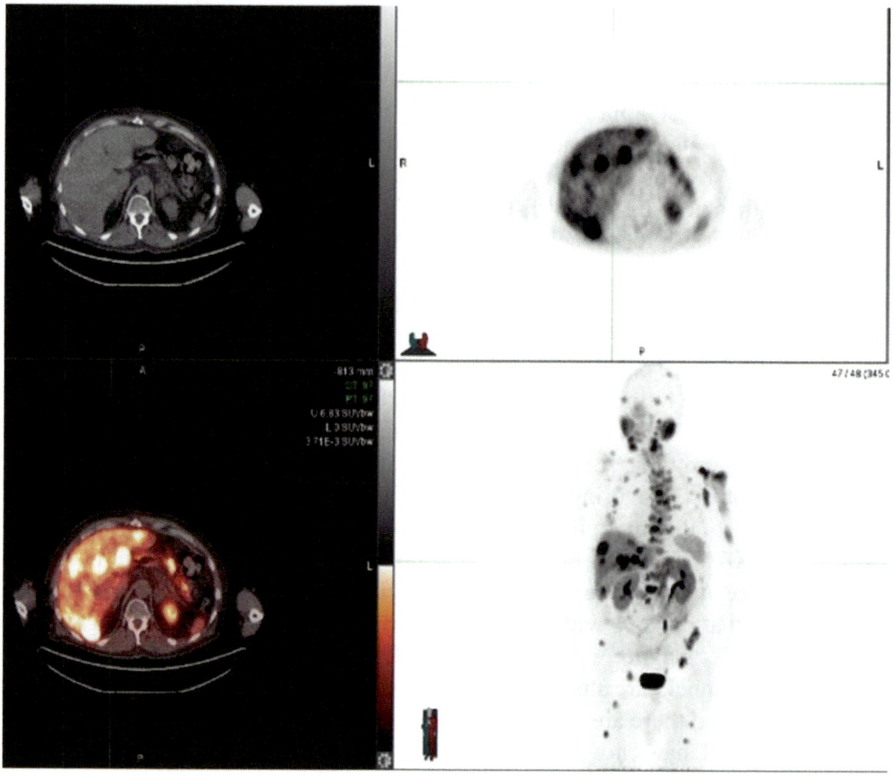

Fig. 6.3 A ^{68}Ga-PSMA-11-PET/CT study of a 62-year-old man with metastatic prostate adenocarcinoma with relapse after initial diagnosis 2 years earlier (T4M1N1, GS8). MIP image (right lower panel) demonstrates skeletal and liver metastases. Axial PET/CT fusion (left lower panel), CT image (left upper panel), and PET image (right upper panel) demonstrate multiple liver metastases. For assessing liver metastases, hydrophilic tracers (e.g., ^{68}Ga-PSMA-11) are better than lipophilic tracers (e.g., ^{18}F-PSMA-1007)

metastases which could be treated, and second relapse had additional liver metastases.

Figure 6.4 represents a ^{68}Ga-PSMA-PET and Na^{18}F-PET studies of a 57-year-old man with prostate cancer which was operated with robot-assisted radical prostatectomy and pelvic lymphadenectomy. His original diagnosis was T3aN0M0, with a Gleason score of 8, and initial S-PSA was 58 μg/l. He was treated additionally with external beam radiotherapy, and S-PSA dropped down to 0.67 μg/l. In the follow-up, S-PSA increased to 2.6 μg/l and thus a biochemical recurrence was suspected. In this case, a strong pathologic uptake was observed in the lower part of thoracic spine in the ^{68}Ga-PSMA-PET study, whereas Na^{18}F-PET study was completely negative. The SUVmax was very high, 27, located in the bone marrow. Presumably, the Na^{18}F-PET study was negative, because this metastasis was just developing (high SUV) without having time to cause any changes in the cortical. Typically, Na^{18}F-PET is the most sensitive method to see skeletal metastases.

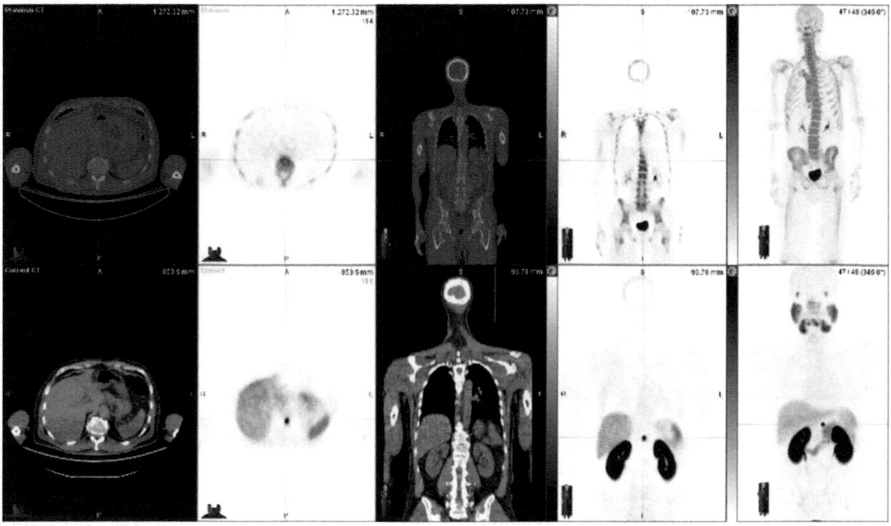

Fig. 6.4 Example of a 57-year-old prostate cancer patient who was initially treated with radical prostatectomy and pelvic lymphadenectomy following subsequent radiation therapy (T3aN0M0, Gleason score 8). Initial S-PSA was 58. In the follow-up, the S-PSA reached the nadir of 0.67 and now 2.6. Where is the biochemical recurrence? The upper row shows Na^{18}F-PET/CT study: one transaxial CT and PET, one coronal CT and PET, and MIP image. The lower row illustrates the same sections in the ^{68}Ga-PSMA-PET study. There are no pathologic uptakes in the Na^{18}F-PET study, normal skeleton. There is a strong pathologic uptake in the ^{68}Ga-PSMA-PET in the lowest part of the thoracic spine, best shown in transaxial and coronal PET sections (lower row), and SUVmax was 27, which is high. These PET tracers show different distributions, i.e., Na^{18}F is targeting cortical bone lesions and ^{68}Ga-PSMA bone marrow disease

Figure 6.5 represents a ^{68}Ga-PSMA-PET study of 67-year-old man with prostate cancer (Gleason score 8) which was operated with transurethral resection of the prostate, treated subsequently with androgen deprivation and external beam radiation therapy. He developed 4 years later mediastinal lymph node metastases. The patient was then treated with docetaxel and abiraterone, but 2 years later, rising PSA was detected (PSA was 3.1 μg/l). Thus, a biochemical recurrence was suspected. A tiny 3 mm perineum metastasis was identified in the ^{68}Ga-PSMA-PET study. It was surgically removed; histology revealed malignant histology consistent with a metastasis of an adenocarcinoma and immunohistochemistry with PSA staining proved it to be of prostate-specific origin (Fig. 6.5).

Figure 6.6 demonstrates how two consecutive ^{68}Ga-PSMA-PET studies can be used for assessing radionuclide therapy response. This 59-year-old man had an aggressive prostate cancer (GS 9) and was successfully treated with ^{177}Lu-PSMA-617 therapy for his third relapse in 9 years. A major response is seen while all the pelvic and retroperitoneal lymph nodes disappear in the later image in 3 months, and the large mediastinal lymph node becomes smaller (Fig. 6.6). This image pair has another lesion: it shows how important it is to distinguish pathologic lymph nodes (blue arrows) from the physiologic urinary uptakes (red arrows). The CT component of PET/CT is often helpful in this respect.

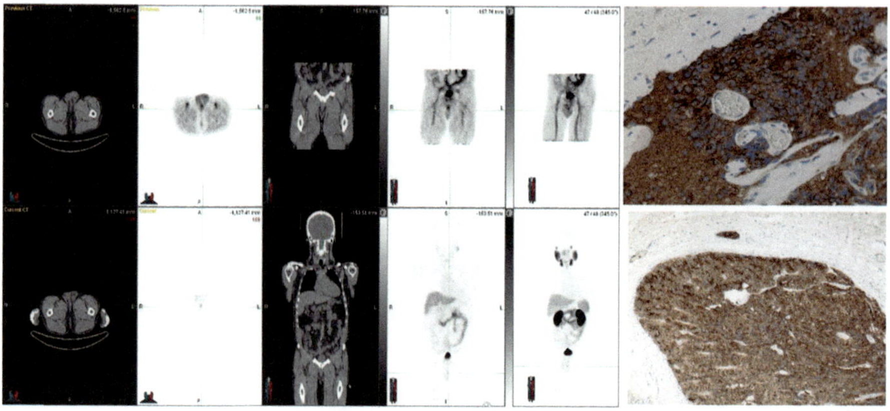

Fig. 6.5 Dual time point imagings with ^{68}Ga-PSMA-11-PET at 15 min (upper row) and at 60 min (lower row): transaxial and coronal CT and PET slices and MIP images. This 67-year-old man had originally Gleason score 8 prostate cancer, initially treated with surgery and hormone and radiation therapy but developed 4 years later lymph node metastases in the nediastinum. Two years after chemotherapy, he developed second relapse with an elevated S-PSA (3.1 μg/l). A small perineum metastasis (diameter 3 mm) was identified, better depicted in the lower row slice images (at the sites of crossings). It was surgically removed; histology (upper right image) revealed malignant histology, and immunohistochemistry (lower right image) with PSA staining proved it to derive from the prostate

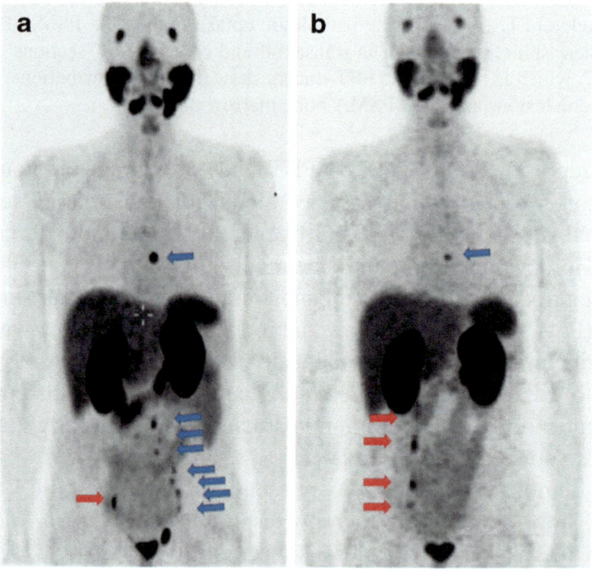

Fig. 6.6 Consecutive imaging with ^{68}Ga-PSMA-11-PET before ^{177}Lu-PSMA-617 therapies (**a**) and after the second cycle 3 months later (**b**). This 59-year-old man had an aggressive prostate cancer (GS 9) and was treated for his third relapse in 9 years. This image pair also shows how important it is to distinguish pathologic lymph nodes (blue arrows) from the physiologic ureter uptakes (red arrows) due to urinary excretion. From these images, it can be seen how the pelvic and retroperitioneal lymph nodes have disappeared, and the mediastinal lymph node has decreased substantially. PET images can be analyzed quantitatively in a more detail manner, but this is even visually a major response

References

1. Hofman MS, Lawrentschuk N, Francis RJ, et al. Prostate-specific membrane antigen PET-CT in patients with high-risk prostate cancer before curative-intent surgery or radiotherapy (proPSMA): a prospective, randomised, multicentre study. Lancet. 2020;395:1208–16.
2. Pienta KJ, Gorin MA, Rowe SP, et al. A phase 2/3 prospective multicenter study of the diagnostic accuracy of prostate specific membrane antigen PET/CT with (^{18})F-DCFPyL in prostate cancer patients (OSPREY). J Urol. 2021;206:52–61.
3. Surasi DS, Eiber M, Maurer T, et al. Diagnostic performance and safety of positron emission tomography with (^{18})F-rhPSMA-7.3 in patients with newly diagnosed unfavourable intermediate- to very-high-risk prostate cancer: results from a phase 3, prospective, multicentre study (LIGHTHOUSE). Eur Urol. 2023;84:361–70.
4. Vogel MME, Dewes S, Sage EK, et al. A survey among German-speaking radiation oncologists on PET-based radiotherapy of prostate cancer. Radiat Oncol. 2021;16:82.
5. Moran S, Cheng HH, Weg E, Kim EH, Chen DL, Iravani A, et al. Prostate-specific membrane antigen-positron emission tomography (PSMA-PET) of prostate cancer: current and emerging applications. Abdom Radiol (NY). 2024;49:1288–305.
6. Cornford P, van den Bergh RCN, Briers E, et al. EAU-EANM-ESTRO-ESUR-ISUP-SIOG guidelines on prostate cancer-2024 update. Part I: screening, diagnosis, and local treatment with curative intent. Eur Urol. 2024;86:P148–63.
7. Schaeffer EM, Srinivas S, Adra N, et al. Prostate cancer, version 4.2023, NCCN clinical practice guidelines in oncology. J Natl Compr Cancer Netw. 2023;21:1067–96.
8. Ost P, Mottet N. PSMA PET-CT, when seeing becomes improving. Int J Radiat Oncol Biol Phys. 2024;120:646–7.
9. Sood A, Kishan AU, Evans CP, et al. The impact of positron emission tomography imaging and tumor molecular profiling on risk stratification, treatment choice, and oncological outcomes of patients with primary or relapsed prostate cancer: an international collaborative review of the existing literature. Eur Urol Oncol. 2024;7:27–43.
10. Kawada T, Yanagisawa T, Rajwa P, et al. Diagnostic performance of prostate-specific membrane antigen positron emission tomography-targeted biopsy for detection of clinically significant prostate cancer: a systematic review and meta-analysis. Eur Urol Oncol. 2022;5:390–400.
11. Evangelista L, Zattoni F, Cassarino G, et al. PET/MRI in prostate cancer: a systematic review and meta-analysis. Eur J Nucl Med Mol Imaging. 2021;48:859–73.
12. Satapathy S, Singh H, Kumar R, et al. Diagnostic accuracy of ^{68}Ga-PSMA PET/CT for initial detection in patients with suspected prostate cancer: a systematic review and meta-analysis. AJR Am J Roentgenol. 2021;216:599–607.
13. Ptasznik G, Moon D, Buteau J, et al. A systematic review of the variability in performing and reporting intraprostatic prostate-specific membrane antigen positron emission tomography in primary staging studies. Eur Urol Open Sci. 2023;50:91–105.
14. Caracciolo M, Castello A, Urso L, et al. The role of [^{68}Ga]PSMA PET/CT for clinical suspicion of prostate cancer in patients with or without previous negative biopsy: a systematic review. Cancer. 2022;14(20):5036.
15. Yadav D, Hwang H, Qiao W, et al. ^{18}F-Fluciclovine versus PSMA PET imaging in primary tumor detection during initial staging of high-risk prostate cancer: a systematic review and meta-analysis. Radiol Imaging Cancer. 2022;4(2):e210091.
16. Zhao Y, Simpson BS, Morka N, et al. Comparison of multiparametric magnetic resonance imaging with prostate-specific membrane antigen positron-emission tomography imaging in primary prostate cancer diagnosis: a systematic review and meta-analysis. Cancer. 2022;14:3497.
17. Wu H, Xu T, Wang X, et al. Diagnostic performance of 68Gallium labelled prostate-specific membrane antigen positron emission tomography/computed tomography and magnetic resonance imaging for staging the prostate cancer with intermediate or high risk before radical prostatectomy: a systematic review and meta-analysis. World J Mens Health. 2020;38:208–19.

18. Hu X, Wu Y, Yang P, et al. Performance of ^{68}Ga-labeled prostate-specific membrane antigen ligand positron emission tomography/computed tomography in the diagnosis of primary prostate cancer: a systematic review and meta-analysis. Int Braz J Urol. 2022;48:891–902.
19. Morigi JJ, Anderson J, De Nunzio C, et al. Prostate specific membrane antigen positron emission tomography/computed tomography and staging high risk prostate cancer: a non-systematic review of high clinical impact literature. Minerva Urol Nephrol. 2021;73:32–41.
20. Ling SW, de Jong AC, Schoots IG, et al. Comparison of ^{68}Ga-labeled prostate-specific membrane antigen ligand positron emission tomography/magnetic resonance imaging and positron emission tomography/computed tomography for primary staging of prostate cancer: a systematic review and meta-analysis. Eur Urol Open Sci. 2021;33:61–71.
21. Jiao J, Zhang J, Li Z, et al. Prostate specific membrane antigen positron emission tomography in primary prostate cancer diagnosis: first-line imaging is afoot. Cancer Lett. 2022;548:215883.
22. Abrams-Pompe RS, Fanti S, Schoots IG, et al. The role of magnetic resonance imaging and positron emission tomography/computed tomography in the primary staging of newly diagnosed prostate cancer: a systematic review of the literature. Eur Urol Oncol. 2021;4:370–95.
23. Woo S, Ghafoor S, Becker AS, et al. Prostate-specific membrane antigen positron emission tomography (PSMA-PET) for local staging of prostate cancer: a systematic review and meta-analysis. Eur J Hybrid Imaging. 2020;4:16.
24. Hernes E, Revheim ME, Hole KH, et al. Prostate-specific membrane antigen PET for assessment of primary and recurrent prostate cancer with histopathology as reference standard: a systematic review and meta-analysis. PET Clin. 2021;16:147–65.
25. Petersen LJ, Zacho HD. PSMA PET for primary lymph node staging of intermediate and high-risk prostate cancer: an expedited systematic review. Cancer Imaging. 2020;20:10.
26. Tu X, Zhang C, Liu Z, et al. The role of ^{68}Ga-PSMA positron emission tomography/computerized tomography for preoperative lymph node staging in intermediate/high risk patients with prostate cancer: a diagnostic meta-analysis. Front Oncol. 2020;10:1365.
27. Lin M, Ta RT, Kairemo K, Le DB, Ravizzini GC. Prostate-specific membrane antigen-targeted radiopharmaceuticals in diagnosis and therapy of prostate cancer: current status and future perspectives. Cancer Biother Radiopharm. 2021;36(2):37–251.
28. Chandekar KR, Singh H, Kumar R, et al. Comparison of 18 F-PSMA-1007 PET/CT with 68 Ga-PSMA-11 PET/CT for initial staging in intermediate- and high-risk prostate cancer. Clin Nucl Med. 2023;48:e1–8.
29. Hoffmann MA, Muller-Hubenthal J, Rosar F, et al. Primary staging of prostate cancer patients with [(^{18})F]PSMA-1007 PET/CT compared with [(^{68})Ga]Ga-PSMA-11 PET/CT. J Clin Med. 2022;11:5064.
30. Evangelista L, Maurer T, van der Poel H, et al. [(^{68})Ga]Ga-PSMA versus [(^{18})F]PSMA positron emission tomography/computed tomography in the staging of primary and recurrent prostate cancer. A systematic review of the literature. Eur Urol Oncol. 2022;5:273–82.
31. Bauknecht M, Lanfranchi F, Albano D, et al. Diverse imaging methods may influence long-term oncologic outcomes in oligorecurrent prostate cancer patients treated with metastasis-directed therapy (the PRECISE-MDT study). J Nucl Med. 2024;65:1202–9.

^{18}F-FLT PET/CT in Prostate Adenocarcinoma

7

Fluorothymidine F-18 (FLT) is a tumor-associated PET tracer and radiopharmaceutical [1–3]. It is a radionuclide analogue of 3′-deoxy-3′-fluorothymidine also known as alovudine. FLT is suitable for monitoring how tumors respond to cytostatic therapy. FLT accumulates in proliferating cells where it indicates the activity of the enzyme thymidine kinase. Cell division can be characterized by the activity of that enzyme. FLT is phosphorylated as though it were thymidine and is subsequently incorporated into DNA. Thymidine is essential for DNA replication. Considering that FLT lacks a 3′-hydroxy group, transcription of DNA is impeded following incorporating of FLT. FLT indicates changes in tumor cell proliferation by tracking the restoration of nucleosides from degenerated DNA.

Experimental Background

Uncontrolled proliferation is a hallmark of malignant processes. Monitoring of proliferation can be based on identification of active biologic processes required for cell growth (carbohydrate metabolism), lipid metabolism, amino acid metabolism, and DNA synthesis.

Tumor growth driven by DNA synthesis was a hallmark for development of [^{18}F]3-deoxy-3-fluorothymidine (^{18}F-FLT), imaging biomarker of cell proliferation in vivo. ^{18}F-FLT, labeled analogue of thymidine, is derived from cytostatic drug zidovudine [2]. Thymidine is nucleoside that is selectively incorporated into DNA, not in RNA, and its retention reflects the level of DNA synthesis and cell replication. Precisely, ^{18}F-FLT uptake in malignant cell correlates with activity of enzyme thymidine kinase-1 (TK1) expressed during S-phase of DNA synthesis [3]. Activity of TK-1 is low in cell resting stage and high in deregulated cancer cell cycle. However, only 8–20% of the cells are in S-phase, so in comparison with glucose metabolism and ^{18}F-FDG accumulation, absolute accumulation of TK-1-catalyzed radioactivity is relatively low. The chemical structure of ^{18}F-FLT is shown in Fig. 7.1.

K. Kairemo, *Prostate Cancer from a Nuclear Oncology Perspective*,
https://doi.org/10.1007/978-3-031-90337-3_7

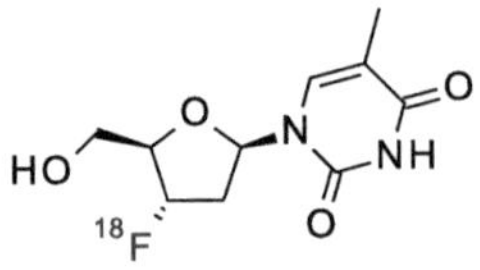

Fig. 7.1 The chemical structure of ^{18}F-FLT, [^{18}F]3-deoxy-3-fluorothymidine

^{18}F-FLT has been designed as a new positron emission tomography imaging agent in year 2000 [4]. Initially FLT was developed as an antiviral agent, but its use was stopped due to the hematologic and hepatic toxicity [5]. In tracer doses, toxicity is not an issue.

Some studies showed significant relationship between ^{18}F-FLT uptake and presence of immunohistochemical cellular marker for proliferation, protein Ki67 [6, 7].

On the other hand, some studies showed conflicting correlation between ^{18}F-FLT uptake and Ki67. Lack of ^{18}F-FLT/Ki67 correlation has been explained by difference in the phosphorylation rate between thymidine and [8] loss of cell cycle TK1 regulation [9] levels of ATP in the cell [9] as well as complex methodology in proliferation tissue vs. imaging biomarker experiments [10]. Factors confounding ^{18}F-FLT uptake in different malignant processes are still not fully understood.

Correlation between ^{18}F-FLT uptake and tumor proliferation has been described in various malignant processes including lymphomas [11], sarcomas [12, 13], melanomas [14], breast cancer [15], colorectal cancer [16], and lung cancer [17–19], but not in prostate cancer before our study [20].

The bone marrow and liver (^{18}F-FLT undergoes glucuronidation in the liver) physiologically accumulates all thymidine tracers, so these areas are more difficult to investigate. In comparison with the bone marrow and liver, there is no physiological ^{18}F-FLT accumulation in the brain, making this tracer suitable for diagnosis of brain metastases [21].

In our pilot study, we evaluated ^{18}F-FLT for PET/CT imaging of prostate cancer in patients undergoing treatment, as a potential imaging biomarker to assess response to treatment [20]. Because ^{18}F-FLT is a structural analog of the DNA component, thymidine, it is trapped in the cell due to phosphorylation by thymidine kinase as a part of the proliferation pathway. Like ^{18}F-FDG, the tracer accumulates in the cell via the same mechanism as the physiological analog, but cannot be further metabolized and is hence “trapped” and continues to accumulate intracellularly. ^{18}F-FLT is a marker of tumor proliferation, and its uptake has been shown to be proportional to the DNA synthesis rate and proliferative indices [21]. Therefore, imaging of cellular proliferation could become an important diagnostic tool to evaluate the tumor growth rates and objectively assess potential response to treatment [22]. Before our study, only preclinical experiments evaluated the ^{18}F-FLT effectiveness in prostate cancer animal models. Pharmacokinetics of ^{18}F-FLT, ^{18}F-FDG and ^{11}C-choline were compared in two hormone independent (PC-3, DU145) and two hormone-dependent (CWR22, PAC120) prostate cancer xenograft mouse models using PET [23]. The highest uptake of both ^{18}F-FLT and ^{18}F-FDG was in PC-3 tumors. Interestingly, uptake of ^{18}F-FLT was insufficient to provide reliable information on response to therapy in CWR22 tumor model [24].

Another study reported a significant decline in ^{18}F-FLT microPET uptake in the 22Rv1 hormone-refractory prostate tumor model, where tumors were implanted in athymic mice after treatment with docetaxel [25]. Therefore, the usefulness of ^{18}F-FLT in the evaluation of treatment response in patients with prostate cancer is largely unknown.

Pilot Study for Early Response in Chemotherapy

We studied the potential of fluorine-18-fluorothymidine positron emission tomography (^{18}F-FLT PET/CT) as a molecular imaging tool for assessing early responses to targeted therapies in patients with advanced prostate adenocarcinoma [20]. The commonly used PET tracer, ^{18}F-FDG, has limitations in prostate cancer evaluation, prompting exploration of alternative tracers like ^{18}F-FLT, which targets tumor cell proliferation by mimicking thymidine, a DNA precursor. This study specifically looks at ^{18}F-FLT PET/CT imaging in patients treated with MET inhibitors, which block the hepatocyte growth factor (HGF)/c-MET pathway known to play a role in prostate cancer progression.

Seven patients with Stage IV prostate adenocarcinoma who were candidates for MET inhibitor therapy participated in the study. Baseline ^{18}F-FLT PET/CT scans were taken before therapy, and follow-up scans were performed approximately 4 weeks after starting treatment. Tumor response was assessed both visually and semiquantitatively using the maximum standardized uptake value (SUVmax). Patients underwent whole-body PET/CT imaging about 60 min after ^{18}F-FLT injection. The imaging focused on the prostate, lymph nodes, skeletal system, and liver to assess changes in tumor activity.

Prostate The SUVmax values in the prostate ranged from 2.5 to 4.2 at baseline. One patient showed mixed results, with a decrease in activity in the left lobe of the prostate (from 3.6 to 2.3) but an increase in the right lobe. Despite the changes, this patient's PSA levels progressed. ^{18}F-FLT PET/CT did not show significant effectiveness for evaluating tumor response in the prostate bed.

Lymph Node Metastases Three patients had detectable lymph node metastases. Of these, only one patient (Patient #3) showed a significant reduction in SUVmax values in the left iliac lymph node (from 4.1 to 2.1), reflecting a 49% decrease in activity. This patient also exhibited a decrease in lymph node size (from 3.6 to 3.1 cm) and showed a PSA response. The other two patients with lymph node involvement did not show any significant (>30%) reduction in SUVmax, correlating with disease progression in both cases.

Skeletal Metastases Three patients demonstrated skeletal metastases, which appeared as defects on the ^{18}F-FLT PET/CT images. These defects were likely due to bone marrow invasion by prostate cancer cells. However, the usefulness of 18F-FLT for detecting skeletal metastases was limited by background activity in the bone marrow. The visualization of cortical bone lesions was not effective with this method.

Liver Metastases Two patients had known liver metastases. In one patient with a single lesion, activity increased post-therapy. For the second patient, multiple liver lesions were visible as defects on the ^{18}F-FLT PET/CT scans, making it difficult to assess activity accurately.

The study concluded that ^{18}F-FLT PET/CT has limited value in assessing early therapy responses in prostate cancer. It might have some utility in evaluating lymph node metastases, but it was not effective in detecting changes in the prostate bed, skeletal metastases, or liver lesions.

Patient Image Examples of Using ^{18}F-FLT PET

Response Evaluation

Three patient cases with advanced prostate cancer are shown who were imaged with ^{18}F-FLT before and 4 weeks after initiating chemotherapy (HGF/c-MET inhibitor). The patient shown in Fig. 7.2 demonstrates a weak response in the left prostate lobe. The patient in Fig. 7.3 shows a visually weak response in left common iliac node—numerically the SUVmax decreased from 4.1 down to 2.4. The patient in Fig. 7.4 had several skeletal metastases which were shown as defects.

Response to Immunotherapy

Scarpelli et al. [26] explored the potential of ^{18}F-FLT-PET/CT imaging as a biomarker for predicting both tumor response and immune-related adverse events in patients undergoing immunotherapy. The study focused on patients with metastatic castration-resistant prostate cancer treated with a combination of pTVG-HP DNA vaccine and pembrolizumab, a PD-1 checkpoint inhibitor [26].

Immunotherapy has revolutionized cancer treatment, but challenges remain in predicting which patients will respond and how to measure that response. Traditional imaging, such as CT or MRI, may not accurately reflect early treatment effects in immunotherapy, where initial tumor growth can sometimes be mistaken for progression. Additionally, specific criteria have been developed for assessing immunotherapy response criteria [27]. Hence, there is a critical need for predictive biomarkers that can monitor tumor responses and potential immune-related adverse effects in real time.

The study investigated whether ^{18}F-FLT-PET/CT can serve as an early biomarker for tumor response, immune activity, and the detection of adverse events during immunotherapy. The study enrolled 17 patients with mCRPC. These patients were treated with a combination of the pTVG-HP DNA vaccine, which targets prostatic acid phosphatase (PAP) to induce immune responses, and pembrolizumab, a

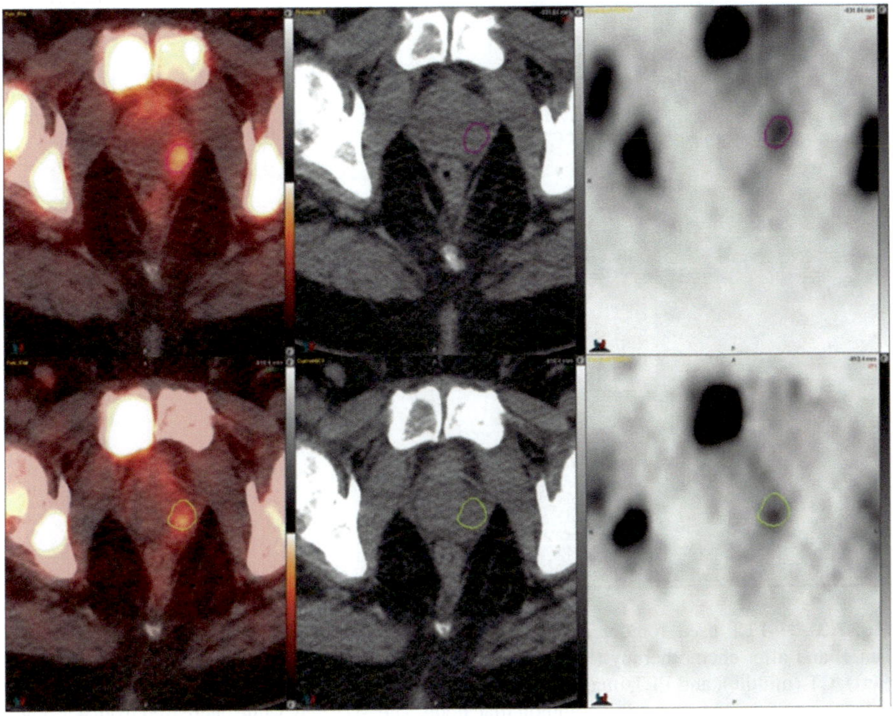

Fig. 7.2 ^{18}F-FLT used for detection of prostate foci before (upper panel) and after chemotherapy (lower panel) in a 67-year-old male. Transaxial PET/CT fusions (left), CT (middle), and PET images (right) are shown. A weak response in the left prostate lobe is seen in 4 weeks [20]

checkpoint inhibitor that prevents immune cells from being deactivated by the tumor [26].

Patients underwent ^{18}F-FLT-PET/CT imaging before starting therapy (baseline) and after 12 weeks of treatment. ^{18}F-FLT uptake was observed in several regions, including tumors, lymph nodes, spleen, bone marrow, pancreas, thyroid. ^{18}F-FLT uptake was quantified as standardized uptake values (SUV), and changes in SUV were analyzed to assess the relationship between cell proliferation, immune response, and progression-free survival (PFS).

Immune Response and ^{18}F-FLT Uptake

Vaccine Draining Lymph Nodes ^{18}F-FLT PET scans showed increased uptake in vaccine-draining lymph nodes compared to non-draining nodes. This suggested a regional immune response to the pTVG-HP vaccine, where immune cells were proliferating. However, this increased ^{18}F-FLT uptake in lymph nodes did not correlate with PFS, indicating it was not predictive of treatment outcome.

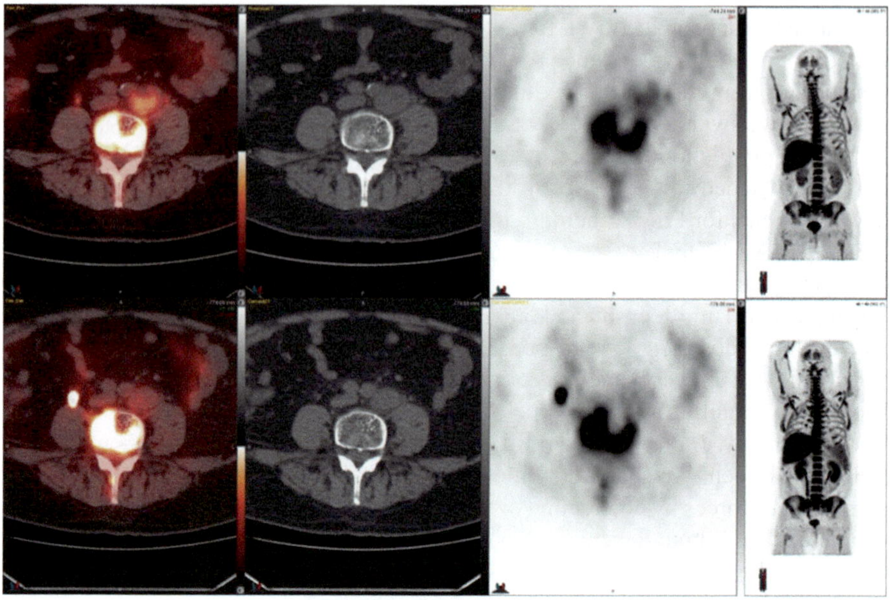

Fig. 7.3 ^{18}F-FLT used for detection of retroperitoneal lymph node metastases before (upper panel) and after chemotherapy (lower panel) in a 65-year-old male. Transaxial PET/CT fusions (left), CT (middle), and PET images (right) are shown and whole-body MIP images (most right). A weak response is seen in a left common iliac node. The SUVmax value decreased from 4.1 down to 2.4 in 4 weeks [20]

Spleen and Bone Marrow Significant increases in spleen ^{18}F-FLT uptake were observed in patients, particularly in those receiving combined vaccine and pembrolizumab therapy (arm 3 of the trial). However, a paradoxical finding was that patients with higher ^{18}F-FLT uptake in the spleen had shorter progression-free survival (PFS). The reason for this remains unclear but may reflect an undesirable immune response.

Tumor Response and ^{18}F-FLT Uptake

Predictive of Progression-Free Survival Changes in ^{18}F-FLT uptake in tumors were strongly predictive of treatment outcomes. Patients whose tumors showed higher ^{18}F-FLT uptake at 12 weeks had significantly shorter PFS (hazard ratio 3.38, $P = 0.05$), indicating that tumor cell proliferation, as measured by FLT PET, was a reliable early marker of disease progression.

Correlation with PSA and RECIST ^{18}F-FLT PET changes were also correlated with traditional measures of tumor response, such as PSA levels and tumor size (measured by RECIST criteria). Patients with increased ^{18}F-FLT uptake in tumors typically showed worse PSA and RECIST responses, further supporting ^{18}F-FLT PET's role as a predictive biomarker.

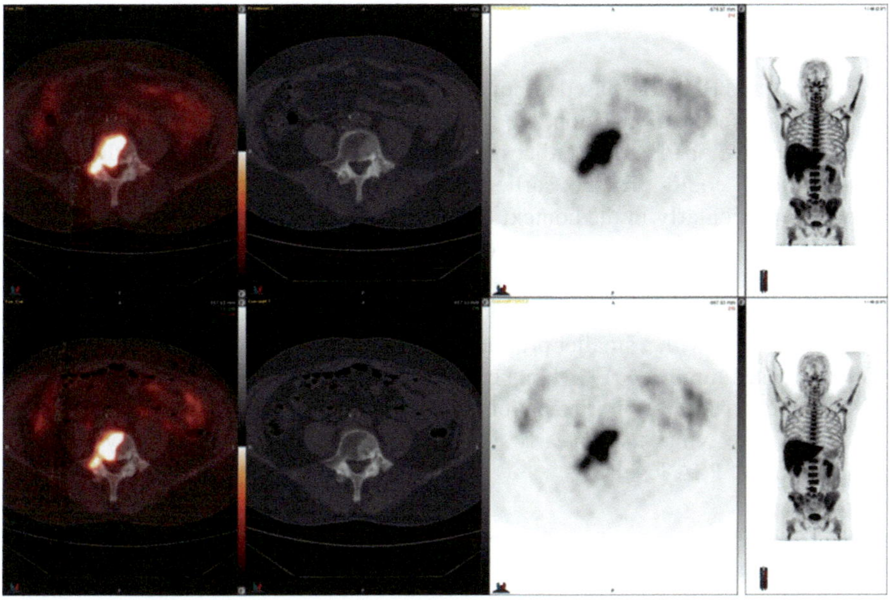

Fig. 7.4 ^{18}F-FLT detection of prostate cancer metastases before and after chemotherapy. The usefulness of ^{18}F-FLT for detection of skeletal metastases is still unclear since visualization of lesions may be hindered by prominent background activity in the bone marrow. The skeletal metastases are visualized most often as defects [20]

FLT Uptake and Immune-Related Adverse Events

Thyroid Events FLT PET also revealed potential predictive capability for immune-related adverse events (irAEs). Patients who had higher baseline FLT uptake in their thyroids were more likely to develop thyroid-related adverse events, such as hyperthyroidism and hypothyroidism, during the course of therapy. The ability of FLT PET to predict these events was highly accurate (AUC = 0.97). This suggests that increased FLT uptake at baseline may identify patients with subclinical thyroid autoimmunity, which pembrolizumab might exacerbate.

Pancreatitis and Other irAEs One patient developed pancreatitis after 12 weeks of treatment, but ^{18}F-FLT PET failed to reliably predict this event, as other patients with higher FLT uptake in the pancreas did not experience adverse effects. Similarly, adrenal insufficiency in another patient was not detected via ^{18}F-FLT PET, indicating limitations in the technology's ability to predict all forms of immune-related adverse events.

Other Biomarkers

While PSA and RECIST-based tumor measurements are standard metrics for assessing prostate cancer progression, the study found that changes in ^{18}F-FLT PET were more predictive of PFS than either of these traditional markers. This indicates that ^{18}F-FLT PET could provide earlier and more reliable insights into treatment response, particularly in the context of immunotherapy, where anatomical changes may not fully reflect therapeutic effects.

Three patients had tumor biopsies that were analyzed for cell proliferation using immunohistochemistry. In one patient, the majority of proliferating cells were prostate cancer cells, with a smaller proportion being immune cells. This finding aligned with increased tumor ^{18}F-FLT uptake, further supporting ^{18}F-FLT PET as a marker of tumor cell proliferation. The patient with the biopsy showed an increase in tumor ^{18}F-FLT uptake, which was an early sign of progression, confirmed later by increased tumor size and PSA levels.

Conclusive Remarks

Chemotherapy Response

From our material we can find only limited applications of FLT in the early response evaluation of chemotherapy in prostate cancer. It may work in the assessment of response in lymph nodes (Fig. 7.3)—it will probably not work in the evaluation of prostate bed (Fig. 7.2), but it will definitely not work in the evaluation of skeletal disease or liver disease. This pilot study shows that ^{18}F-FLT PET/CT has only limited application for early response evaluation in prostate cancer therapy. While it may offer some utility in monitoring lymph node metastases, its effectiveness in the prostate bed, skeletal disease, and liver lesions is minimal. More research is needed to explore other imaging biomarkers and tracers for better treatment monitoring in prostate cancer.

The study highlighted that, unlike ^{18}F-FDG, which accumulates in both tumor and inflamed tissues, ^{18}F-FLT specifically accumulates in proliferating tumor cells and not in inflammatory tissues [28]. This could make ^{18}F-FLT a more specific marker of tumor activity, particularly in distinguishing tumors from inflammation post-therapy. However, the limited response seen in this pilot study suggests that ^{18}F-FLT may not be a reliable biomarker for early response in prostate cancer, particularly in advanced disease stages with skeletal and liver metastases.

Immunotherapy Response

In patients undergoing immunotherapy, ^{18}F-FLT PET/CT imaging shows promise as a biomarker for predicting both tumor progression and certain immune-related adverse events (irAEs). The study suggested that FLT PET could provide an early indicator of treatment efficacy by measuring tumor and immune cell proliferation, which could guide clinical decisions more effectively than traditional imaging or PSA measurements.

The ability of ^{18}F-FLT PET to predict thyroid-related adverse events offers a new tool for monitoring potential irAEs in immunotherapy patients, allowing for early intervention and potentially avoiding severe complications.

Both the pilot studies [20, 27] were limited by their small sample sizes (7 and 17 patients) and the inability to evaluate bone metastases due to high ^{18}F-FLT uptake in normal bone marrow. Further research is needed to refine the timing of ^{18}F-FLT PET scans and to better understand the biological mechanisms behind increased ^{18}F-FLT uptake in immune organs like the spleen.

In summary, FLT PET/CT imaging holds potential as a noninvasive method to assess both tumor response and immune activity during cancer immunotherapy. It may serve as a valuable tool for early detection of treatment failure and adverse effects, leading to more personalized and adaptive treatment strategies in prostate cancer.

References

1. McKinley ET, Ayers GD, Smith RA, et al. Limits of [18F]-FLT PET as a biomarker of proliferation in oncology. PLoS One. 2013;8(3):e58938.
2. Drontle DP, Wagner CR. Designing a pronucleotide stratagem: lessons from amino acid phosphoramidates of anticancer and antiviral pyrimidines. Mini-Rev Med Chem. 2004;4:409–19.
3. Rasey JS, Grierson JR, Wiens LW, et al. Validation of FLT uptake as a measure of thymidine kinase-1 activity in A549 carcinoma cells. J Nucl Med. 2002;43:1210–7.
4. Grierson JR, Shields AF. Radiosynthesis of 3′-deoxy-3′-[(^{18})F]fluorothymidine: [(^{18})F]FLT for imaging of cellular proliferation in vivo. Nucl Med Biol. 2000;27:143–56.
5. Matthes E, Lehmann C, Scholz D, Rosenthal HA, Langen P. Phosphorylation, anti-HIV activity and cytotoxicity of 3′-fluorothymidine. Biochem Biophys Res Commun. 1988;153:825–31.
6. Avril N, Menzel MJ, Dose J, et al. Glucose metabolism of breast cancer assessed by 18F-FDG PET: histologic and immunohistochemical tissue analysis. J Nucl Med. 2001;42:9–16.
7. Vesselle H, Schmidt RA, Pugsley JM, et al. Lung cancer proliferation correlates with [F-18] fluorodeoxyglucose uptake by positron emission tomography. Clin Cancer Res. 2000;6:3837–44.
8. van Westreenen HL, Cobben DC, Jager PL, et al. Comparison of ^{18}F-FLT PET and ^{18}F-FDG PET in esophageal cancer. J Nucl Med. 2005;46:400–4.
9. Kameyama R, Yamamoto Y, Izuishi K, et al. Detection of gastric cancer using ^{18}F-FLT PET: comparison with 18F-FDG PET. Eur J Nucl Med Mol Imaging. 2009;36(3):382–8.
10. Chalkidou A, Landau DB, Odell EW, Cornelius VR, O'Doherty MJ, Marsden PK. Correlation between Ki-67 immunohistochemistry and ^{18}F-fluorothymidine uptake in patients with cancer: a systematic review and meta-analysis. Eur J Cancer. 2012;48:3499–513.
11. Wagner M, Seitz U, Buck A, et al. 3′-[^{18}F]Fluoro-3′-deoxythymidine ([^{18}F]-FLT) as positron emission tomography tracer for imaging proliferation in a murine B-cell lymphoma model and in the human disease. Cancer Res. 2003;63:2681–7.
12. Cobben DC, Elsinga PH, Suurmeijer AJ, et al. Detection and grading of soft tissue sarcomas of the extremities with ^{18}F-3′-fluoro-3′-deoxy-L-thymidine. Clin Cancer Res. 2004;10:1685–90.
13. Kairemo K, Santos EB, Macapinlac HA, Patel S, Conley AP, Hong DS, Subbiah AV. Molecular imaging with 3′-deoxy-3′[(^{18})F]-fluorothymidine (^{18}F-FLT) PET/CT for early response to targeted therapies in sarcomas: a pilot study. Diagnostics (Basel). 2020;10:125.

14. Cobben DC, Jager PL, Elsinga PH, et al. 3′-^{18}F-Fluoro-3_deoxy-L-thymidine: a new tracer for staging metastatic melanoma? J Nucl Med. 2003;44:1927–32.
15. Contractor KB, Kenny LM, Stebbing J, et al. Biological basis of [(^{11})C]choline-positron emission tomography in patients with breast cancer: comparison with [(^{18})F]fluorothymidine positron emission tomography. Nucl Med Commun. 2011;32:997–1004.
16. Francis DL, Visvikis D, Costa DC, et al. Potential impact of [^{18}F]3_-deoxy-3_-flurorothymidine versus [^{18}F]fluoro-2-deoxy-D-glucose in positron emission tomography for colorectal cancer. Eur J Nucl Med Mol Imaging. 2003;30:988–94.
17. Buck AK, Schirrmeister H, Hetzel M, et al. 3-Deoxy-3-[^{18}F]fluorothymidine positron emission tomography for noninvasive assessment of proliferation in pulmonary nodules. Cancer Res. 2002;62:3331–4.
18. Yap CS, Czernin J, Fishbein MC, et al. Evaluation of thoracic tumors with ^{18}F-fluorothymidine and ^{18}F-fluorodeoxyglucosepositron emission tomography. Chest. 2006;129:393–401.
19. Kairemo K, Santos EB, Macapinlac HA, Subbiah V. Early response assessment to targeted therapy using 3′-deoxy-3′[(^{18})F]-fluorothymidine (^{18}F-FLT) PET/CT in lung cancer. Diagnostics (Basel). 2020;10:26.
20. Kairemo K, Ravizzini GC, Macapinlac HA, Subbiah V. An assessment of early response to targeted therapy via molecular imaging: a pilot study of 3′-deoxy-3′[(^{18})F]-fluorothymidine positron emission tomography ^{18}F-FLT PET/CT in prostate adenocarcinoma. Diagnostics (Basel). 2017;7(2):20.
21. Buck AK, Bommer M, Stilgenbauer S, et al. Molecular imaging of proliferation in malignant lymphoma. Cancer Res. 2006;66:11055–61.
22. Nimmagadda S, Shields AF. The role of DNA synthesis imaging in cancer in the era of targeted therapeutics. Cancer Metastasis Rev. 2008;27:575–87.
23. Kukuk D, Reischl G, Raguin O, et al. Assessment of PET tracer uptake in hormone-independent and hormone-dependent xenograft prostate cancer mouse models. J Nucl Med. 2011;52:1654–166.
24. Oyama N, Ponde DE, Dence C, Kim J, Tai YC, et al. Monitoring of therapy in androgen-dependent prostate tumor model by measuring tumor proliferation. J Nucl Med. 2004;45:519–25.
25. Oyama N, Hasegawa Y, Kiyono Y, Kobayashi M, Fujibayashi Y, et al. Early response assessment in prostate carcinoma by (^{18})F-fluorothymidine following anticancer therapy with docetaxel using preclinical tumour models. Eur J Nucl Med Mol Imaging. 2011;38:81–9.
26. Scarpelli M, Zahm C, Perlman S, McNeel DG, Jeraj R, Liu G. FLT PET/CT imaging of metastatic prostate cancer patients treated with pTVG-HP DNA vaccine and pembrolizumab. J Immunother Cancer. 2019;7:23.
27. Subbiah V, Chuang HH, Gambhire D, Kairemo K. Defining clinical response criteria and early response criteria for precision oncology: current state-of-the-art and future perspectives. Diagnostics (Basel). 2017;7:E10.
28. van Waarde A, Cobben DC, Suurmeijer AJ, et al. Selectivity of ^{18}F-FLT and ^{18}F-FDG for differentiating tumor from inflammation in a rodent model. J Nucl Med. 2004;45:695–700.

^{18}F-FDHT-PET Imaging in the Management of Hormone-Dependent Prostate Cancer

8

I have written recently a review entitled “Androgen Receptor Imaging in the Management of Hormone-Dependent Cancers with Emphasis on Prostate Cancer” together with professor Marina Hodolic (2023) providing a detailed review of the role of androgen receptor (AR) imaging in the diagnosis and management of hormone-dependent cancers, especially in prostate cancer [1]. Here is a brief summary.

Prostate cancer progression is heavily influenced by androgens like testosterone. These hormones promote tumor growth by binding to androgen receptors in prostate cells. Traditional treatments have involved endocrine therapies that either reduce hormone production or block these receptors. However, the effectiveness of these therapies varies among patients, necessitating personalized treatment approaches.

We reviewed on the use of ^{18}F-FDHT-PET, a specific PET imaging agent, which is a radiolabeled androgen that binds to ARs. The structure of compound is show in Fig. 8.1. This imaging modality is used to assess the presence of ARs in tumors, which can help predict the response to endocrine therapies.

Our review also describes the history of the tracer development: Briefly, initial studies using radiolabeled androgens faced challenges with poor stability and uptake [1]. Over time, ^{18}F-FDHT-PET was developed and has shown better stability and uptake in prostate tissues, making it a promising tool for clinical use.

^{18}F-FDHT-PET has been used in various studies to diagnose and manage prostate cancer. It has helped in assessing metastatic spread and evaluating the biological activity of tumors.

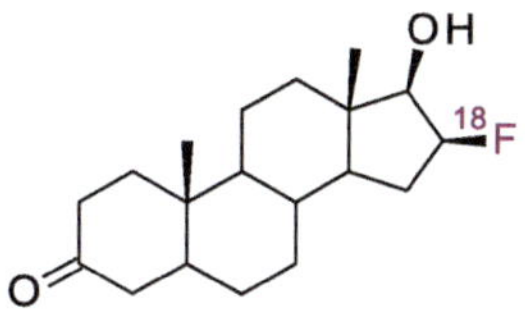

Fig. 8.1 The chemical structure of ^{18}F-FDHT, 16α-18F-fluoro-5α-dihydrotestosterone

K. Kairemo, *Prostate Cancer from a Nuclear Oncology Perspective*,
https://doi.org/10.1007/978-3-031-90337-3_8

More importantly, it has predictive power: Imaging results with ^{18}F-FDHT-PET have been correlated with clinical outcomes such as patient survival rates and response to treatments, suggesting its utility as a predictive biomarker.

We also extended the discussion to the use of ^{18}F-FDHT-PET beyond prostate cancer. In other hormone-dependent cancers, such as breast cancer, ARs may also play a significant role [2]. The imaging technique has potential applications in evaluating treatment efficacy and guiding therapy decisions across various cancers. Anecdotally, it has been used for assessing ARs in high grade glioblastoma [3].

Despite its benefits, ^{18}F-FDHT-PET faces challenges such as variability in tumor uptake and the need for improved imaging protocols to enhance sensitivity and specificity.

Our review highlights the need for further studies to refine AR-targeted imaging techniques, develop new imaging agents, and integrate these tools into routine clinical practice to improve the management of hormone-dependent cancers. The studies in the literature are listed in Table 8.1.

These documents center on advanced prostate cancer, particularly metastatic castration-resistant prostate cancer (mCRPC), discussing various diagnostic techniques, particularly PET/CT imaging, and therapeutic strategies involving novel androgens and radiotracers. The use of imaging to assess androgen receptor (AR) expression and glycolytic activity as biomarkers for prognosis and therapeutic targeting forms a significant focus of these studies.

In the first published article in 2004, Steven M. Larson et al. [4] aimed to assess the effectiveness of 16α-18F-fluoro-5α-dihydrotestosterone (^{18}F-FDHT) PET imaging for detecting androgen receptor expression in metastatic prostate cancer patients, compared to 18F-FDG PET scans and traditional imaging techniques. Seven male patients with clinically confirmed progressive metastatic prostate cancer underwent dual imaging with ^{18}F-FDG and ^{18}F-FDHT PET scans, in addition to standard imaging protocols (one patient example is shown in Fig. 8.2). Metabolism and tissue distribution of ^{18}F-FDHT were studied, focusing on its rapid uptake and prolonged retention at tumor sites. The study also involved lesion-by-lesion comparison across imaging methods. Conventional imaging detected 59 lesions. ^{18}F-FDG PET scans identified 57 of these lesions (97% detection rate), whereas ^{18}F-FDHT PET scans detected 46 lesions (78% detection rate) [4].

^{18}F-FDHT exhibited rapid metabolism with significant conversion to radiolabeled metabolites that bind to plasma proteins, which circulated post-administration. Changes in ^{18}F-FDHT uptake were observed post testosterone treatment, indicating a dynamic and responsive AR signaling pathway. While ^{18}F-FDG was generally more sensitive in detecting lesions, ^{18}F-FDHT provided critical insights into the functional status of AR, especially in lesions that are difficult to biopsy [4].

Pat B. Zanzonico et al. [5] aimed at optimizing the dosage of [^{18}F]-FDHT to maximize imaging efficacy while minimizing exposure to radiation. They found in ten PET studies using ^{18}F-FDHT conducted on seven prostate cancer patients that maximum administered activity of 331 MBq keeps the radiation dose to the bladder wall under recommended threshold. Normal organ uptakes are shown in Table 8.2 according to the measurements from [11].

Table 8.1 Clinical studies with ^{18}F-FDHT in patients with prostate cancer presented in the literature

First author, year, [ref]	No of patients with PCa	Objective of the study	[^{18}F] FDHT PET	SUV_{max}	Conclusion
Larson 2004 [4]	7	To assess AR status		Average SUV(max) = 5.28	[^{18}F]FDHT PET/CT localizes prostate cancer
Zanzonico 2004 [5]	7	To derive estimates of normal tissue absorbed doses for [^{18}F]FDHT			331 MBq (5 cGy/[0.0151 cGy/MBq]) is recommended for [^{18}F]FDHT
Dehdashti 2005 [6]	20	To evaluate the feasibility of [^{18}F] FDHT PET/CT and to assess the binding selectivity of [^{18}F]FDHT to AR			[^{18}F]FDHT uptake is a receptor-mediated process. Positive PET studies were associated with higher PSA levels and thus, presumably, with greater tumor burden
Fox 2011 [7]	20	Correlation between imaging signals of [^{18}F] FDG and [^{18}F] FDHT by readers	[^{18}F] FDHT [^{18}F] FDG	1.8–2.6 for the response assessment	99% concordance of identifying [^{18}F]FDG and [^{18}F]FDHT negative sites and positive-site agreement was 83% for [^{18}F]FDG and 85% for [^{18}F] FDHT. New method for response assessment
Vargas 2014 [8]	38	To determine associations between [^{18}F] FDHT PET/CT and overall survival			Patients with higher SUVmax on [^{18}F] FDHT PET/CT had significantly shorter overall survival
Fox 2018 [9]	133	To determine combined value of [^{18}F]FDG and [^{18}F]FDHT as prognosticator	[^{18}F] FDHT [^{18}F] FDG	Bone 5.5, lymph nodes 6.4, prostate 7.6	Three phenotypes—AR_1Glyc_1, AR_1Glyc_0, and AR_0Glyc_1—were identified. If AR is negative and FDG positive, it has negative impact on survival
Al Jalali 2023 [10]	10	Correlation between imaging signals of [^{68}Ga] PSMA and [^{18}F] FDHT	[^{18}F] FDHT PET/MRI [^{68}Ga] PSMA		Tumor detection rate of the [^{68}Ga]PSMA was 90%, but only 40% for the [^{18}F] FDHT PET/CT

Modified from Ref. [1]

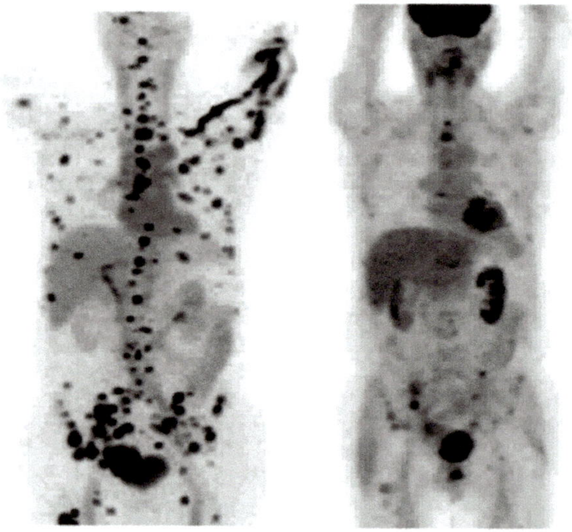

Fig. 8.2 ^{18}F-FDHT-PET (left) and ^{18}F-FDG (right) PET of patient with prostate cancer, demonstrating major differences in the uptakes. This cancer is AR-positive but FDG-avid only to a limited extent. (These pictures are provided by Steven M. Larson (MSKCC, New York, NY, USA))

Table 8.2 ^{18}F-FDHT PET uptakes in different organs

^{18}F-FDHT	SUV_{max}	SUV_{mean}	Uptake variability
Liver	5.12 (3.65–7.08)	4.10 (2.83–6.06)	14.6%
Blood pool	5.24 (3.06–7.2)	4.71 (2.45–6.67)	21.2%
Thoracic vertebra	1.95 (1.12–3.91)	1.36 (0.86–3.32)	21.6%
Muscle	1.14 (0.62–3.1)	0.76 (0.47–2.72)	23.1%
Lumbar vertebra	2.18 (1.17–4.14)	1.60 (0.89–3.56)	23.6%
Lung basally	1.61 (0.71–3.57)	1.00 (0.51–2.96)	28.6%*
Lung apically	1.36 (0.31–3.32)	0.90 (0.26–2.86)	39.3%*

Modified from Ref. [11]

Vargas et al. [8] assessed the repeatability of ^{18}F-FDHT uptake metrics under consistent conditions and reproducibility under variable conditions across different centers [8]. The research was conducted at 3 prominent institutions, enrolling 27 mCRPC patients who underwent 2 consecutive ^{18}F-FDHT PET/CT scans over 2 days. The metrics evaluated included standardized uptake values (SUVs), androgen receptor-positive tumor volumes (ARTV), and total lesion uptake (TLU). The metrics' reproducibility was analyzed across various predefined anatomical regions. The study established that ^{18}F-FDHT PET/CT is a robust method for monitoring mCRPC, with particularly strong repeatability for SUV measurements: intraclass correlation coefficients exceeded 0.92, interobserver reproducibility coefficient was 0.98 [8]. This supports the potential of ^{18}F-FDHT as a biomarker for evaluating the effects of AR-directed therapies, crucial for mCRPC treatment. However, variability in ARTV and TLU suggests that SUV metrics are more reliable for consistent clinical use [8].

Diagnostic Imaging and Prognostic Biomarkers

The book chapter by Steven M. Larson [12] details the utility of PET/CT-based assessments of AR expression and glycolytic activity using fluorodihydrotestosterone (^{18}F-FDHT) and fluoro-2-D-deoxyglucose (^{18}F-FDG) in mCRPC. The study, involving 133 patients, indicated that imaging phenotypes could predict patient prognosis and highlight heterogeneity in tumor biology, potentially guiding personalized therapy. Notably, different imaging phenotypes—specifically AR-positive and AR-negative lesions—correlated with survival outcomes, suggesting that these markers could refine prognostic accuracy beyond traditional clinical parameters.

The study, first published in 2018, evaluated whether ^{18}F-FDHT to detect androgen receptor (AR) expression and ^{18}F-FDG for glycolysis can serve as prognostic biomarkers for metastatic castration-resistant prostate cancer (mCRPC) [9]. The research assesses if distinct imaging phenotypes based on these biomarkers can predict patient prognosis and guide treatment strategies.

This cohort study involved 133 mCRPC patients who underwent ^{18}F-FDHT and ^{18}F-FDG PET/CT scans at Memorial Sloan Kettering Cancer Center between 2007 and 2012. Imaging data categorized lesions into three types based on their AR and glycolytic status: AR1Glyc1 (both markers positive), AR1Glyc0 (only AR-positive), and AR0Glyc1 (only glycolysis positive). The study aimed to correlate these imaging phenotypes with patient survival and treatment outcomes [9].

The PET/CT scans identified varying phenotypes of lesions that correlated with different prognostic outcomes:

AR1Glyc1: Most common phenotype, suggesting initial responsiveness to AR signaling inhibitors.

AR1Glyc0 and AR0Glyc1: Indicated potential for resistance to AR signaling inhibitor treatments.

Multivariate analysis showed that AR0Glyc1 lesions had the strongest negative impact on survival, followed by AR1Glyc1 and AR1Glyc0.

The distribution of imaging phenotypes within a patient helps classify mCRPC into distinct groups, which could inform prognosis and potential treatment paths [9]:

1. *Concordant*: Predominantly AR_1Glyc_1 lesions, associated with the best prognosis.
2. *AR Predominant*: Mixture of AR_1Glyc_1 and AR_1Glyc_0, intermediate prognosis.
3. *Glyc Predominant*: Mixture of AR_1Glyc_1 and AR_0Glyc_1, poorer prognosis.
4. *Mixed*: All three types of lesions, variable prognosis.

The data is summarized in Table 8.3. These results offer a viable method for prognostic assessment in mCRPC by identifying patient-specific metabolic and AR expression profiles. These imaging biomarkers provide insights into tumor

Table 8.3 Lesion phenotypes segregated by imaging of [^{18}F]-FDG and [^{18}F]-FDHT[a]

	~Fraction	HR[b]	95% CI	*p*
AR_1GLYC_0	13%	1.03	1.003–1.047	0.038
AR_0GLYC_1	4%	1.11	1.060–1.16	<0.001
AR_1GLYC_1	83%	1.05	1.03–1.064	<0.001

Modified from Ref. [12]

[a]Lesion description with positive or negative [^{18}F]FDG uptake was "$Glyc_1$" or "$Glyc_0$," respectively, as [^{18}F]FDG uptake is based on glycolysis. Similarly, lesions that were ^{18}F-FDHT-positive or ^{18}F-FDHT-negative become "AR_1" and "AR_0," respectively, as FDHT is based on AR binding

[b]Each additional AR_1Glyc_0 lesion increases risk of death by 3%, AR_0Glyc_1 by 11% and AR_1Glyc_1 by 5% when the number of the lesion phenotypes is held constant

heterogeneity and potential resistance to conventional therapies, highlighting the need for personalized treatment strategies based on individual imaging phenotypes. The study supports the use of molecular imaging to guide therapeutic decisions and improve outcomes in mCRPC patients [9, 12].

Pharmaceutical Development

ARN-509, a novel androgen receptor (AR), was designed to treat mCRPC more effectively by inhibiting AR nuclear translocation and binding to androgen response elements, without the agonist properties seen in older treatments like bicalutamide [13].

The first-in-human phase I trial included 30 patients with progressive metastatic CRPC, published in 2013 [13]. They were given daily oral doses of ARN-509 ranging from 30 to 480 mg, following a single-dose administration and a 1-week observation period to assess pharmacokinetics. The primary goal was to determine the safety, pharmacokinetic profile, and the recommended dose for phase II trials.

Blood samples were taken at multiple intervals post-dosing to measure ARN-509 levels. ^{18}F-FDHT PET/CT imaging was used to monitor changes in AR binding in tumors. ARN-509 displayed linear and dose-proportional pharmacokinetics. Optimal AR saturation was observed at 120 mg, but a dose of 240 mg daily was identified as providing the best balance of safety and efficacy, termed the maximum efficacious dose (MED) [13].

The drug was generally well tolerated with the most common adverse effect being grade 1/2 fatigue. No maximum tolerated dose was identified as dose-limiting toxicities were minimal.

Approximately 47% of patients experienced a greater than 50% reduction in PSA levels at 12 weeks. Antitumor activity was consistent across all doses, and ^{18}F-FDHT uptake reduction confirmed effective AR targeting [13]. This drug has got later a marketing approval with name apalutamide (Erleada®).

There are multiple new therapeutic advances in prostate cancer, particularly those targeting the AR pathway. New agents like abiraterone acetate and enzalutamide have shown promise in extending survival for mCRPC patients. Our review highlighted the critical role of the AR in the progression of prostate cancer, underscoring ongoing efforts to develop AR signaling inhibitors (that could offer new treatment avenues) [1]. A key theme across the reviewed documents is the integration of advanced imaging techniques into the treatment strategy for prostate cancer. Imaging biomarkers like ^{18}F-FDHT uptake have been linked to tumor characteristics and responses to AR-targeted therapies. Such biomarkers provide a noninvasive means to monitor disease progression and response to treatment, offering a dynamic tool to guide clinical decision-making. A review with PRISMA criteria [14] was published half a year after our review [1] focusing on prostate and breast cancer. The data was basically identical. A key theme across these reviews [1, 14] is the integration of advanced imaging techniques into the treatment strategy for prostate cancer. Imaging biomarkers like ^{18}F-FDHT uptake have been linked to tumor characteristics and responses to AR-targeted therapies. Such biomarkers provide a noninvasive means to monitor disease progression and response to treatment, offering a dynamic tool to guide clinical decision-making.

Finally, the role of molecular imaging in advancing personalized medicine is a prominent discussion. Molecular imaging allows for the visualization of biological processes that are pivotal in cancer progression. By linking imaging findings with molecular and genetic data, clinicians can better understand the biological underpinnings of each patient's tumor, leading to more effective and personalized treatment plans.

Conclusive Remarks

This chapter concludes that ^{18}F-FDHT-PET is a valuable tool for visualizing androgen receptors and could significantly impact the treatment of prostate and other hormone-dependent cancers by providing a noninvasive method to assess receptor status and guide therapy choices.

This comprehensive summary captures the key aspects of the article, emphasizing the importance of ^{18}F-FDHT-PET in advancing personalized medicine for cancer treatment based on hormonal dynamics. Androgen receptor (AR) signaling plays a crucial role in the progression of prostate cancer, especially in castrate-resistant stages where conventional biopsy methods are less feasible due to metastatic spread primarily to bones.

The ongoing research and development in imaging and therapy for prostate cancer hold promise for transforming patient outcomes. As these technologies evolve and become more integrated into clinical practice, they offer the potential to significantly improve diagnostic accuracy, treatment efficacy, and patient survival. ^{18}F-FDHT-PET combined with ^{18}F-FDG can act as a prognostic biomarker. Continued advancements in this field are critical to overcoming current limitations and fully realizing the benefits of these innovative approaches in the treatment of prostate cancer. This synthesis underscores the importance of a multidisciplinary approach to prostate cancer care, leveraging cutting-edge technologies to optimize patient management and therapeutic outcomes.

References

1. Kairemo K, Hodolic M. Androgen receptor imaging in the management of hormone-dependent cancers with emphasis on prostate cancer. Int J Mol Sci. 2023;24:8235.
2. Venema CM, Mammatas LH, Schröder CP, et al. Androgen and estrogen receptor imaging in metastatic breast cancer patients as a surrogate for tissue biopsies. J Nucl Med. 2017;58(12):1906–12.
3. Orevi M, Shamni O, Zalcman N, et al. [^{18}F]-FDHT PET/CT as a tool for imaging androgen receptor expression in high-grade glioma. Neurooncol Adv. 2021;3:vdab019.
4. Larson SM, Morris M, Gunther I, et al. Tumor localization of 16beta-18F-fluoro-5alpha-dihydrotestosterone versus 18F-FDG in patients with progressive, metastatic prostate cancer. J Nucl Med. 2004;45:366–73.
5. Zanzonico PB, Finn R, Pentlow KS, et al. PET-based radiation dosimetry in man of ^{18}F-fluorodihydrotestosterone, a new radiotracer for imaging prostate cancer. J Nucl Med. 2004;45:1966–71.
6. Dehdashti F, Picus J, Michalski JM, et al. Positron tomographic assessment of androgen receptors in prostatic carcinoma. Eur J Nucl Med Mol Imaging. 2005;32:344–50.
7. Fox JJ, Autran-Blanc E, Morris MJ, et al. Practical approach for comparative analysis of multilesion molecular imaging using a semiautomated program for PET/CT. J Nucl Med. 2011;52:1727–32.
8. Vargas HA, Kramer GM, Scott AM, et al. Reproducibility and repeatability of semiquantitative ^{18}F-fluorodihydrotestosterone uptake metrics in castration-resistant prostate cancer metastases: a prospective multicenter study. J Nucl Med. 2018;59:1516–23.
9. Fox JJ, Gavane SC, Blanc-Autran E, et al. Positron emission tomography/computed tomography-based assessments of androgen receptor expression and glycolytic activity as a prognostic biomarker for metastatic castration-resistant prostate cancer. JAMA Oncol. 2018;4:217–24.
10. Al Jalali V, Wasinger G, Rasul S, et al. Consecutive prostate-specific membrane antigen (PSMA) and antigen receptor (AR) PET imaging shows positive correlation with AR and PSMA protein expression in primary hormone-Naïve prostate cancer. J Nucl Med. 2023 Jun;64(6):863–8.
11. Jansen BHE, Kramer GM, Cysouw MCF, et al. Healthy tissue uptake of ^{68}Ga-prostate-specific membrane antigen, ^{18}F-DCFPyL, ^{18}F-fluoromethylcholine, and ^{18}F-dihydrotestosterone. J Nucl Med. 2019;60:1111–7.
12. Larson SM. Cancer biology of molecular imaging. In: Volterrani D, Erba PA, Strauss HW, Mariani G, Larson SM, editors. Nuclear oncology. Cham: Springer; 2022. https://doi.org/10.1007/978-3-031-05494-5_1.
13. Rathkopf DE, Morris MJ, Fox JJ, et al. Phase I study of ARN-509, a novel antiandrogen, in the treatment of castration-resistant prostate cancer. J Clin Oncol. 2013;31:3525–30.
14. Filippi L, Urso L, Schillaci O, Evangelista L. [^{18}F]-FDHT PET for the imaging of androgen receptor in prostate and breast cancer: a systematic review. Diagnostics (Basel). 2023;13:2613.

9 Immunoscintigraphy and Radioimmunotherapy of Prostate Cancer Including Own Personal Journey: Anti-PAP and Anti-PSMA Antibodies

Early attempts with monoclonal antibodies (MAb) against prostatic acid phosphatase were active in Finland in the late 1980s and early 1990s. Prostatic acid phosphatase (PAP) was isolated and characterized immunohistochemically in the late 1970s [1, 2]. First clinical anti-PAP experiments were performed with polyclonal antibodies by Goldenberg et al. in 1983 [3]. They used ^{131}I-labeled rabbit antibody IgG against PAP and performed total-body photoscans with a gamma scintillation camera in two patients. Surprisingly, they could show indirectly that the lung accumulations were due to prostate origin [4]. Thus, these findings initiated the antibody imaging (also called radioimmunodetection or immunoscintigraphy) of primary prostate cancers and non-bone metastases, even allowing differential diagnostics between lung tumors of prostatic and pulmonary origin.

At the same time, the group in Oulu, Finland, reported the use of ^{99m}Tc-labeled polyclonal antibodies raised in rabbits against human prostate-specific acid phosphatase which was used to detect metastases of prostatic carcinoma in all of the studied four patients [5]. After this work, they started to develop monoclonal anti-PAP antibodies which were then tested in xenografts, although most of the data was published much later [6, 7]. We in Helsinki started to use these monoclonal antibodies already in 1987 with an ^{111}In label. Our main approach was to inject the monoclonal antibody (MoAb) into the prostate lobes—in practice, the injections were given by an experienced urologist.

In Paris, another anti-PAP-MAb 227 A was used [8]. They published the results of 15 patients with various stages of histologically proven prostatic cancer. They were using immunolymphoscintigraphy (ILS) in order to detect lymph node metastases before treatment. These patients had stage A–D tumors. Iodine-123 (^{123}I)-labeled F(ab')$_2$ fragments (100–400 µg) were injected directly into the periprostatic area 3 days before lymphadenectomy for histologic examination [8]. In five cases, scintigraphy suggested the presence of lymph node invasion by prostatic cancer which was confirmed by histology in three of the five cases. Ten patients had no findings [8]. Therefore, they concluded that ILS appears to be capable of

K. Kairemo, *Prostate Cancer from a Nuclear Oncology Perspective*,
https://doi.org/10.1007/978-3-031-90337-3_9

detecting lymph node metastases in prostatic cancer, because of sensitivity of 100% and specificity of 83% [8].

We in Helsinki, were actually disappointed with all our immunoscintigraphic results in prostate cancer [9]. The ^{111}In-labeled monoclonal anti-prostatic acid phosphatase (PAP) monoclonal antibody F(ab')2 fragment (FC 3001) was used for the radioimmunodetection of prostate cancer in two different patient groups: 15 patients with surgically verified T1–2 prostate cancer were imaged prior to staging lymphadenectomy and total prostatectomy using lymphatic administration (intraprostatic (ipr) injection), and 15 patients with verified metastatic prostatic cancer were imaged after intravenous (i.v.) injection [9]. The extirpated tissues were counted for radioactivity and studied immunohistochemically (IHC) and histologically. The anti-PAP MAb was labeled with high efficiency (87–99%), and it demonstrated good immunoreactivity (90–95%) and a high affinity to the target antigen. In the excised prostates, cut into 12–18 smaller pieces, there was a clear correlation between the PAP content (as detected by IHC) and absolute radioactivity (% ID of ^{111}In anti-PAP/g prostate). However, there was no correlation between radioactivity and the amount of cancer tissue (% of histological slices) inside the removed prostate tissue [9]. In the pharmacokinetic studies, maximum activity in the serum was obtained within 3–5 h after ipr injection; after that the kinetic behavior was similar to that after i.v. injection.From the intravenous administration of FC 3001, the pharmacokinetics revealed two components; the half-lives for mean distribution and elimination were 0.62 and 35.6 hrs, respectively. The mean distribution half-life as well as the AUC from the pharmacokinetic curves correlated significantly with serum PAP ($p < 0.05$) [9]. This labeled antibody FC3001 was tested in 15 prostate cancer patients who underwent staging pelvic lymphadenectomy; nine of them received labeled antibody alone, whereas six received simultaneous injections of labeled and unlabeled antibody with two dose levels (40 or 80 mg) [9]. A similar study with cold antibody blockade, but with systemic injection, had been done at MD Anderson Cancer Center in the United States: A total of 25 patients with histologically proven adenocarcinoma of the prostate received increasing doses of PAY 276, an anti-PAP monoclonal antibody for radioimmunological imaging [10]. The patients were divided into five groups of five patients. Groups 1 through 5 received an infusion of 5, 10, 20, 40, or 80 mg of MAb, respectively, 1 mg of which was labeled to 5 mCi of ^{111}indium, while stable monoclonal antibody was added to achieve the desired antibody concentration [10]. The monoclonal antibody scan visualized at least 1 lesion in 19 of 25 patients (76%): 4 in groups 1 and 2 and all 15 in groups 3–5. The detection of metastatic lesions increased as the concentration of unlabeled monoclonal antibody increased [10]. Figure 9.1 demonstrates how the added cold antibody changes the pharmacokinetic behavior of the FC3001 monoclonal antibody [11].

In our study, after intraprostatic injection, biodistribution data obtained by direct blood measurements and imaging procedures indicated that simultaneous injection of unlabeled antibody reduced both the blood elimination rate and the accumulation in the liver. Accumulation of the radionuclide in pelvic lymph node metastases was observed in some patients, but in a couple of patients, accumulation was noted also in normal lymph nodes. At that time, we concluded that the method cannot in its

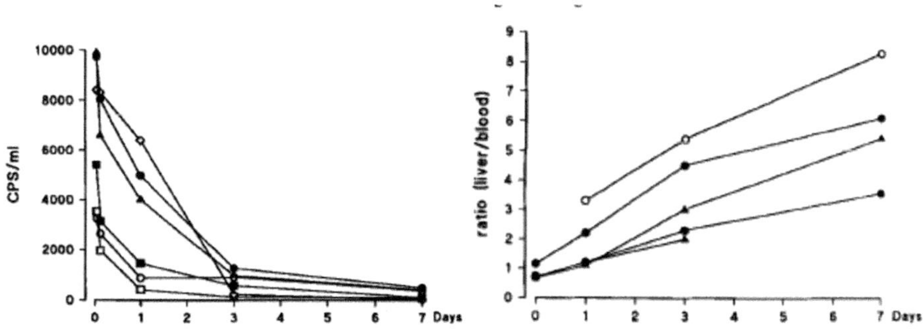

Fig. 9.1 ^{111}In concentration in serum (cps/ml) after ^{111}In-FC3001 MAb injection (on the left). The curves with solid symbols refer to patients who were coinjected with 40 mg or 80 mg of unlabeled Mab. The curves with open symbols (circles or squares) refer to patients who recieved no unlabeled MAb. The curves on the right represent liver-to-blood ratios as measured from whole body imaging data. The ratio is higher in the patient (open circles) who did not receive unlabeled Mab as compared to those patients who received 40 mg (solid circles) or 80 mg (solid triangles) unlabeled Mab (right). (The data is presented in [11])

present design replace staging pelvic lymphadenectomy, and further studies are needed for elaboration of clinically useful radioimmunodetection methods [11]. Further studies were never done.

I defended my doctoral dissertation in 1993 and it dealt with the use of MAbs in cancer diagnostics, but prostate cancer was not included in this thesis. I personally was very much interested of radioimmunodetection and radioimmunotherapy [12, 13] and started clinical radioimmunotherapy in Helsinki in 1993. I had also learned that MAbs were utilized for differentiating between malignant and benign prostate tissue. These included antibodies against prostatic acid phosphatase, prostate-specific antigens, and the 7Ell-C5 glycoprotein [14]. Some MAbs had been developed against prostate cancer cell antigens, such as EMBP, KR-P8, D83.21, P6.2, PEQ 226, and Turp 27, and also against androgen receptors [12, 14]. EMBP is discussed in this book in Chap. 2 in a detailed manner. However, there was only one report of treatment of metastatic prostate carcinoma with a radiolabeled antibody in the 1990s. Meredith et al. [15] treated 15 patients with hormone-resistant cancer in a phase II trial using 75 mCi/m2 I3lI-anti-TAG-72 high-affinity antibody CC49. Six out of ten symptomatic patients had bone pain relief, but no patient met the radiographic or PSA criteria for objective response. Positive imaging of bone and/or soft-tissue lesions was noted for 13 patients.

In New York, at the Memorial Sloan-Kettering Cancer Center (MSKCC), professor Olof Alfthan introduced me to the urology professor William H. Fair, when professor Alfthan came to visit me in New York with his wife. At that time I personally was aware of the discovery of "PSMA." The first tracer was developed by Horoszewicz et al. in the form of 7E11-C5 monoclonal antibody (capromab) from mice immunized with the human prostate cancer-derived cell line, LNCaP, in 1987 [16]. 7E11-C5 recognized an antigen restricted to normal and malignant prostate epithelium and was present in some sera of prostate cancer patients [16].

Horoszewicz et al. described this as "new antigenic marker may be of clinical potential in prostate cancer" [16]. Using the MAb 7E11-C5, Warren "Skip" Heston with William Fair at MSKCC cloned the PSMA gene in 1993 [17, 18]. PSMA, also known as folate hydrolase I (FOLH1) and glutamate carboxypeptidase II (GCP-II), is a 750-amino-acid, 100kD, type II transmembrane protein, with a short N-terminal intracellular domain and a large C-terminal extracellular domain (2). I also learned to know Skip Heston and discussed with him and professor Fair about my Finnish antibodies. I also got own antibodies to New York (delivered by Juha Ellmen from Farmos, Turku), but we only made limited tumor targeting tests with Dr. Craig Zippe using mouse xenograft models. At that time, the major interest at MSKCC lied on PSMA which I did not know. I understood that PSMA is predominantly expressed in the prostate and a subset of proximal renal tubules, with lower level expression in small bowel, salivary glands, etc. [16–20]. In 1993, Heston concluded that "as an integral membrane protein unique to prostatic epithelial cells, the antigen or perhaps a specific PSMA ligand may serve as an excellent site for imaging and/or targeting of metastatic deposits," setting the stage for PSMA as a theranostic target [17].

I went back to Helsinki in 1993. In 1994 and 1995, Fair and Heston described PSMA as a folate hydrolase highly expressed in prostate cancer [21], further detailed its tissue distribution [20], and mapped its genomic organization on chromosome 11p11-12 [18, 22]. PSMA expression was observed in the vast majority (~95%) of primary prostate cancer and lymph node metastases, consistent with observed 7E11-C5 immunoreactivity [23, 24]. PSMA was also expressed on neovasculature of epithelial malignancies including renal cell, bladder, and colon cancers [20].

Development of 7E11-C5 as a theranostic agent began prior to identification of PSMA as its target [25, 26]. In 1996, ^{111}In-capromab pendetide (ProstaScint®) became the first US Food and Drug Administration (FDA)-approved molecular imaging agent for prostate cancer. 7E11-C5 targets an intracellular epitope of PSMA [16, 27], binding only dying or dead cells. This fact limited ProstaScint® performance as an imaging agent, particularly in well-vascularized bone metastases. The first antibodies to the extracellular domain of PSMA were developed in 1997 by Neil Bander et al. at Weill Cornell Medical College [28]. J591, the lead antibody, enabled studies of PSMA in viable cells. Bander's team demonstrated that PSMA is constitutively internalized, and antibody-binding increased the rate of internalization by severalfold [29]. This property according to the authors "should aid the development of novel therapeutic methods to target the delivery of toxins, drugs, or short-range isotopes specifically to the interior of prostate cancer cells" [29].

David Scheinberg from MSKCC started to develop alpha particle-emitting antibody radionuclide therapy constructs for prostate cancer. I was in this team a short time when we started to develop labeling for Bi-212 and Bi-213, mainly for M195 antibody for hematologic malignancies. This was in spring 1993. My son was born in July 1993 and I never returned back to New York although I was following what was happening in NYC. In collaboration with Bander, Scheinberg et al. demonstrated preclinical activity for ^{213}Bi-J591 and ^{225}Ac-J591 conjugates [30, 31]. Bander et al. further demonstrated promising antitumor efficacy of beta-emitting conjugates ^{90}Y-J591 and ^{177}Lu-J591 in preclinical models [32]. Humanized J591 (huJ591) was developed to increase its clinical potential [33] and advanced to prostate cancer theranostics trials.

The first PSMA-targeted radiopharmaceutical tested as a therapeutic agent in prostate cancer patients was 7E11-C5.3 (^{90}Y-capromab pendetide) [34]. However, significant bone marrow toxicity and no objective clinical responses were observed in phase I and II trials [34, 35].

In the early 2000s, Bander et al. from the Weill Cornell Medical College initiated a series of phase I/II trials testing huJ591-based molecular radionuclide therapy in advanced prostate cancer. These studies represented the first clinical use of ^{177}Lu as a systemically administered agent and demonstrated safety, accurate targeting of metastatic prostate cancer sites, and preliminary antitumor activity for ^{90}Y-huJ591 and ^{177}Lu-huJ591, providing the first direct clinical evidence supporting the potential of PSMA-targeted radionuclide therapy [36–38].

Bander's team also demonstrated safety, feasibility, and promising activity with dose-fractionated 177Lu-huJ591, with higher cumulative doses associated with longer median overall survival (OS) and increased myelosuppression [39]. In another trial, fractionated ^{177}Lu-huJ591 administered concurrently with standard docetaxel was tolerable and feasible, with no dose-limiting toxicities observed and preliminary efficacy indicated [40]. This was the first trial testing PSMA-targeted radionuclide therapy in combination with chemotherapy. Now there are multiple anti-PSMA MAbs under clinical development.

Multiple anti-PSMA antibodies have also been developed for diagnostic purposes, such as ^{89}Zr-J591. This agent together with Indium-111 capromab pendetide showed promise in improving the accuracy of cancer detection, by enhancing the visualization of cancer spread to lymph nodes and metastatic sites, potentially guiding surgical resection and assessing the extent of disease.The specificity of PSMA-based imaging and therapy poses challenges. PSMA expression is not exclusive to prostate cancer cells; it has been detected in various tissues and certain other cancer types, which could lead to false-positive results and impact the accuracy of both diagnostic imaging and targeted therapies. Additionally, the expression of PSMA in nonmalignant tissues like the ganglionic cells of the neurovascular bundle complicates the use of PSMA-targeted imaging agents in surgical settings. The expression of PSMA in nontarget tissues limits intraoperative use in tumor margin assessments.

References

1. Choe BK, Pontes EJ, Bloink S, Rose NR. Human prostatic acid phosphatases: I. Isolation. Arch Androl. 1978;1:221–6.
2. Choe BK, Pontes EJ, McDonald I, Rose NR. Immunochemical studies of prostatic acid phosphatase. Cancer Treat Rep. 1977;61:201–4.
3. Goldenberg DM, DeLand FH, Bennett SJ, et al. Radioimmunodetection of prostatic cancer: in vivo use of radioactive antibodies against prostatic acid phosphatase for diagnosis and detection of prostatic cancer by nuclear imaging. JAMA. 1983;250:630–5.

4. Goldenberg DM, DeLand FH. Clinical studies of prostatic cancer imaging with radiolabeled antibodies against prostatic acid phosphatase. Urol Clin North Am. 1984;11:277–81.
5. Vihko P, Heikkilä J, Kontturi M, Wahlberg L, Vihko R. Radioimaging of the prostate and metastases of prostatic carcinoma with ^{99m}Tc-labelled prostatic acid phosphatase-specific antibodies and their Fab fragments. Ann Clin Res. 1984;16:51–2.
6. Perälä-Heape M, Vihko P, Vihko R. Effect of unlabelled monoclonal antibodies on the biodistribution of 111In-labelled anti-prostate-specific acid phosphatase monoclonal antibodies in the mouse model. Anticancer Res. 1991;11:1327–31.
7. Perälä-Heape M, Vihko P, Pelkonen I, Laine A, Vihko R. Effect of conjugation on the biodistribution of 111In-labelled anti-PAP and anti-PSA monoclonal antibodies examined in nude mice with PC-82 human tumor xenografts. In Vivo. 1991;5:159–65.
8. Leroy M, Teillac P, Rain JD, Saccavini JC, Le Duc A, Najean Y. Radioimmunodetection of lymph node invasion in prostatic cancer. The use of iodine 123 (^{123}I)-labeled monoclonal anti-prostatic acid phosphatase (PAP) 227 A F(ab')$_2$ antibody fragments in vivo. Cancer. 1989;64:1–5.
9. Kairemo KJ, Rannikko S, Nordling S, Savalainen S, Ahonen A, Taavitsainen MJ, Alfthan OS. In vivo behavior of 111In-labeled monoclonal anti-prostatic acid phosphatase antibody after intraprostatic and intravenous injections. J Nucl Biol Med (1991). 1994;38(4 Suppl 1):151–5.
10. Babaian RJ, Murray JL, Lamki LM, Haynie TP, Hersh EM, Rosenblum MG, Glenn HJ, Unger MW, Carlo DJ, von Eschenbach AC. Radioimmunological imaging of metastatic prostatic cancer with 111indium-labeled monoclonal antibody PAY 276. J Urol. 1987;137:439–43.
11. Ahonen A, Kairemo K, Karnani P, et al. Radioimmunodetection of prostate cancer by ^{111}In-labeled monoclonal antibody against prostatic acid phosphatase. Acta Oncol. 1993;32:723–7.
12. Kairemo KJA, Liewendahl K. Radioimmunodetection of solid tumors. Invited review. Scand J Clin Lab Invest. 1994;54:569–83.
13. Kairemo KJA. Radioimmunotherapy of solid cancers. A review. Acta Oncol. 1996;35:343–55.
14. Schellhammer PF, Wright GL Jr. Biomolecular and clinical characteristics of PSA and other candidate prostate tumor markers. Urol Clin North Am. 1993;20:597–606.
15. Meredith RF, Bueschen AJ, Khazaeli MB, et al. Treatment of metastatic prostate carcinoma with radiolabeled antibody CC49. J Nucl Med. 1994;35:1017–22.
16. Horoszewicz JS, Kawinski E, Murphy GP. Monoclonal antibodies to a new antigenic marker in epithelial prostatic cells and serum of prostatic cancer patients. Anticancer Res. 1987;7:927–35.
17. Israeli RS, Powell CT, Fair WR, Heston WD. Molecular cloning of a complementary DNA encoding a prostate-specific membrane antigen. Cancer Res. 1993;53:227–30.
18. O'Keefe DS, Su SL, Bacich DJ, et al. Mapping, genomic organization and promoter analysis of the human prostate-specific membrane antigen gene. Biochim Biophys Acta. 1998;1443:113–27.
19. Israeli RS, Powell CT, Corr JG, Fair WR, Heston WD. Expression of the prostate-specific membrane antigen. Cancer Res. 1994;54:1807–11.
20. Silver DA, Pellicer I, Fair WR, Heston WD, Cordon-Cardo C. Prostate-specific membrane antigen expression in normal and malignant human tissues. Clin Cancer Res. 1997;3:81–5.
21. Pinto JT, Suffoletto BP, Berzin TM, et al. Prostate-specific membrane antigen: a novel folate-hydrolase in human prostatic carcinoma cells. Clin Cancer Res. 1996;2:1445–51.
22. Rinker-Schaeffer CW, Hawkins AL, Su SL, et al. Localization and physical mapping of the prostate-specific membrane antigen (PSM) gene to human chromosome 11. Genomics. 1995;30:105–8.
23. Lopes AD, Davis WL, Rosenstraus MJ, Uveges AJ, Gilman SC. Immunohistochemical and pharmacokinetic characterization of the site-specific immunoconjugate CYT-356 derived from antiprostate monoclonal antibody 7E11-C5. Cancer Res. 1990;50:6423–9.
24. Wright GL Jr, Haley C, Beckett ML, Schellhammer PF. Expression of prostate-specific membrane antigen in normal, benign, and malignant prostate tissues. Urol Oncol. 1995;1:18–28.

25. Kahn D, Williams RD, Seldin DW, et al. Radioimmunoscintigraphy with 111indium labeled CYT-356 for the detection of occult prostate cancer recurrence. J Urol. 1994;152:1490–5.
26. Wynant GE, Murphy GP, Horoszewicz JS, et al. Immunoscintigraphy of prostatic cancer: preliminary results with 111In-labeled monoclonal antibody 7E11-C5.3 (CYT-356). Prostate. 1991;18:229–41.
27. Troyer JK, Feng Q, Beckett ML, Wright GL Jr. Biochemical characterization and mapping of the 7E11-C5.3 epitope of the prostate-specific membrane antigen. Urol Oncol. 1995;1:29–37.
28. Liu H, Moy P, Kim S, et al. Monoclonal antibodies to the extracellular domain of prostate-specific membrane antigen also react with tumor vascular endothelium. Cancer Res. 1997;57:3629–34.
29. Liu H, Rajasekaran AK, Moy P, et al. Constitutive and antibody-induced internalization of prostate-specific membrane antigen. Cancer Res. 1998;58:4055–60.
30. McDevitt MR, Barendswaard E, Ma D, et al. An alpha-particle emitting antibody ([213Bi]J591) for radioimmunotherapy of prostate cancer. Cancer Res. 2000;60:6095–100.
31. McDevitt MR, Ma D, Lai LT, et al. Tumor therapy with targeted atomic nanogenerators. Science. 2001;294:1537–40.
32. Smith-Jones PM, Vallabhajosula S, Navarro V, Bastidas D, Goldsmith SJ, Bander NH. Radiolabeled monoclonal antibodies specific to the extracellular domain of prostate-specific membrane antigen: preclinical studies in nude mice bearing LNCaP human prostate tumor. J Nucl Med. 2003;44:610–7.
33. Nanus DM, Milowsky MI, Kostakoglu L, et al. Clinical use of monoclonal antibody HuJ591 therapy: targeting prostate specific membrane antigen. J Urol. 2003;170:S84–8.
34. Deb N, Goris M, Trisler K, et al. Treatment of hormone-refractory prostate cancer with ^{90}Y-CYT-356 monoclonal antibody. Clin Cancer Res. 1996;2:1289–97.
35. Kahn D, Austin JC, Maguire RT, Miller SJ, Gerstbrein J, Williams RD. A phase II study of [^{90}Y] yttrium-capromab pendetide in the treatment of men with prostate cancer recurrence following radical prostatectomy. Cancer Biother Radiopharm. 1999;14:99–111.
36. Milowsky MI, Nanus DM, Kostakoglu L, Vallabhajosula S, Goldsmith SJ, Bander NH. Phase I trial of yttrium-90-labeled anti-prostate-specific membrane antigen monoclonal antibody J591 for androgen-independent prostate cancer. J Clin Oncol. 2004;22:2522–31.
37. Bander NH, Milowsky MI, Nanus DM, Kostakoglu L, Vallabhajosula S, Goldsmith SJ. Phase I trial of 177lutetium-labeled J591, a monoclonal antibody to prostate-specific membrane antigen, in patients with androgen-independent prostate cancer. J Clin Oncol. 2005;23:4591–601.
38. Tagawa ST, Milowsky MI, Morris M, et al. Phase II study of Lutetium-177-labeled anti-prostate-specific membrane antigen monoclonal antibody J591 for metastatic castration-resistant prostate cancer. Clin Cancer Res. 2013;19:5182–91.
39. Tagawa ST, Vallabhajosula S, Christos PJ, et al. Phase 1/2 study of fractionated dose lutetium-177-labeled anti-prostate-specific membrane antigen monoclonal antibody J591 ((177) Lu-J591) for metastatic castration-resistant prostate cancer. Cancer. 2019;125:2561–9.
40. Batra JS, Niaz MJ, Whang YE, et al. Phase I trial of docetaxel plus lutetium-177-labeled anti-prostate-specific membrane antigen monoclonal antibody J591 (177Lu-J591) for metastatic castration-resistant prostate cancer. Urol Oncol. 2020;38:848.e849–16.

Briefly About Radiation Therapy 10

External beam radiotherapy (EBRT) plays an essential role in the management of prostate cancer [1, 2]. The use of positron emission tomography (PET) targeting radiation therapy planning has been discussed comprehensively in Chap. 11. PSMA PET demonstrated higher diagnostic performances than conventional imaging (CT, MRI, bone scan) and other PET tracers (choline, fluciclovine) to localize PCa lesions [3–7] and thus can guide radiotherapy planning [8, 9]. Radiation has been used for the treatment of cancer for over 100 years, but the last decade has seen great technical advances that make it more focused on the target (the prostate), with improved cure rates. Radiation therapy is used to either attempt to cure the prostate cancer or to help symptoms when a cure is not possible. This chapter reviews briefly methods for radiation therapy in prostate cancer.

Radiation therapy, also called *radiotherapy*, is the use of high-energy X-rays to kill cancer cells. The high-energy X-rays penetrate through normal tissues to the site of the cancer. Radiotherapy works by damaging the cells so that they eventually die. Radiotherapy will damage any type of cell, either normal or cancerous, that lies in the path of the beam. Therefore, great care must be taken to aim the beam only at the affected part of the body and avoid treatment of as much healthy tissue as possible.

Fortunately, normal cells repair themselves from radiation damage more completely than cancer cells do. Thus, by giving the radiation in a series of small treatments, usually once a day, the normal cells can recover between treatments while the cancer cells die. There are two commonly used types of radiotherapy: external beam radiation therapy (EBRT), which is given by liner accelerators, and brachytherapy (sometimes called *brachy* or *seed treatment*), where radioactive seeds are inserted either permanently or temporarily into the prostate. Which is best for the selection of the therapy form is dependent on the cancer characteristics, prostate size, body shape, general health, and personal preference (doctor = radiation oncologist and/or patient).

K. Kairemo, *Prostate Cancer from a Nuclear Oncology Perspective*,
https://doi.org/10.1007/978-3-031-90337-3_10

With EBRT, typically multiple beams of radiation are used to focus on the cancer. In this way the normal parts of the body do not receive a high enough amount to cause damage, while the tumor gets the full dose. Cancer cells are more sensitive to the effects of radiation and lack the ability of the normal cells to repair the damage that occurs. Radiation therapy is also sometimes combined with hormone therapy.

Radiotherapy can be used for all stages of prostate cancer, including in men who have already had a radical prostatectomy but for whom the pathology indicates that cancer may have been left behind or when there are signs that the cancer may have recurred. Figure 10.1 gives as example how radiation therapy can be given in different stages/risk groups of prostate cancer. There are only a few situations where it would not be possible to give the treatment. These situations include men who have had high-dose radiotherapy to the prostate or the surrounding region before (e.g., radiotherapy is used for rectal cancer, and the overlap of radiation treatments could cause side effects) and, rarely, in those with ulcerative colitis or previous extensive surgery to the bowel.

Radiation therapy has a possibility for side effects. There is a possibility for early side effects (within 3–6 months of treatment) and late side effects (which can come on as long as several years after treatment). Side effects of external beam radiation therapy and brachytherapy differ because of the amount of radiation that the prostate and urethra (higher with brachytherapy) and rectum (higher with external beam radiation therapy) receive. Most men get some degree of early side effects, but the chance of late side effects is low. Patient age, strength of erections, general health, and the presence of previous urinary or bowel problems also affect the side effects to be expected.

GS 6, T1-2, low PSA, long PSADT
VMAT RapidArc RT
Hydrogel protection **(prostate** ↦ rectum)
Fiducial markers (prostate)
60 - **62 Gy in 20 fractions**

OR

HDR Brachytherapy
Hydrogel protection
Iridium (^{192}Ir)source
3 x 11 Gy with 2 wk intervals

GS7-10, T3, high PSA, short PSADT
Hydrogel protection + fiducial markers
Short hormone therapy
(LHRH antagonists +/- antiandrogen)
VMAT RapidArc RT
Pelvic LNs 20 x 2.2 Gy
PSMA-**positive** LNs 20 x 3 Gy
Prostate + SVs 20 x 2.47 Gy

\+

HDR Brachytherapy
2 x 10 Gy with 2 interval

Fig. 10.1 Combinations of external beam radiation therapy (VMAT), brachytherapy, and hormone therapy in different conditions of prostate cancer, PSA values, PSA doubling time (PSADT), T (tumor)-stage, and Gleason score (GS). (This example comes from Helsinki, Finland, updated from [10])

External Beam Radiation Therapy

In external beam radiation therapy (EBRT), the beams of radiation are focused on the prostate gland from a *linear accelerator*. Sophisticated shielding devices allow multiple beams—typically three to seven—to be individually shaped according to the size and position of the prostate target. The simplest form of modern radiation is three-dimensional conformal radiation. The name conformal radiation describes the way the treatment is planned to "conform" closely to the prostate target, when viewed in three dimensions from a CT scan.

Intensity-modulated radiation therapy (IMRT) is a newer version of three-dimensional conformal radiation. Each of the radiation beams is shaped to conform to the target, and they are also additionally shielded (modulated) to produce radiation doses that spare more of the normal body parts. This allows a higher dose of radiation to be safely delivered, and as a result cure rates are higher.

A course of radiation is typically given as 30–40 once daily treatments (called fractions). By getting a little bit of radiation treatment each day, the body can heal the effects of the previous day's treatment and gradually the cancer cells are destroyed. The unit of measurement of radiation is Gray.

Radiation therapy is very much a team effort. The first step is planning the treatment. This may require the insertion of three marker seeds into the prostate under ultrasound, similar to the biopsy procedure, but much less invasive. These marker seeds are called *fiducial markers*, not to be confused with brachytherapy seeds. The marker seeds act as a daily reference point for the precise position of the prostate gland, which can actually move by up to a centimeter (Fig. 10.2). Alternatively, the same accuracy can be obtained by using the treatment machine itself to check the

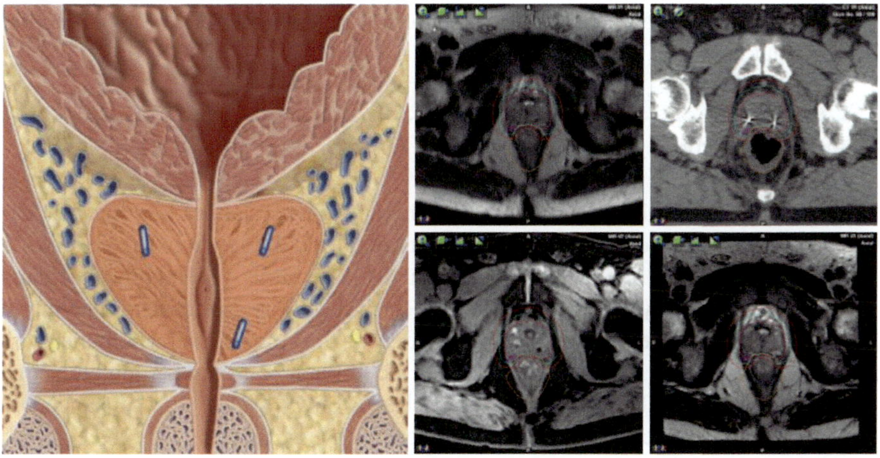

Fig. 10.2 An example of placement of fiducial markers for EBRT technique. The schematic picture on the left presents three fiducial markers inside the prostate. These markers can be identified in morphologic imaging (MRI and CT), and they will guide prostate positioning during external beam radiation therapy cycle

prostate position by taking a quick scan of the prostate before the treatment (called cone beam imaging). Then a planning CT scan will be done in the radiation department.

The scan images are processed by a computer, and then a radiation oncologist and medical physicist come up with a treatment plan for the best number and direction of radiation beams, as well as the dose and duration of treatment. A typical total radiation dose is 68–78 cGy given over 28–40 fractions. The treatment is scheduled 5 days per week, so the entire course can take 6–8 weeks.

Typically 2–3 weeks into treatment, there will be increasing irritation of the rectum (sometimes giving symptoms such as hemorrhoids or loose stools), as well as increased frequency and urgency to urinate. This is due to the lining of the rectum, bladder, and urethra reacting to the radiation therapy and causing local swelling and irritation. The symptoms are usually mild and, if needed, medication is given to help. These symptoms typically peak around the end of the treatment course and then subside over the next few weeks.

Late (longer-term) side effects occur in 20% (mild) to 5% (more significant) of men. Change in bowel habits is common, with increased bowel movements and occasional spotting of blood. As these are also early symptoms of a bowel cancer, it is important to have bleeding investigated with a colonoscopy.

Urinary symptoms can indicate the development of a narrowing of the urethra (urethral stricture), for which a minor procedure called *dilatation* may be helpful. Rarely, these strictures may be severe enough to require more intensive treatment. Incontinence is relatively unusual after external beam radiation therapy—only about 1% of men will have severe incontinence, and 10% of men have occasional drips. Impotence (also called *erectile dysfunction*), which is defined as the inability to have an erection strong enough for intercourse, is common after all forms of prostate cancer treatment. With radiation though, erectile dysfunction tends to come on gradually over 2–5 years, rather than the more immediate erectile dysfunction typical after surgery.

Brachytherapy

Brachytherapy is another form of radiation therapy that uses about 120 tiny radioactive pellets (also called brachy or seeds) that are placed directly into the prostate.

Brachytherapy is a one-time treatment usually done under general or spinal anesthetic but occasionally under local anesthetic. The seeds are positioned in about 25 needles that are inserted through the skin under the scrotum, behind where the prostate is. As the needle is pulled out, the seeds are left in place in and around the edge of the prostate gland. The radiation from each seed only travels a small distance, but as there are so many concentrated in one area, the radiation dose there is very high (much higher than can be given by external beam radiation therapy), and the radiation dose in the normal parts of the body is much reduced because the radiation does not need to go through the body on its way to the prostate target. In high-dose brachytherapy, the radiation source is kept in the needle predefined time in the planned location of the prostate and then pulled out (an example is given in Chap. 18).

An advantage of brachytherapy is that the higher dose leads to high cure rates, and treatment is done in 1 day—a considerable time saving. The disadvantage of brachytherapy is that the radiation is so localized that it does not cover the local lymph nodes that external beam radiation therapy (EBRT) can also treat, which may be needed for high-risk cancers. Sometimes brachy and EBRT are combined together, with initial treatment by EBRT covering a wide area and then a boost to the prostate only from the brachy seeds. Another disadvantage is that men with very large prostate glands cannot be treated with brachytherapy, as it may not be possible to position all the needles due to the pelvic bones getting in the way. If this is the case, hormonal therapy or other medication can be used to shrink the prostate size down to the 60 cc or so that is the maximum that can be treated.

Like external beam radiation therapy, brachytherapy starts with a consultation with a radiation oncologist who is specially trained in the procedure. The first step in planning the treatment is to have a prostate ultrasound. It is like the one at your prostate biopsy, but this time the images are used by the oncologist and medical physicist in the planning computer to determine the number of seeds required and their precise position (and no biopsies are taken). The use of PET for radiation therapy planning is discussed in Chap. 11.

The actual treatment only takes an hour. Under anesthetic (usually general anesthetic but occasionally under local), a catheter is inserted into the bladder, an ultrasound probe is placed in the rectum, and an X-ray machine above you is used to see the seed placements. The needles containing the radioactive seeds are then inserted through the patch of skin under the scrotum, because the prostate is located behind here. The seed placement takes about 30–40 min.

Much of the information about external beam radiation therapy side effects also apply to brachytherapy, but there are some important differences. The early urinary side effects tend to be worse with brachytherapy. The radiation dose that the prostate and urethra receive is much higher, and typically there will be a fairly intense onset of urinary difficulties starting about 7–10 days after treatment, which will gradually improve over several weeks to months. About 1 in 15 men will need a catheter due to inability to urinate during this early period. Most men who need a catheter only have it in place for a day or two, but about one-third of men will have it in place for several weeks, and rarely (1–2%) long term. Rectal irritation is less common with brachytherapy than with external beam radiation therapy in the early phase. The chance of erectile dysfunction after brachytherapy is similar to the chance of erectile dysfunction after external beam radiation.

Overall the late side effects of brachytherapy are similar to the side effects of EBRT. The risk of narrowing of the urethra (urethral stricture) is higher with brachytherapy, but the longer-term bowel side effects are less common. There is a very serious but rare (1 in 400) chance that there will be a fistula between the rectum and prostate.

The PSA is the key to monitor progress after radiation therapy. Unlike with surgery, where the PSA should go to zero, with radiation the PSA gradually falls, after an initial steep drop, and takes 3–4 years to reach its minimum level. With external beam radiation therapy, a typical result 4 years after treatment is 0.5 μg/l and after brachy it is 0.1 μg/l. If the PSA subsequently rises above 2 μg/l, there is a good chance that the cancer is returning.

One concern often raised about radiation therapy is that once a man has been treated with radiation, second-line treatment (also known as salvage treatment) with surgery or more radiation is usually not possible if there is a concern that not all of the cancer cells have been killed. This is because radiation can cause scar tissue to form, especially after brachy. If a man has had surgery and there is concern about ongoing local cancer deposits, radiation can be used more safely for second-line treatment.

However, after radiation treatment, only a few men will run into life-threatening trouble because of the inability to have further prostate treatment. With brachytherapy, typically 5–10% of men will be found to have a rising PSA 5–10 years after treatment, and for half of these men, the cancer will have spread beyond the prostate (metastasized), which is likely to have occurred unknown, before treatment. So about 2.5–5% of men will have a recurrence only within the prostate. These are the men who are potential candidates for surgery. For some of these men, the cancer will be growing very slowly and not require treatment, and in others it can be managed with hormone therapy.

Other Refinements of Radiation Therapy

External beam radiation therapy and brachy come in many forms, and refinements are constantly being explored. A comparison of different types of radiation therapy, with or without hormone therapy, is shown in Table 10.1. The EBRT techniques develop, and new methods and new equipment with sophisticated properties will appear all along. Some of the new refinements have been listed here briefly.

Hypofractionation

This is a technique where the number of daily treatments is reduced from conventional fractionation of 30–40 treatments down to 28, 20, or even once or twice a week for 5–10 treatments (called *extreme hypofractionation*). The results of these approaches are not yet proven to be as effective as giving 30–40 daily treatments over 7–8 weeks, but early results are promising. The concern is that the side effects may be somewhat worse and the cure rates not quite as good. Only after studying men treated with these regimes for 5–10 years will we know if it is a good option.

Table 10.1 Comparison of different types of radiation therapy, with or without hormone therapy

	EBRT	Brachytherapy	Hormone therapy + EBRT	Hormone therapy + EBRT + brachytherapy
Suitable for which risk group	Any	Low and intermediate	High and selected intermediate	High
Duration of treatment course	6–8 weeks	Single day	6 months to 3 years HT including 7–8 week EBRT/IMRT	6 months to 3 years' HT including 4 weeks EBRT + single brachy treatment
Urinary side effects	Few	More	Few	More
Bowel side effects	More	Least	Less	More
Impotence	About 50%	About 50%	100% while on HT, about 50% long term	100% while on HT, about 50% long term
Cure rate	Good	Excellent	HT improves EBRT results	HT improves EBRT + brachy results
Contraindications	None	Very large prostate gland those unfit for anesthesia	HT may be a problem with prior cardiac disease in older men	HT may be a problem with prior cardiac disease in older men

Modified from Ref. [2]

ERBT external beam radiation therapy, *HT* hormone therapy, *IMRT* intensity-modulated radiation therapy

Volumetric-Modulated Arc Therapy

Volumetric-modulated arc therapy (e.g., RapidArc®) is a refinement of intensity-modulated radiation therapy (IMRT).

The treatment is delivered as a single rotation of the treatment machine around the patient, rather than with many separate IMRT beams. The advantage is that the treatment is delivered in a minute rather than about 10 min. An example of the principle is shown in Fig. 10.3.

Cyberknife and Tomotherapy

Cyberknife and tomotherapy are clever forms of IMRT that focus very tightly on the prostate cancer. They are often combined with extreme hypofractionation. Studies have not yet proven any advances as compared to conventional IMRT. These are briefly discussed in the therapy planning (Chap. 11).

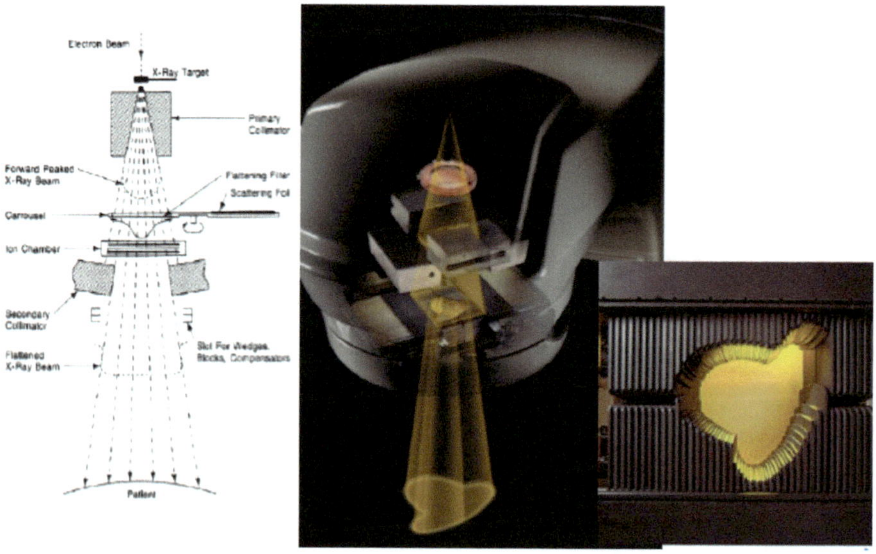

Fig. 10.3 Principle of the volumetric-modulated arc therapy (VMAT) radiation therapy technique. This novel radiation technique (since 2007) has continuous modulation of the multileaf collimators (MLCs) (for field shaping, shown in the lower panel on the right), along with the dose rate and gantry speed rotation utilized to deliver highly conformal dose distributions simultaneously, in a minimal time period. In VMAT, the aperture (defined by the MLCs) of a conventional accelerator changes dynamically, while gantry rotation speed and dose rate remain (principle of the structure on the left and schematic presentation in the middle)

Proton Therapy

Proton therapy uses particles of radiation that differ from X-rays. They are not widely available as the machines required to produce these particles are immensely expensive. Proton beam therapy enables a dose of high-energy protons to be precisely targeted at a tumor, reducing the damage to surrounding healthy tissues and vital organs. This is an advantage in certain groups of patients or where the cancer is close to a critical part of the body.

References

1. Roy Berger E, Lewis J Jr. Updated guidelines for surviving prostate cancer. 1st ed. Jericho: Health Education Literary Publisher; 2004. 464 p. ISBN 1-4107-9127-0.
2. Larry Goldenberg S, Pickles T, Chi KN. Intelligent patient guide to prostate cancer. 4th ed. Granville Island Publishing Ltd; 2014. 318 p. ISBN 978-0-9811599-2-8.
3. Tan N, Oyoyo U, Bavadian N, et al. PSMA-targeted radiotracers versus (^{18})F fluciclovine for the detection of prostate cancer biochemical recurrence after definitive therapy: a systematic review and meta-analysis. Radiology. 2020;296:44–55.
4. Hope TA, Eiber M, Armstrong WR, et al. Diagnostic accuracy of ^{68}Ga-PSMA-11 PET for pelvic nodal metastasis detection prior to radical prostatectomy and pelvic lymph node dissection: a multicenter prospective phase 3 imaging trial. JAMA Oncol. 2021;7:1635–42.
5. Fendler WP, Calais J, Eiber M, et al. Assessment of 68Ga-PSMA-11 PET accuracy in localizing recurrent prostate cancer: a prospective single-arm clinical trial. JAMA Oncol. 2019;5:856–63.
6. Pienta KJ, Gorin MA, Rowe SP, et al. A phase 2/3 prospective multicenter study of the diagnostic accuracy of prostate specific membrane antigen PET/CT with (^{18})F-DCFPyL in prostate cancer patients (OSPREY). J Urol. 2021;206:52–61.
7. Calais J, Ceci F, Eiber M, et al. (^{18})F-fluciclovine PET-CT and (68)Ga-PSMA-11 PET-CT in patients with early biochemical recurrence after prostatectomy: a prospective, single-centre, single-arm, comparative imaging trial. Lancet Oncol. 2019;20:1286–94.
8. Hofman MS, Lawrentschuk N, Francis RJ, et al. Prostate-specific membrane antigen PET-CT in patients with high-risk prostate cancer before curative-intent surgery or radiotherapy (proPSMA): a prospective, randomised, multicentre study. Lancet. 2020;395:1208–16.
9. Sonni I, Dal Pra A, O'Connell DP, et al. (^{68})Ga-PSMA PET/CT-based atlas for prostate bed recurrence after radical prostatectomy: clinical implications for salvage radiation therapy contouring guidelines. J Nucl Med. 2023;64:902–9.
10. Kairemo KJA. PET/computed tomography for radiation therapy planning of prostate cancer. PET Clinics. 2017;12:257–67.

PET/CT for Radiation Therapy Planning of Prostate Cancer

11

Summary

This chapter reviews the use of PET/CT in the radiation therapy planning of prostate cancer. The successful history of PET imaging in prostate cancer is rather short, maximally two decades, and its use in routine practice is even shorter, maximally 5 years. Because of approval of new potential imaging agents, prostate cancer staging with PET has become increasingly well-adapted. This had led to better and earlier diagnosis which requires precise treatment. Oligometastatic or oligorecurrent disease can be treated with modern targeted therapies, including multiple external beam radiation therapy methods. Here, the history of PET/CT in radiation therapy planning has been reviewed in local or more disseminated disease tracer by tracer, including ^{11}C/^{18}F-choline, ^{11}C-acetate, ^{68}Ga-PSMA, multiple ^{18}F-PSMA tracers, ^{18}F-FACBC, and ^{18}F-fluoride. Additionally, a few cases who have been successfully treated with own PET based radiation therapy planning are presented, both in primary and oligorecurrent situation.

Introduction

Radical prostatectomy (RP) and definite radiotherapy are two main treatments for locoregional prostate cancer (PCa). RP may be limited to prostatectomy, but also extended to pelvic lymph node dissection (PLND). Radiotherapy involves external beam radiotherapy (EBRT) or brachytherapy or their combinations. Brachytherapy gives little radiation to surrounding normal organs.

EBRT is developed from conventional two-dimensional EBRT to three-dimensional conformal radiotherapy (3D-CRT), image-guided radiotherapy (IGRT), intensity-modulated radiotherapy (IMRT), and volumetric-modulated arc therapy (VMAT). High-risk patients are often treated with combinatory therapies in addition to RP and EBRT, such as androgen deprivation therapy (ADT). This article describes how PET imaging is applied in radiation therapy planning.

K. Kairemo, *Prostate Cancer from a Nuclear Oncology Perspective*,
https://doi.org/10.1007/978-3-031-90337-3_11

Radiotherapy Methods in Prostate Cancer

Method Selection

The new radiotherapy technology which should be selected is dependent on disease, because oligometastatic prostate cancer encompasses a heterogenous group of clinical entities defined by the timing of the development of metastases. These include de novo oligometastatic, oligorecurrent, and oligoprogressive PCa: (I) de novo or synchronous, oligometastatic disease at the time of presentation of the primary; (II) oligorecurrent or metachronous, limited metastatic recurrence after treatment of primary; and (III) oligoprogressive: well-controlled metastatic disease with disease progression seen in a limited number of metastases [1]. There is evidence supporting the use of stereotactic ablative radiotherapy (SABR) to the oligometastases to improve patient outcomes, e.g., in STOMP [2], ORIOLE [3], SABR-COMET [4], and POPSTAR [5] trials.

Typically, the treatments are individual, and thus it is hard to rank the technologies. In a recent study, different techniques such as Cyberknife, helical tomotherapy, and RapidArc for PCa were compared dosimetrically within the same margins in simultaneous integrated boost—stereotactic body radiotherapy [6]. In this study RapidArc achieved better target dose distribution and sparing of critical structures as compared to Cyberknife and helical tomotherapy [6].

Trial Results

STOMP A multicenter randomized phase II trial of oligorecurrent PCa, with 3 or fewer lesions, enrolled 62 men and offered salvage SABR to the lesions versus surveillance. The trial was described as "Surveillance or Metastasis-Directed Therapy for Oligometastatic PrCa recurrence," or STOMP trial. As expected, those men offered surveillance required ADT within 13 months versus 21 months in the intervention group. The comparator arm of the trial was surveillance, which at the time reflected the European guidelines for asymptomatic patients. For most clinicians, the use of ADT would have been a better reflection of real-world practice. The STOMP trial was a hypothesis generating trial, opening the way for future randomized controlled clinical trials [2].

SABR-COMET SABR-COMET was an international randomized phase II trial in which 99 patients with 1–5 metachronous oligometastases from different primary cancer sites were randomized to receive stereotactic ablative therapy to all oligometastases or palliative standard of care. A median overall survival (OS) benefit of 22 months which translated to an absolute survival benefit of 24.6% at 5 years was observed in patients who received stereotactic ablative treatment [4].

ORIOLE In the ORIOLE trial, men with recurrent metastatic hormone sensitive prostate cancer (mHSPC) (no ADT for at least 6 months) and oligometastatic disease (defined as less than three metastases) were randomized to salvage SABR or observation [3]. At 6 months, 19% of men treated with SABR progressed compared to 61% of those on observation [3]. This trial would have been more applicable to current practice if the results had been compared with those of ADT.

Despite the multitude of trials showing a progression-free survival benefit, there is only one trial that has shown the OS advantage, that is, the SABR-COMET trial [4]. According to a Markov model assessment of the cost of radiotherapy, based on the results of the COMET-SABR trial, the salvage SABR approach in oligometastatic PCa is cost-effective. The analysis looked at the different treatment options, and for one lesion, the cost was $28,000 per quality adjusted life year (QALY) [7].

Biologic studies support the use of metastasis directed therapy in oligometastatic PCa. Modern imaging techniques such as PSMA PET/CT, fluciclovine PET/CT, and whole-body MRI are fundamental to implement such an approach given the high diagnostic yield at low PSA values [8, 9]. Most of the data available on metastasis directed therapy concerns retrospective trials, although three prospective randomized trials, such as STOMP and ORIOLE, have assessed the safety and feasibility of metastasis targeted treatment. Overall, it appears that metastasis directed therapy delays significantly PCa progression and time to systemic therapy.

POPSTAR In the POPSTAR trial, patients with bone metastases in a prospective trial treated with single fraction SABR received a ^{18}F-NaF PET/CT scan prior to and 6 months post-SABR [5]. The SUV_{max} values in the tumors were determined before and after SABR. Reduction in SUV_{max} was observed in 29 of 33 lesions 6 months after SABR [mean absolute decrease in SUV_{max} was 17.7 (95% CI 25.8 to − 9.4), $p = 0.0001$] [5].

Role of Prostatectomy

The promise of salvage prostatectomy is not attractive in de novo or synchronous cases, because of the variability of outcomes and risk of severe toxicity. The evidence is based on retrospective trials, with 27 single or multicenter trials showing a risk of urinary incontinence from 30% to 70%, anastomotic urethral stenosis from 10% to 20%, and rectal injury from 5% to 10%. The biochemical control rate was noted as between 30% and 100% [10].

Role of Molecular Imaging

Molecular imaging is the only way of defining biological target volume (BTV) for EBRT and may be used for advanced targeting in dose planning and dose painting

[11, 12]. In the literature, there are only a few reports about the EBRT response when dose planning is based on BTV target definition in prostate cancer [13].

In treatment planning for prostate cancer, detecting intra- and extra-prostatic tumor foci is essential. A review of the value of PET imaging in radiation therapy reported that most studies in the last 5 years showed that PET imaging with a prostate-specific membrane antigen (PSMA) tracer allows more sensitivity and specificity in the detection of prostate cancer lesions than other imaging techniques [14]. Hofman et al. [15] reported the results of the proPSMA study, a phase III randomized trial on whether novel imaging using prostate-specific membrane antigen (PSMA) PET-CT might improve accuracy and affect management. They reported that the application of PSMA-PET/CT has higher accuracy for detecting lymph nodes and bone metastases than CT or bone scan, therefore having a relevant impact on patient management [15]. Karagiannis et al. [16], in a study of 43 patients, showed that PSMA-PET/CT influences radiotherapy choice, adjuvant therapy regimens, and treatment decisions in the treatment of prostate cancer [16]. In that study, the final treatment choice was affected by PSMA-PET/CT outcome in 60.5% of cases, and only 39.5% of the patients who underwent PSMA-PET/CT were treated according to their initial treatment plans [16]. More clinical trials are underway to concretize the role of PET/CT in prostate cancer.

External Beam Radiation Therapy (EBRT)

Definitive EBRT is radiotherapy with a curative intention. EBRT for an intermediate-risk patient mainly involves IGRT, IMRT, ADT, and a high radiation dose of 75–86 Gy [17]. EBRT mainly uses a conventional fractionation schedule, a dose of 1.8–2.0 Gy for each fraction, and five fractions each week. Patients with low and intermediate risk had a better PSA recurrence-free survival after high-dose IMRT than high-risk patients [18], and controlled trials of EBRT showed that a high radiation dose for localized prostate cancer increased PSA recurrence-free survival.

EBRT may be given as an adjuvant after surgery (RP and PLND). Previously, patients with lymph node negative disease were given adjuvant EBRT after RP, if the risk of occult metastases in regional lymph nodes was estimated to be higher than 15% based on clinical findings [19].

Staging with PET/CT is a noninvasive alternative to PLND. Retrospective studies indicated that survival increased if adjuvant EBRT was added to the treatment of patients with pelvic lymph node metastases given RP, PLND, and ADT [20]; adjuvant EBRT after RP improved survival in a controlled trial of patients with localized prostate cancer.

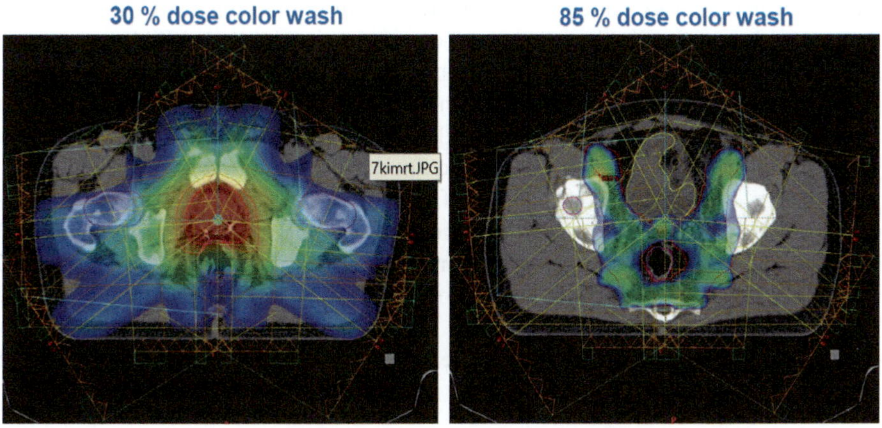

Fig. 11.1 An example of external beam dose planning using a seven-field IMRT technique. The picture on the left presents 30% color wash and the picture on the right 85% color wash. In this case, the total dose to the prostate is 78 Gy, to the seminal vesicles 50 Gy, and to the pelvic lymph nodes 45 Gy

Intensity-Modulated Radiotherapy (IMRT) or Volumetric-Modulated Arc Therapy (VMAT) with RapidArc

VMAT, e.g., RapidArc, needs shorter treatment time than IMRT for each fraction. A short treatment time reduces the risk for organ movements during treatment allowing smaller margins around the gross tumor volume (GTV). Plans for IMRT and VMAT give similar dose-volume histograms. In Fig. 11.1, the differences in the dose distributions between IMRT and VMAT are shown. In this example, the dose to urinary bladder differs marginally, and these methods have been compared in the literature for treating prostate cancer: an article compared EBRT planning for IMRT, intensity-modulated proton therapy, and RapidArc, and the authors preferred RapidArc [21]. Macdougall et al. [22] compared Cyberknife and RapidArc, and did not find advantages from choosing Cyberknife for RapidArc. Tomotherapy and RapidArc have also been compared in the management of prostate cancer [23]. Ost et al. [24] compared IMRT and VMAT for a boost for GTV_{PET}, and VMAT allowed an increased median dose boost for GTV_{PET} of 93 Gy with better sparing of radiation to the rectum. CT data from PET/CT scans could be transferred directly to CT planning systems for radiotherapy.

EBRT and Brachytherapy

The new radiotherapy technologies allow a high radiation dose to the planned target volume (PTV) and a low radiation dose to surrounding normal organs. Radiotherapy may also be improved otherwise: randomized trials showed a better PSA recurrence-free survival from combined IMRT and brachytherapy, already a long time ago [25].

Also intermediate-risk patients could benefit from combining IMRT and brachytherapy with increased radiation dose; the combination improves PSA recurrence-free survival as compared with IMRT alone [26]. The bimodal radiotherapy added a little toxicity. Brachytherapy as monotherapy also has less toxicity than EBRT. Toxicity may be reduced by installing a gel to increase the distance between gross intraprostatic tumor volume and rectum during the radiotherapy.

Recently, a retrospective analysis of 21 unfavorable intermediate or high−/very high-risk patients were assessed and received one treatment with interstitial HDR brachytherapy after external beam radiotherapy (46 Gy): the prescribed HDR doses were 10 Gy to the whole prostate, 12 Gy to the peripheral zone and 15 Gy to the areas at risk [27]. So far, no biochemical nor radiological recurrences, including PSMA-PET, have been recorded in patients who were treated in 2014–2022 [27].

Method Example of External Beam Radiation Therapy Contouring

A practical example is given here, how contouring can be done. The rectum is contoured with its contents, as recommended by quantitative analysis of normal tissue effects in the clinic [28] and the bladder using a single CT simulation image. To minimize bladder volume variation, patients should empty the bladder and drink approximately 200 mL of water 30 min prior to all imaging and treatment sessions.

$PTV_{prostate}$ is contoured using the MR (T2-weighted) image (CTV) with a 5-mm margin. PTV_{sv} is most often painted according to the CT image (CTV) with a 5-mm margin. PTV_{ln} is based on the CT image and can be contoured according to the Radiation Therapy Oncology Group consensus [29]. PTV_{ln} covers all visible lymph node metastases in CT, MR imaging, or PET/CT. Bone metastases are most often drawn using the PET images, fused with dose planning CT and MR imaging. PTV_{bone} has typically a 5-mm margin for GTV_{bone}. The RapidArc VMAT technique can be applied in all patients individually using two full arcs, but for some patients with complex PTVs, a complementary arc can be introduced. Treatment planning can be done, e.g., using the Eclipse dose calculation analytical anisotropic algorithm (Varian). Radiation therapy course begins with large fields, including lymph nodes, metastases, seminal vesicles, and prostate. After 50–56 Gy (e.g., in 25–28 fractions), $PTV_{prostate}$ will be the only target. The total dose to prostate varies between 76 and 80 Gy with 2 Gy/day fractionation. An example of PET/CT planning is shown in Fig. 11.2 in an oligorecurrent disease.

PTV_{sv} is similarly fractionated as the prostate, whereas PTV_{ln} fractionation is 1.8 Gy/d. For bone metastases, the fractionation varies: typically, PTV_{bone} is the same as PTV_{ln} during the first 5 weeks (45 Gy/25 fractions) and then boosted to higher doses, with variable fractions (1.8–3.5 Gy) for bone metastases ranging from

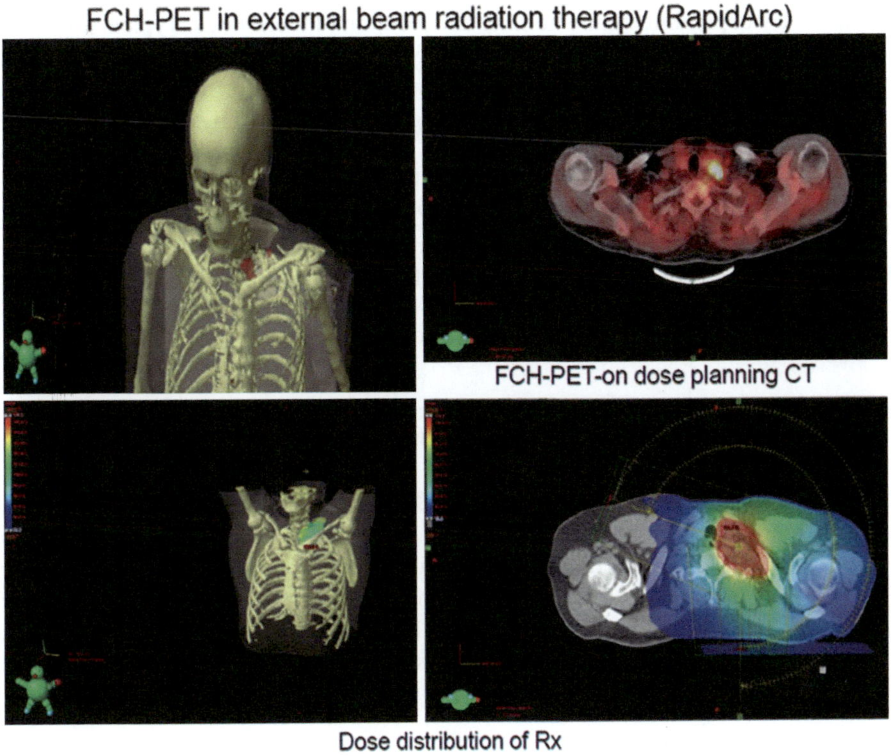

Fig. 11.2 An example of a patient case, where EBRT dose planning using is based on a PET finding in an oligorecurrent metastatic disease. The upper panel on the left demonstrates the PET finding in 3D (skeleton) and a soft tissue uptake in the left supraclavicular fossa and in the upper right panel the corresponding finding on a fusion PET/CT image. In the lower panel, on the left the RapidArc dose in the supraclavicular lymph node metastasis (85% color wash) and in the picture on the right, 30% color wash is shown on the dose planning CT

Table 11.1 Summary of target delineation principle and planned doses in high-risk prostate cancer [9]

	High-risk prostate cancer		
Parameters	Prostate	SV + regional LN	Metastases
GTV	Fusion MRI, PET	PET, MRI	PET, MRI, CT
CTV	CT	CT	CT
PTV = CTV + treatment [margins (5–10 mm)]	78–86 Gy	45–56 Gy (SV) +45–50 Gy (LN)	45–78 Gy

Abbreviations: *CTV* clinical target volume, *GTV* gross target volume, *LN* lymph nodes, *PTV* planned target volume, *SV* seminal vesicles

39 to 76 Gy depending on the number and location of metastases. Typical doses are summarized in Table 11.1, but there is wider variation in the literature—this is just to give an idea. Patients will be treated with a linear accelerator equipped with online imaging. Orthogonal X-ray imaging will be used daily to match prostate fiducial markers (e.g., gold anchors) with the digitally reconstructed radiograph image. Cone-beam CT imaging will be used in first three fractions to check bladder and rectum filling and its influence on the PTVs. Even large (>5-mm) table corrections based on the fiducial markers can be accepted in the routine, if target coverage is confirmed with cone-beam CT imaging. If there is a difference between the bones and the markers, the PTV_{bone} margin will be increased in concordance with the daily prostate movement.

PET/CT for Radiation Therapy Planning of Prostate Cancer

Molecular imaging may be used for advanced targeting in dose planning of EBRT [11, 12]. As seen earlier, biologic studies support the use of metastasis directed therapy in oligometastatic PCa. Modern imaging techniques as gozetotide PET/CT, fluciclovine PET/CT, and whole-body MRI are fundamental to implement such an approach given the high diagnostic yield at low PSA values. Most of data consists retrospective trials, although four prospective randomized trials [2–5] demonstrate metastasis targeted therapy delays significantly PCa progression and time to systemic therapy.

PET Tracers

Centers with departments for nuclear medicine and access to a cyclotron increasingly use PET/CT for imaging of prostate cancer. The United States mainly used in the beginning ^{18}F-NaF and ^{18}F-fluorodeoxyglucose (^{18}F-FDG) PET/CT and then ^{18}F-FACBC which got FDA approval in June 2016—commercial trade name is Axumin®. In the beginning, Europe preferred ^{11}C- and ^{18}F-choline PET/CT [30], because choline was a registered radiopharmaceutical in more than 15 EU countries. Radiolabeled choline PET/CT scans give a whole-body staging and delineate gross tumor volumes in a single test. Previous meta-analyses summarized the clinical use of radiolabeled choline PET/CT for prostate cancer [31]. However, the situation changed when PSMA tracers got their approvals for clinical use, F-18-PSMA compound ^{18}F-piflufolastat as known as ^{18}F-DCFPyL (Pylarify® in the United States or Pylclari® in Europe) and ^{68}Ga-PSMA-11 compound as known as ^{68}Ga-gozetotide with tradenames Illuccix® and Locametz®. The latest approved compound is the hybrid theranostic tracer ^{18}F-rhPSMA7.3 (Posluma®). The newest compounds, which are commercially available, are listed in Table 11.2. In Table 11.2, also the start of PET tracers in own EBRT planning is reported. This was possible, because all these tracers were produced locally and got a local authorization from the Medical Agency for compassionate use in single patients. A summary of PET tracers is presented in Table 11.3. All these can be used for EBRT planning. The pros and cons are discussed here in detail.

Table 11.2 The commercial compounds available for prostate cancer imaging

Compound	Trade name	Own start in EBRT planning	FDA approval	Indication
^{18}F fluorocholine, fluoromethylcholine	Iaso-Choline®	2011		Prostate cancer, parathyroid
^{18}F-fluciclovine, ^{18}F-FACBC	Axumin®	2013	V-2016	Prostate cancer
^{68}Ga-PSMA-11		2015	XII-2020	Prostate cancer
^{68}Ga-gozetotide, ^{68}Ga-PSMA-11	Illuccix®	2015	XII-2021	Prostate cancer
^{68}Ga-gozetotide, ^{68}Ga-PSMA-11	Locametz®	2015	III-2022	Prostate cancer
^{18}F-piflufolastat, ^{18}F-DCFPyL	Pylarify® Pylclari® (EMA)	2016	V-2022	Prostate cancer
^{18}F-flotufolastat, ^{18}F-rhPSMA7.3	Posluma®		V-2023	Prostate cancer

Abbreviations: *DCFPyL* piflufolastat, *EBRT* external beam radiation therapy, *EMA* European Medical Agency, *FACBC* fluciclovine, *FDA* Food and Drug Administration (US authority), *PCa* prostate cancer, *PSMA* prostate-specific membrane antigen

Table 11.3 PET tracers suitable for target delineation in prostate cancer, updated from [9]

	Tracer characteristics		
Target	Event	Radiopharmaceutical	Significance
glut1, *glut3*, hexokinase Choline kinase L- amino acid transport Androgen receptor PSMA Acetyl-Co-A DNA	Glycolysis Membrane synthesis Amino acid transport Hormone receptor Transmembrane protein Lipid synthesis Cell proliferation	^{18}F-FDG ^{18}F-FCH; ^{11}C-CHO ^{18}F-FACBC; ^{11}C-Met ^{18}F-FDHT ^{68}Ga-PSMA-11; ^{18}F-PSMA- 1007;^{18}F-DCFBC; ^{18}F-DCFPyL; ^{18}F-rhPSMA7.3 ^{11}C-acetate ^{18}F-FLT	Prognostic, aggressive disease (T)NM staging (T)N(M) staging AR status TNM staging (T)NM staging Proliferation activity, response evaluation
Hydroxy apatite	Bone formation	Na ^{18}F	Skeletal disease localization

Abbreviations: *AR* androgen receptor, *^{11}C-CHO* carbon-11-choline, *^{11}C-Met* carbon-11-methionine, *^{18}F-FACBC* anti-trans-1-amino-3-^{18}F-fluorocyclobutanecarboxylic-acid or ^{18}F-fluciclovine, *^{18}F-FCH* ^{18}F-fluorocholine, *^{18}F-DCFBC* *N*-[*N*-[(*S*)-1,3-dicarboxypropyl]carbamoyl]-4-^{18}F-fluorobenzyl-l-cysteine, *^{18}F-DCFPyL* 2-(3-(1-carboxy-5-[(6-^{18}F- fluoropyridine-2-carbonyl)-amino]-pentyl)-ureido)-pentanedioic acid or ^{18}F-piflufolastat, *^{18}F-FDG* ^{18}F-fluorodeoxyglucose, *^{18}F-FDHT* 16β-^{18}F-fluoro-5α-dihydrotestosterone, *^{18}F-FLT* ^{18}F-fluorothymidine, *Na ^{18}F* sodium ^{18}F-fluoride, *PSMA* prostate-specific membrane antigen

Current Imaging for Oligometastatic PCa

PSMA Tracers

^{68}Ga-PSMA-11

PSA has been the main trigger of treatment initiation in case of recurrent PCa for the past 30 years. The inherent definition of a "biochemical recurrence" underlines the importance of such serum marker in defining such a pathologic state. However, metastasis targeted therapy clearly requires a precise definition of the metastatic active lesions which need treatment. Standard imaging techniques as CT scan or bone scintigraphy are unable to detect oligorecurrent disease in an early phase in which targeted treatments could be administered. As such, novel highly sensible imaging techniques have entered clinical practice.

PSMA-PET/CT is able to detect PCa recurrences even at low PSA levels of <0.5 ng/mL [32, 33]. The test relies on the overexpression of PSMA by PCa cells [34]. PSMA is a transmembrane type II glycoprotein also called folate hydrolase or glutamate carboxypeptidase II, which has a 19-amino-acid intracellular portion, a 24-amino-acid transmembrane portion, and a 707-amino-acid extracellular portion [35]. The preference of this dual enzyme function is dependent on the location in the body, i.e., where folate or glutamate metabolism should be activated. Although multiple ligands of PSMA have been tested, the inhibitor Glu-NH-CO-NH-Lys(Ahx)-HBED-CC(^{68}Ga-PSMA-HBED-CC) is the most commonly used and is being throughout fully investigated. After ligation to PCa, the tracer is internalized in the cell, while a rapid clearance in healthy tissue is observed [36]. As such, although PSMA accumulates in the salivary glands, liver, and urinary tract, little compound is taken up in the retroperitoneal fatty tissue, benign lymphatic tissue, and bone, making it an appealing option to localize PCa metastases [36]. In the setting of recurrent PCa, the largest study to date has been published by Afshar-Oromieh et al. [37], exploring the results of PSMA 1007 patients with recurring disease. PSMA-PET was positive in 79.5% of patients [37]. Eiber et al. retrospectively evaluated 248 men with PCa recurrence after radical prostatectomy; 90% had at least one suspicious lesion, and a positive correlation with serum PSA was also found. For PSA values of 0.2 to <0.5 ng/mL, 0.5–1 ng/mL, 1–2 ng/mL, and ≥2 ng/mL, detection rates were 57.9%, 72.7%, 93.0%, and 96.8%, respectively [33]. Raveenthiran et al. [38] analyzed 276 men undergoing a PSMAPET/CT due to a recurrence after definitive radiotherapy. Overall detection rate was 86%, with a local recurrence being the most frequent finding (57%) [38]. Farolfi et al. [39] retrospectively review a multicentric cohort of patients with persistent PSA after radical prostatectomy. Interestingly, already 33% of these men had extrapelvic disease, although 8 of 33 patients who had available PET imaging before and after surgery did show new PET lesions so early after surgery [39].

In a systematic review, Kimura et al. reported the diagnostic accuracy of PSMAPET/CT before salvage node dissection [40]. The pooled sensitivity using lesion-based and field-based analyses was 0.84 (95% CI 0.61–0.95) and 0.82 (95% CI 0.72–0.89), respectively, making PSMA an excellent examination to identify candidates for salvage node dissection. ^{68}Ga PSMA-PET/CT was compared to bone scintigraphy by Pyka et al. [41] for detection of bone metastases. In their study exploring 126 men, of which 76 were diagnosed with metastatic bone disease, PSMA-PET/CT significantly outperformed bone scintigraphy, with overall sensitivity and specificity of 98.7–100% and 88.2–100%, compared to 86.7–89.3% sensitivity and a 60.8–96.1% specificity of bone scintigraphy ($P < 0.001$) [41]. Bluemel et al. [42] performed a sequential imaging study, offering PSMA-PET/CT to 125 patients with recurring PCa in whom ^{11}C-choline PET was negative. They report an increase in detection rates from 74.4% with only ^{11}C-choline PET to 85.6% when adding PSMA [42]. PSMA-PET can also be incorporated to an MRI in order to improve soft-tissue visualization and in particular help in gaining details on local recurrences. In a retrospective trial analyzing 66 patients with biochemical recurrence (≤0.5 ng/mL), Kranzbühler et al. [43] reported a positive scan in 36 of 66 patients (54.5%). Of note, in 26 of 66 patients (39.4%), PSMA-positive lesions were located outside a standard salvage radiotherapy volume, making the examination fundamental to define adequate salvage therapy [43].

The performance of ^{68}Ga-PSMA PET/CT has been analyzed in multiple systematic reviews—it has been turned out to be superior to bone scintigraphy in a systematic review of 37 studies [44] and in a meta-analysis of 6 studies consisting 546 patients [45].

Systematic reviews have demonstrated superiority to conventional imaging for primary staging of high-risk prostate cancer (Corfield et al. [46]; 322 patients in 12 studies), biochemical recurrence (Eissa et al. [33]; 37 studies), and lymph node detection preoperatively (e.g., Kimura et al. [40]: 462 patients in 14 studies; Petersen et al. [47]: 969 patients in 18 studies). There is evidence that ^{68}Ga-PSMA PET/CT is also effective for recurrence localization with extremely low PSA levels such as <0.5 ng/ml (Eissa et al. [33])—it has clinical significance in detecting the recurrence site in patients with PSA values smaller than 1.0 ng/ml after radical prostatectomy [48]. Von Eyben et al. [48] conducted a meta-analysis to evaluate ^{68}Ga-PSMA PET/CT or PET/MRI for PCa staging, diagnostic test accuracy, and biochemical recurrence in a total of 1256 patients in 15 studies. After this study, several meta-analyses have been published in lymph node staging for patients with moderate- or high-risk prostate cancer, for example, Peng et al. ([49]; 701 patients in 10 studies) and Tu et al. ([50]; 904 patients in 11 studies). A large meta-analysis by Hope et al. [51] confirmed the excellent diagnostic value of ^{68}Ga-PSMA-11 PET for initial staging and biochemical recurrence with histological confirmations in 29 studies. The superiority of ^{68}Ga-PSMA-11 PET to MRI has been confirmed by two meta-analyses: Wu et al. [51] and Wang et al. [52]. PET is more sensitive than MRI in detecting metastases in moderate- and high-risk cancer in an analysis of 1597 patients in 13 studies and can detect better lymph node metastases before surgery [51]. Similar findings were observed in another analysis where multiparametric MRI was compared with ^{68}Ga-PSMA-11 PET for pelvic lymph node staging prior to radical prostatectomy and pelvic lymph node dissection [52]. Overall, sensitivities and specificities up to 97–98% have been reported in these multiple studies depending on the study setup; in general, accuracies higher than 90% were reported in almost every study. Therefore, this tracer ^{68}Ga-PSMA-11 got marketing authorization (Table 11.2) in 2021 and is commercially available with tradenames Illuccix® and Locametz® as shown in Table 11.2.

The advantages of ^{68}Ga-PSMA-11 and PSMA tracers are obvious in prostate cancer detection and lesion delineation [53, 54]. Some of the skeletal lesions may be visualized earlier with Na^{18}F [55], but ^{68}Ga-PSMA-11 PET may play an essential role in lesion characterization in EBRT. ^{68}Ga-PSMA-11 PET/CT has been used for delineating clinical target volumes (CTVs), prostate bed recurrence, or biochemical recurrence after radical prostatectomy by Sonni et al. [56]. In their study of 226 patients, 127 patients had PSMA recurrence limited to the prostate bed, 30 had pelvic nodal disease, 32 had extrapelvic disease, and 37 had both pelvic nodal disease and extrapelvic disease. Positive prostate recurrences were completely covered by the CTV in 68 of 127 patients (53%), partially covered in 43 of 127 (34%), and not covered in 16 of 127 (13%). This indicates that PET should be part of guiding salvage radiation therapy planning directed to the prostate bed in the setting of postoperative biochemical recurrence or persistence and should be a part of future guidelines [56]. In a recent biology-guided radiotherapy study, ^{68}Ga-PSMA-11 PET/CT was used to identify dominant intraprostatic lesion and measure GTVs using PSMA-avid subvolume in the prostate region [57]. They found in 83 patients that PSMA-PET is feasible to identify GTVs suitable for targeted radiotherapy in the prostate. These GTVs were characterized by a strong signal-to-background ratio and a surrounding tissue free of PSMA uptake [57]. A recent trial evaluated the effect of PSMA-PET/computed tomography (CT)-guided boost of radiation therapy on patient outcomes in 253 patients [58]. New lesions were detected in 45.5% of oligometastatic patients, 39.5% of high-risk patients, 14.3% of salvage post radiotherapy patients, and 51.6% of salvage therapy after radical prostatectomy. Overall, PSMA-PET/CT led to intensification of radiotherapy in more than half of patients (52.0%), with minimal intensification of systemic therapy (4.0%), resulting in a minimal increased toxicity in 2.5% patients [58]. The information is limited so far. In a PROPER 1 trial, radiotherapy was adapted after 50 Gy, when nonresponders (PSA still $\geq$0.15 ng/mL) received sequential lymph node irradiation with a boost to PSMA-PET positive lesions, whereas responders (PSA $<$ 0.15 ng/mL) continued radiotherapy as planned [59]. PET findings were only taken into consideration for treatment planning in case of PSA nonresponse after 50 Gy, but high tumor control rate was observed in both responders and nonresponders [59], indicating a clinically significant effect in patients with otherwise poor prognosis. In a study of 63 patients with 89 metastases (68 in lymph nodes and 21 in bones) identified by ^{68}Ga-PSMA-11 PET/CT, the patients received either 50 Gy (25 fractions) or 30 Gy (10 fractions) [60]. In 33 patients (52%), a distant progression was observed. The first tumor-related event was in average in 16.6 months, and 22.2% of patients had no tumor-related clinical events after 3-year follow-up [60]. Thus, local control may be achieved, but the conditions have to be identified in prospective randomized trials. This is a problem in a trial design, because typically diseases and treatment plans are very individual.

^{18}F-PSMAs

There are multiple, fluorinated PSMA tracers, and the most important of those are ^{18}F-PSMA-1007, ^{18}F-DCFPyL, ^{18}F-DCFBC, and ^{18}F-rhPSMA7.3. At this moment, ^{18}F-DCFPyL and ^{18}F-rhPSMA7.3 have marketing authorization (Table 11.2). However, most widely used tracer is ^{18}F-PSMA-1007 which was discovered later than the other two; this agent is more lipophilic, is not excreted into the urinary system, and has been widely tested in Europe, very much under compassionate use. ^{18}F-DCFPyL and ^{18}F-DCFBC have been used more in the United States and almost only in clinical trials. Therefore, almost all of the systematic reviews deal with ^{18}F-PSMA-1007. The original meta-analysis was performed by Treglia et al. [61] concerning biochemical recurrence in 645 patients in 6 studies. After that, a few other "meta-analyses" have been published, for example, Huang et al. ([62]; 12 studies/540 patients) and Liu et al. ([63]; 11 studies/799 patients). Importantly, a meta-analysis regarding PET-targeted biopsy has been published by Kawada et al. [64]. In their analysis of 497 patients in 5 studies, a very good diagnostic accuracy was observed for clinically significant PCa, and when combining with MRI its performance will even improve [64]. In general, the performance characteristics do not essentially differ from those of ^{68}Ga-PSMA-11.

Recently, ^{18}F-DCFBC and ^{18}F-DCFPyL were studied in 34 patients after failure of a group of post-prostatectomy patients who received adjuvant or salvage radiation therapy and subsequently experienced biochemical recurrence [65]. ^{18}F-DCFBC is chemically (N-[N-[(S)-1,3-dicarboxypropyl] carbamoyl]-4-^{18}F-fluorobenzyl-L-cysteine), and it was one of the first fluorinated compounds taken into clinical studies. Distant recurrence was the predominant pattern of failure, and local recurrence was noted in approximately one-fifth of patients which should be kept in mind when planning radiotherapy after prostatectomy [65].

In a North American study, both PSMA PET/MRI and multiparametric MRI were used for planning focal intraprostatic boosts for stereotactic radiation therapy (SBRT) [66]. They used 2-(3-(1-carboxy-5-[(6-^{18}F-fluoro-pyridine-2-carbonyl)-amino]-pentyl)-ureido)-pentanedioic acid as PET tracer—this tracer is known as ^{18}F-DCFPyL with its commercial name Pylarify® (and later Pylclari® in Europe) and its generic name piflufolastat (Table 11.2). They evaluated 13 patients with local prostate prospectively before therapies, and most of the lesions (21/39, 53.8%) were discordant between MRI and PET, with more lesions seen by PET alone (12) than MRI alone (9) [66]. They concluded that using both MRI- and PSMA-directed PET may better identify all areas of gross disease within the prostate. It is known that the accurate detection and segmentation of the intraprostatic GTV is pivotal for radiotherapy in PCa. In a European study, multiparametric MRI was compared with ^{18}F-PSMA-1007 PET for intraprostatic GTV detection and delineation [67]. In this study of 93 patients in 2 German cities, intraprostatic GTV segmentation based on ^{18}F-PSMA-1007 PET resulted in more and larger GTVs compared to MRI [67]. The clinical significance of this should be studied in prospective trials. Whole-body MRI is gaining success in PCa imaging given its ability to directly visualize the metastatic lesions, the absence of radiation exposure, and the possibility to evaluate response to treatment. A key advantage of MRI is its ability to visualize bone lesions and, incorporating multiple sequences, accurately distinguish benign from malignant skeletal disease. Various MRI techniques can be combined in one single examination to explore the various compartments of bony structures, such as the marrow (exploring bone marrow water and fat composition with T_1-weighed, T_2-weighted, and STIR sequences), the vascularization (via DCE-MRI), and the trabecular bone (ultrashort echo time MRI and susceptibility weighted MRI). Moreover, a key sequence is diffusion-weighted MRI, which analyzes free water movement at a microscopic level. Generally, a reduced apparent diffusion coefficient well correlates to cancerous tissue cytoarchitectural disorganization [68].

Maybe, all the benefits and limitations from the imaging modalities PET/CT/MRI should be taken into account in radiation therapy planning [69]. Interobserver variation is less important when multiple methods are combined [70], and the future may reveal new radiomic parameters for characterizing the disease [71]. In this book, I present a case which was studied both with ^{18}F-PSMA-1007 and ^{18}F-DCFPyL prior therapies (Chap. 18). In this case, the treatment planning was dose according to the PET with two intraprostatic lesions where the smaller lesion was not identified by multiparametric MRI nor CT.

Fluciclovine

Fluciclovine (Axumin®) is a rather new tracer, currently implemented in recurrent PCa—it was known as trans-1-Amino-3-^{18}F-fluorocyclobutanecarboxylic acid (anti-^{18}F-FACBC) [72]. Fluciclovine has minimal urinary excretion and minimal brain uptake which allows excellent imaging of the cerebrum, retroperitoneum, and pelvis. In a multicenter phase IIb clinical trial, ^{18}F-fluciclovine PET/CT was compared to conventional imaging with CT and bone scan [73]. The overall accuracies were similar for ^{18}F-fluciclovine PET/CT and conventional imaging (85.5% vs. 87.3%). However, ^{18}F-fluciclovine PET/CT was positive in 5–9 mm lymph nodes that were not detected by conventional imaging [73]. In a prospective study, Nanni et al. [74] compared the performance of fluciclovine PET-CT to 11 C-choline PET-CT and demonstrated statistically superior sensitivity of fluciclovine, particularly significant in the lowest PSA subgroup (<1 ng/mL; 21% vs. 14%). Pernthaler et al. [75] compared fluciclovine to PSMA in a prospective trial exploring results in 58 patients with BCR after definitive treatment for PCa. The overall detection rate for PCa recurrence was 79.3% in ^{18}F-fuciclovine and 82.8% in ^{68}Ga-PSMA-11 (P = 0.64). Local recurrence was detected in 37.9% on 18F-fuciclovine and in 27.6% on Ga-PSMA-11 (P = 0.03) [75]. Local pelvic lymph node recurrence was detected on ^{18}F-fuciclovine versus Ga-PSMA-11 in 46.6% versus 50%, in extrapelvic lymph node metastases in 41.4% versus 51.7%, and in bone metastases in 25.9% versus 36.2%, respectively. Thus, fluciclovine appears appealing in defining local recurrences, given its better visualization of the urinary system compared to PSMA. However, Calais et al. [76] recently performed a comparative single centric study in 50 men with a BCR after radical prostatectomy and PSA values of 0.2–2 ng/mL. These patients underwent ^{68}Ga-PSMA and ^{18}F-fluciclovine PET/CT. Metastasis detection was significantly higher in the PSMA arm (56% vs. 26%, P = 0.0026), supporting the superiority of PSMA [76]. In the most recent EMPIRE-1 study, patients were randomized to radiation therapy planning via either conventional imaging only (bone scanning plus abdominopelvic CT or MRI) or conventional imaging plus ^{18}F-fluciclovine PET/CT [77]. They found that including ^{18}F-fluciclovine PET/CT to radiation therapy planning leads to survival benefits in patients with a PSA < 2 ng/mL but not in patients with a PSA > 2 ng/mL [77].

Cholines

When the use of PET was introduced into radiotherapy planning, most of the articles reported radiolabeled choline PET/CT-guided planning in EBRT [12]. Six articles evaluated localized prostate cancer and reported 178 patients with PET/CT-guided planning of a boost to GTV_{PET} [12]. Pinkawa et al. [12] simultaneously integrated a boost with 80 Gy for the GTV_{PET} with a dose of 76 Gy for the whole prostate, their first study was published in 2010 [78]. The small boost did not increase toxicity for normal organs at risk. Four articles evaluated pelvic lymph node metastases and reported 254 patients with PET/CT-guided planning of EBRT for the pelvic lymph nodes [12]. In a study by Picchio et al. [79], 66 of 94 (70%) treatments gave a greater than 50% PSA reduction for 83 patients after helical tomotherapy for recurrent prostate cancer with lymph node metastases; 36 of the 83 patients (47%) did not develop a second recurrence during the first short phase of follow-up; and 4 of 12 patients remained in partial PSA remission for 1 year [79]. In a study of 93 patients with sites of recurrence in lymph nodes, patients had a better biochemical recurrence-free survival if they had been treated with salvage lymph node dissection combined with radiotherapy than if they had been treated with only salvage lymph node dissection [80].

Even though radiolabeled choline turned out to be an excellent tracer in meta-analysis in more than 3000 patients [30], it has been replaced by PSMA tracers since the mid-2010s, especially because of better sensitivity. However, the basics of PET guidance in radiation therapy planning were made by choline. One of the challenges was the presence of liver metastases, where hydrophilic tracers perform better as compared to lipophilic tracers—dual-phase imaging can be a solution, if a hydrophilic PET tracer is not available [81].

Other Tracers

Table 11.3 represents the PET tracers which can be used for radiation therapy planning. Table 11.3 is an updated version from my earlier review with demonstrative cases from [9]. In this chapter, a few practical cases are shown and a few new ideas are given.

In the literature, one of first PET demonstrations of the whole concept was given by carbon-11-acetate PET/CT-based planning in dose escalated IMRT by Seppälä et al. [82]. They gave a simultaneously integrated boost of 90 Gy to the GTV_{PET} combined with 78 Gy to the prostate.

^{18}F-FDG has not been used in radiation therapy planning for prostate cancer, even though it has been used to exclude patients who would respond to targeted therapies [15]. One could assume that FDG-positive targets which are associated with a poor prognosis might respond to higher radiation doses. Similarly, hypoxia could be identified and could be selection of patients who respond to radiation therapy [83]. Actually, the Warburg effect differentiates malignant cells from benign cells: anaerobic glycolysis occurs only in malignant cells. Thus, combination of FDG and hypoxia imaging could be a solution of radiation resistance as well. However, it remains elusive if the combinatory imaging can be applied for therapy planning.

In prostate cancer, the lack of androgen receptors and the FDG positivity is a poor prognostic factor [84]. On the other hand, the presence of androgen receptors is a sign of a good prognosis, and it may be used in the clinics, because androgen receptor status can be imaged. Proliferation is a prognostic factor as well, but FLT-imaging is in the assessment chemotherapy response of PCa failed [85]. Therefore, probably fluorothymidine imaging will not work in radiation therapy planning either.

Metastatic prostate cancer is approximately present in 80% cases in the skeleton. We have demonstrated that, targeting skeletal lesions contemporaneously with two PET tracers, the distribution may differ dramatically; this is the case with $Na^{18}F$ and ^{18}F-fluorocholine [86] and with $Na^{18}F$ and ^{68}Ga-PSMA-11 [55]. The bone-seeking $Na^{18}F$ is detecting active osteoblasts around cancer cells, i.e., in the cortical bone and the oncotropic tracers (cholines and PSMAs) are targeting cancer cells, e.g. in bone marrow. Therefore the combined volumes should be taken in consideration in EBRT planning. $Na^{18}F$ seems to be very sensitive, and we use it very often in radiation therapy planning. The POPSTAR trial gave excellent results when judging responses with $Na^{18}F$ [5].

Case Presentations

Here, some practical cases are presented, where PET has been applied in dose delineation.

Case 1 This 72-year-old patient had originally a Gleason score 8 prostate cancer, and it was originally treated with EBRT combined with androgen deprivation therapy. A biochemical relapse was observed, and imaging revealed a local relapse in the prostate and pelvic bone metastases. ^{18}F-FCH/$Na^{18}F$-PET studies for VMAT external beam radiation therapy planning (RapidArc) are shown in Fig. 11.3. On the left, FCH-PET demonstrates pelvic soft-tissue disease (prostate) and oligometastatic skeletal disease and NaF-PET skeletal disease in same locations. On the right, examples of treatment plans are shown. Salvage treatment with VMAT was given to this oligometastatic disease with an excellent response (Fig. 11.3).

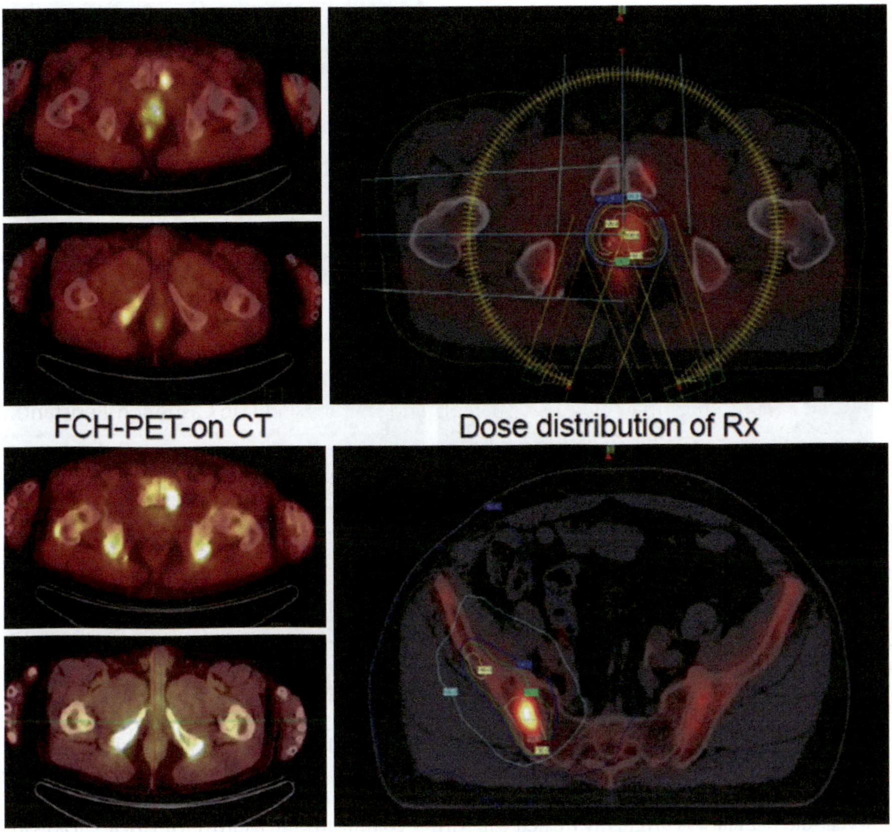

Fig. 11.3 An example of a patient case, where EBRT dose planning using is based on two PET studies in an oligoprogressive disease. The upper panel on the left demonstrates FCH-PET study with two skeletal metastases and a recurrence in the left lobe of the prostate, the upper right panel the dose distribution in the prostate on CT which is based on FCH-PET. The lower left panel shows skeletal metastases in a $Na^{18}F$-PET study at two levels and the lower right panel dose distribution in a skeletal metastasis at a third level based on $Na^{18}F$-PET. This 72-year-old patient had been treated originally with radiation therapy and ADT. Now five lesions were treated with RapidArc outside the previously treated regions, and the prostate target region got an extra booster dose. (Presented in [9])

Case 2 This 68-year-old patient was originally treated with EBRT combined with androgen deprivation therapy for a GS 6 disease 10 years earlier. A biochemical relapse was observed in the left presacral node, and S-PSA value was 1.85. Treatment with VMAT was given to this disease with a complete response.

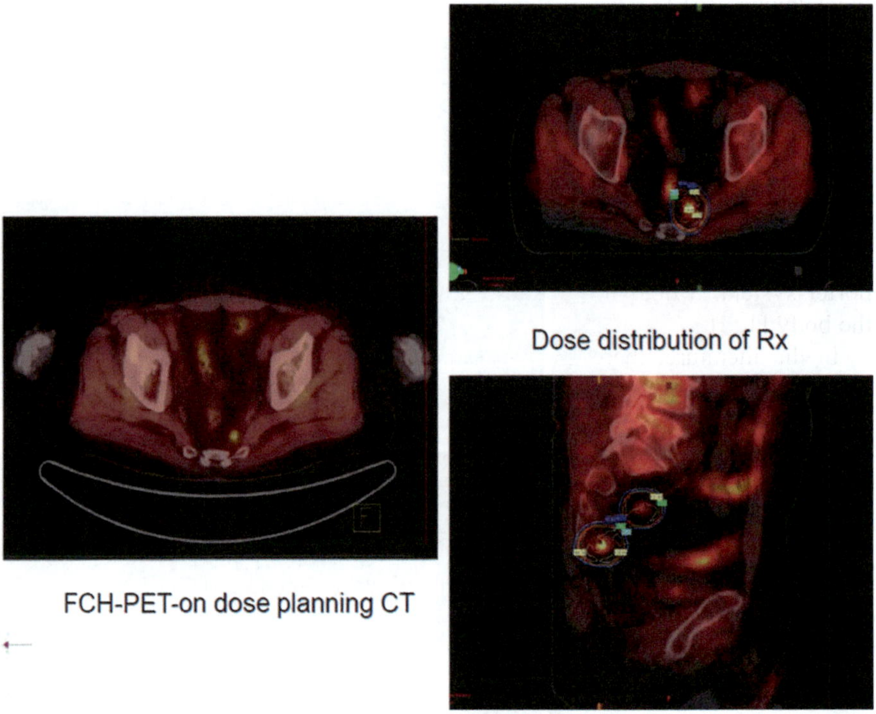

Fig. 11.4 FCH-PET studies in for VMAT external beam radiation therapy planning (RapidArc). On the left, FCH-PET/CT image demonstrates pelvic lymph node disease (presacral node on the patient's left side). On the right, examples of treatment plans from two directions are shown. This 68-year-old patient was originally treated with EBRT combined with androgen deprivation therapy for a GS 6 disease 10 years earlier. A biochemical relapse was observed in the left presacral node. S-PSA value was 1.85. Treatment with VMAT was given to this disease with a complete response

In Fig. 11.4 on the left, FCH-PET/CT-image demonstrates pelvic lymph node disease (presacral node on the patient's left side). On the right, examples of treatment plans from two directions are shown (Fig. 11.4).

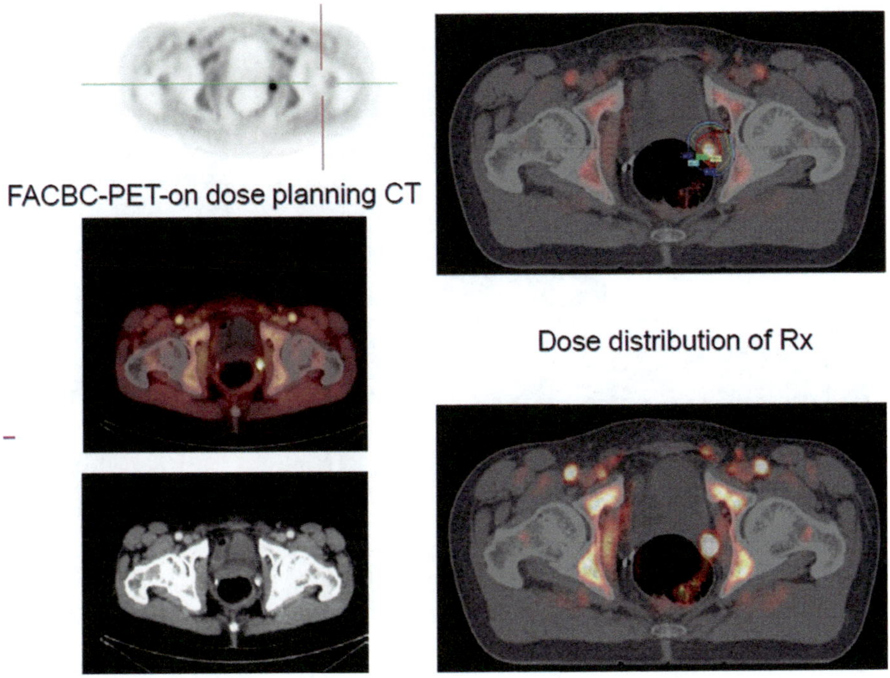

Fig. 11.5 ^{18}F-fluciclovine-PET studies for VMAT external beam radiation therapy planning (RapidArc). On the left, ^{18}F-fluciclovine-PET demonstrates soft-tissue disease in a lymph node. On the right, examples of treatment plans are shown. This 55-year-old patient with PCa (Gleason 9) was treated radical prostatectomy and hormone therapy. A biochemical relapse was observed in soft tissue. S-PSA was then 0.3. Treatment with VMAT was given with a good response. (Presented in [9])

Case 3 This 55-year-old patient with PCa (Gleason 9) was treated radical prostatectomy and hormone therapy. A biochemical relapse was observed in soft tissue. S-PSA was then 0.3. Treatment with VMAT was given with a good response.

^{18}F-fluciclovine-PET studies for VMAT external beam radiation therapy planning (RapidArc) (Fig. 11.5). On the left, ^{18}F-fluciclovine-PET demonstrates soft-tissue disease in a lymph node. On the right, examples of treatment plans are shown (Fig. 11.5).

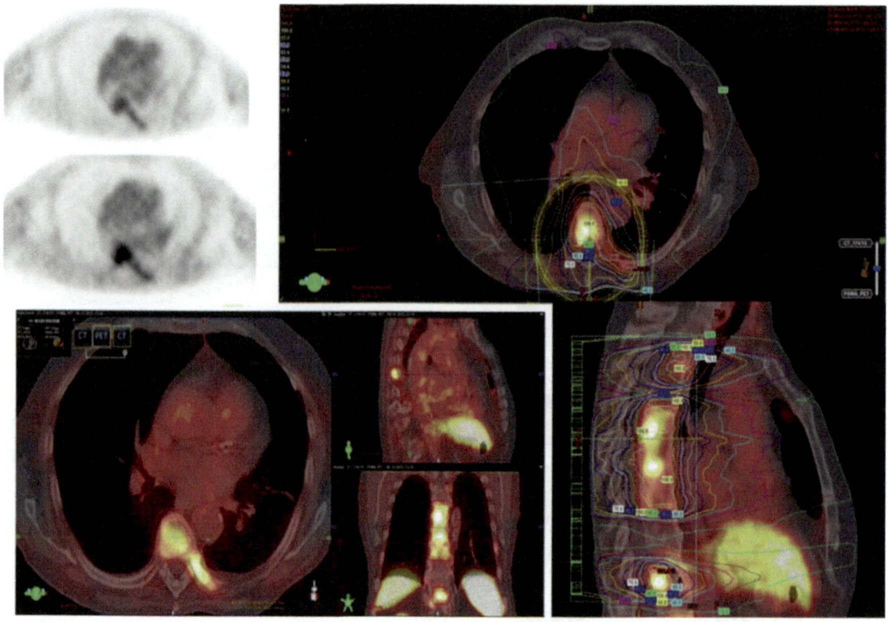

Fig. 11.6 ^{68}Ga-PSMA-11-PET/CT studies for VMAT EBRT planning (RapidArc®). On the left, ^{68}Ga-PSMA-11-PET demonstrates thoracic skeletal disease in multiple locations (upper left corner). PET/CT fusion images are shown in the lower left corner (transaxial, sagittal, and coronal projections). These demonstrate disease in the transverse process besides vertebral body. On the right, examples of treatment plans are shown (transaxial view [upper panel]; sagittal view [lower panel]). This patient was treated with EBRT because of back pain. Palliation treatment with VMAT was given to this oligometastatic disease with excellent response to tumor burden and pain. (Presented in [9])

Case 4 This 85-year-old patient with PCa (Gleason 6) was originally treated with hormone therapy and active surveillance. During the 10-year follow-up, he developed metastatic disease with a maximum S-PSA of 200 μg/l—he was treated with locoregional EBRT and docetaxel and S-PSA decreased down to 9 μg/l. He developed a new biochemical relapse and had pain between shoulder blades. A ^{68}Ga-PSMA-11-PET was performed, and the imaging findings are shown in Fig. 11.6. A new palliative treatment for skeletal disease was planned according to PSMA-PET findings and the patient responded well.

Rationale for Metastasis Directed Therapy in Oligorecurrent Disease

For decades, surveillance or androgen deprivation therapy was offered for patients suffering from clinical recurrence after radical prostatectomy or radiation therapy. The aim of surveillance was to delay the onset of ADT and its adverse events. Although more than 90% of clinical recurrences respond to androgen deprivation therapy, patients on average developed resistance to systemic therapy within 2–3 years [87]. These results suggest room for improved disease management, particularly for individuals with oligorecurrent metastatic disease.

We have learned here from the trials briefly reviewed, STOMP [2], ORIOLE [3], SABR-COMET [4], and POPSTAR [5], that multimodal, sequential, or combination therapies can improve patient outcomes. Although the clinical data are convincing, the underlying mechanisms leading to potentially improved outcome receiving metastasis directed therapy remain still speculative.

Although PET/CTs using novel tracers hold great potential, the widespread availability of them is still limited, and their value and impact on management and survival of men with advanced prostate cancer has not been proven. Nearly all of the studies using PET/CT with new tracers are single-center protocols, neither prospective nor randomized, with questionable definition of reference standard, thus leading to lack of evidence to allow recommending such procedures for everyday practice.

In regard to the management of men with oligometastatic castration-naïve prostate cancer, this is an area where research should be conducted to define optimal management strategies. The available data on treatment of men with oligometastatic prostate cancer are sparse and heterogeneous regarding definitions, patient populations, imaging methods, and treatment approaches applied.

VMAT is a new radiation treatment technique that can create highly conformal dose distribution in a short time. Despite wide use of this technique, a majority of published data on VMAT are dosimetric planning studies with limited clinical outcome data. VMAT enables optimization and delivery of a complex dose painting treatment plans [9]. The author's own retrospective analysis found that the patients with advanced prostate cancer using PET/CT-based EBRT dose planning had lower incidence for biochemical relapse, fewer clinical manifestations of disease, and longer duration of disease-free period and biochemical stability compared with patients whose dose planning was based on conventional imaging.

In this review, multiple PET tracers suitable for EBRT planning are shown. Only a few of them have been used in clinical routine practice. This is just beginning. Luckily the technique was tested earlier, mainly with choline tracers, and the results were very encouraging. The field is completely open, and the results could be even better with new more accurate tracers. Because PSMA tracers are already part of international and national guidelines, their use should be implemented as part of individual treatment routines in oligometastatic prostate cancer. The real-world cases shown here all have got excellent response to EBRT, lasting up several years.

The international approval only awaits for intelligent randomized trials where the benefit can be confirmed in statistically significant numbers.

References

1. Mikropoulos C, Saxby H, Boussios S. Prostate cancer—what about oligometastatic disease and stereotactic ablative radiotherapy?—a narrative review. Ann Palliat Med. 2023;12:646–52.
2. Ost P, Reynders D, Decaestecker K, et al. Surveillance or metastasis-directed therapy for oligometastatic prostate cancer recurrence: a prospective, randomized, multicenter phase II trial. J Clin Oncol. 2018;36:446–53.
3. Phillips R, Shi WY, Deek M, et al. Outcomes of observation vs stereotactic ablative radiation for oligometastatic prostate cancer: the ORIOLE phase 2 randomized clinical trial. JAMA Oncol. 2020;6:650–9.
4. Palma DA, Olson R, Harrow S, et al. Stereotactic ablative radiotherapy versus standard of care palliative treatment in patients with oligometastatic cancers (SABR-COMET): a randomised, phase 2, open-label trial. Lancet. 2019;393:2051–8.
5. Hardcastle N, Hofman MS, Lee CY, et al. NaF PET/CT for response assessment of prostate cancer bone metastases treated with single fraction stereotactic ablative body radiotherapy. Radiat Oncol. 2019;14:164.
6. Bijina TK, Ganesh KM, Pichandi A, Muthuselvi CA. Cyberknife, helical tomotherapy and rapid arc SIB-SBRT treatment plan comparison for carcinoma prostate. Asian Pac J Cancer Prev. 2020;21:1149–54.
7. Qu XM, Chen Y, Zaric GS, Senan S, Olson RA, Harrow S, et al. Is SABR cost-effective in oligometastatic cancer? An economic analysis of the SABR-COMET randomized trial. Int J Radiat Oncol Biol Phys. 2021;109:1176–84.
8. Albisinni S, Van Damme J, Aoun F, Bou Kheir G, Roumeguère T, De Nunzio C. A systematic review of imaging-guided metastasis-directed therapy for oligorecurrent prostate cancer: revolution or devolution? Minerva Urol Nephrol. 2020;72:279–91.
9. Kairemo KJA. PET/computed tomography for radiation therapy planning of prostate cancer. PET Clin. 2017;12:257–67.
10. Matei DV, Ferro M, Jereczek-Fossa BA, et al. Salvage radical prostatectomy after external beam radiation therapy: a systematic review of current approaches. Urol Int. 2015;94:373–82.
11. Kairemo K, Rasulova N, Kiljunen T, Partanen K, Kangasmäki A, Joensuu T. PET/CT dose planning for volumetric modulated arc radiation therapy (VMAT)- comparison with conventional approach in prostate cancer patients. Curr Radiopharm. 2015;8:2–8.
12. von Eyben FE, Kairemo K, Kiljunen T, Joensuu T. Planning of external beam radiotherapy for prostate cancer guided by PET/CT. Curr Radiopharm. 2015;8:19–31.
13. Mallum A, Mkhize T, Akudugu JM, Ngwa W, Vorster M. The role of positron emission tomography and computed tomographic (PET/CT) imaging for radiation therapy planning: a literature review. Diagnostics (Basel). 2022;13:53.
14. Lapa C, Nestle, Albert NL, et al. The value of PET imaging for radiation therapy. Strahlenther Onkol. 2021;197:1–23.
15. Hofman MS, Lawrentschuk N, Francis RJ, et al. Prostate-specific membrane antigen PET-CT in patients with high-risk prostate cancer before curative-intent surgery or radiotherapy (proPSMA): a prospective, randomised, multicentre study. Lancet. 2020;395:1208–16.
16. Karagiannis V, Wichmann V, Saarinen J, Eigeliene N, Andersen H, Jekunen A. Radiotherapy treatment modification for prostate cancer patients based on PSMA-PET/CT. Radiat Oncol. 2022;17:19.
17. Zelefsky MJ, Lee WR, Zietman A, et al. Evaluation of adherence to quality measures for prostate cancer radiotherapy in the United States: results from the quality research in radiation oncology (QRRO) survey. Pract Radiat Oncol. 2013;3:2–8.

18. Spratt DE, Pei X, Yamada J, et al. Long-term survival and toxicity in patients treated with high-dose intensity modulated radiation therapy for localized prostate cancer. Int J Radiat Oncol Biol Phys. 2013;85:686–92.
19. Wiegel T, Bottke D, Steiner U, et al. Phase III postoperative adjuvant radiotherapy after radical prostatectomy compared with radical prostatectomy alone in pT3 prostate cancer with postoperative undetectable prostate-specific antigen: ARO 96-02/AUO AP 09/95. J Clin Oncol. 2009;27(2):924–30.
20. Abdollah F, Karnes RJ, Suardi N, et al. Predicting survival of patients with node-positive prostate cancer following multimodal treatment. Eur Urol. 2014;65:554–62.
21. Weber DC, Wang H, Cozzi L, et al. RapidArc, intensity modulated photon and proton techniques for recurrent prostate cancer in previously irradiated patients: a treatment planning comparison study. Radiat Oncol. 2009;4:34.
22. Macdougall ND, Dean C, Muirhead R. Stereotactic body radiotherapy in prostate cancer: is rapidarc a better solution than cyberknife? Clin Oncol (R Coll Radiol). 2014;26:4–9.
23. Rong Y, Tang G, Welsh JS, Mohiuddin MM, Paliwal B, Yu CX. Helical tomotherapy versus single-arc intensity modulated arc therapy: a collaborative dosimetric comparison between two institutions. Int J Radiat Oncol Biol Phys. 2011;81:284–96.
24. Ost P, Speleers B, De Meerleer G, et al. Volumetric arc therapy and intensity modulated radiotherapy for primary prostate radiotherapy with simultaneous integrated boost to intraprostatic lesion with 6 and 18 MV: a planning comparison study. Int J Radiat Oncol Biol Phys. 2011;79:920–6.
25. Sathya JR, Davis IR, Julian JA, et al. Randomized trial comparing iridium implant plus external-beam radiation therapy with external-beam radiation therapy alone in node-negative locally advanced cancer of the prostate. J Clin Oncol. 2005;23:1192–9.
26. Spratt DE, Zumsteg ZS, Ghadjar P, et al. Comparison of high-dose (86.4 Gy) IMRT vs combined brachytherapy plus IMRT for intermediate-risk prostate cancer. BJU Int. 2014;114:360–7.
27. Tagliaferri L, Alemanno G, Fionda B, et al. Multiparametric imaging guided HDR interventional radiotherapy (brachytherapy) boost in localized prostate cancer: a multidisciplinary experience. Eur Rev Med Pharmacol Sci. 2023;27(9):4175–84.
28. Michalski J, Gay H, Jackson A, Tucker SL, Deasy JO. Radiation dose–volume effects in radiation-induced rectal injury. Int J Radiat Oncol Biol Phys. 2010;76(Suppl 3):S123–9. https://doi.org/10.1016/j.ijrobp.2009.03.078.
29. Lawton C, Michalski J, El-Naqa I, et al. Radiation oncology specialists reach consensus on pelvic lymph node volumes for high-risk prostate cancer. Int J Radiat Oncol Biol Phys. 2009;74(2):383–7. https://doi.org/10.1016/j.ijrobp.2008.08.003.
30. von Eyben FE, Kairemo K. Meta-analysis of $(^{11})$C-choline and $(^{18})$F-choline PET/CT for management of patients with prostate cancer. Nucl Med Commun. 2014;35:221–30.
31. von Eyben FE, Kairemo K. Acquisition with $(^{11})$C-choline and $(^{18})$F-fluorocholine PET/CT for patients with biochemical recurrence of prostate cancer: a systematic review and meta-analysis. Ann Nucl Med. 2016;30(6):385–92.
32. Eiber M, Maurer T, Souvatzoglou M, et al. Evaluation of hybrid 68Ga-PSMALigand PET/CT in 248 patients with biochemical recurrence after radical prostatectomy. J Nucl Med. 2015;56:668–74.
33. Eissa A, Elsherbiny A, Coelho RF, et al. The role of ^{68}Ga-PSMA PET/CT scan in biochemical recurrence after primary treatment for prostate cancer: a systematic review of the literature. Minerva Urol Nephrol. 2018;70:462–78.
34. Maurer T, Eiber M, Schwaiger M, Gschwend JE. Current use of PSMA-PET in prostate cancer management. Nat Rev Urol. 2016;13:226–35.
35. Leek J, Lench N, Maraj B, et al. Prostate-specific membrane antigen: evidence for the existence of a second related human gene. Br J Cancer. 1995;72:583–8.
36. Afshar-Oromieh A, Malcher A, Eder M, et al. PET imaging with a [68Ga]gallium-labelled PSMA ligand for the diagnosis of prostate cancer: biodistribution in humans and first evaluation of tumour lesions. Eur J Nucl Med Mol Imaging. 2013;40:486–95.

37. Afshar-Oromieh A, Holland-Letz T, Giesel FL, et al. Diagnostic performance of 68Ga-PSMA-11 (HBED-CC) PET/CT in patients with recurrent prostate cancer: evaluation in 1007 patients. Eur J Nucl Med Mol Imaging. 2017;44:1258–68.
38. Raveenthiran S, Yaxley J, Gianduzzo T, et al. The use of 68Ga-PET/CT PSMA to determine patterns of disease for biochemically recurrent prostate cancer following primary radiotherapy. Prostate Cancer Prostatic Dis. 2019;22:385–90.
39. Farolfi A, Gafita A, Calais J, et al. 68Ga-PSMA-11 positron emission tomography detects residual prostate cancer after prostatectomy in a multicenter retrospective study. J Urol. 2019;202:1174–81.
40. Kimura S, Abufaraj M, Janisch F, Iwata T, Parizi MK, Foerster B, et al. Performance of [(^{68})Ga] Ga-PSMA 11 PET for detecting prostate cancer in the lymph nodes before salvage lymph node dissection: a systematic review and meta-analysis. Prostate Cancer Prostatic Dis. 2020;23:1–10.
41. Pyka T, Okamoto S, Dahlbender M, et al. Comparison of bone scintigraphy and ^{68}GaPSMAPET for skeletal staging in prostate cancer. Eur J Nucl Med Mol Imaging. 2016;43:2114–21.
42. Bluemel C, Krebs M, Polat B, et al. ^{68}Ga-PSMA-PET/CT in patients with biochemical prostate cancer recurrence and negative ^{18}F-choline-PET/CT. Clin Nucl Med. 2016;41:515–21.
43. Kranzbühler B, Müller J, Becker AS, et al. Detection rate and localization of prostate cancer recurrence using 68Ga-PSMA-11 PET/MRI in patients with low PSA values ≤ 0.5 ng/mL. J Nucl Med. 2020;61:194–201.
44. Zacho HD, Nielsen JB, Haberkorn U, Stenholt L, Petersen LJ. (^{68})Ga-PSMAPET/CT for the detection of bone metastases in prostate cancer: a systematic review of the published literature. Clin Physiol Funct Imaging. 2017; https://doi.org/10.1111/cpf.12480.
45. Zhao G, Ji B. Head-to-head comparison of (^{68})Ga-PSMA-11 PET/CT and (^{99m})Tc-MDP bone scintigraphy for the detection of bone metastases in patients with prostate cancer: a meta-analysis. AJR Am J Roentgenol. 2022;219:386–95.
46. Corfield J, Perera M, Bolton D, Lawrentschuk N. (^{68})Ga-prostate specific membrane antigen (PSMA) positron emission tomography (PET) for primary staging of high-risk prostate cancer: a systematic review. World J Urol. 2018;36:519–27.
47. Petersen LJ, Zacho HD. PSMA PET for primary lymph node staging of intermediate and high-risk prostate cancer: an expedited systematic review. Cancer Imaging. 2020;20:10.
48. von Eyben FE, Picchio M, von Eyben R, Rhee H, Bauman G. (^{68})Ga-labeled prostate-specific membrane antigen ligand positron emission tomography/computed tomography for prostate cancer: a systematic review and meta-analysis. Eur Urol Focus. 2018;4:686–93.
49. Peng L, Li J, Meng C, et al. Can (^{68})Ga prostate specific membrane antigen positron emission tomography/computerized tomography provide an accurate lymph node staging for patients with medium/high risk prostate cancer? A diagnostic meta-analysis. Radiat Oncol. 2020;15:227.
50. Tu X, Zhang C, Liu Z, et al. The role of (68)Ga-PSMA positron emission tomography/computerized tomography for preoperative lymph node staging in intermediate/high risk patients with prostate cancer: a diagnostic meta-analysis. Front Oncol. 2020;10:1365.
51. Hope TA, Goodman JZ, Allen IE, Calais J, Fendler WP, Carroll PR. Meta analysis of(68) Ga-PSMA-11 PET accuracy for the detection of prostate cancer validated by histopathology. J Nucl Med. 2019;60:786–93.
52. Wu H, Xu T, Wang X, et al. Diagnostic performance of (^{68})gallium labelled prostate-specific membrane antigen positron emission tomography/computed tomography and magnetic resonance imaging for staging the prostate cancer with intermediate or high risk prior to radical prostatectomy: a systematic review and meta-analysis. World J Mens Health. 2020;38:208–19.
53. Wang X, Wen Q, Zhang H, Ji B. Head-to-head comparison of (68)Ga-PSMA-11 PET/CT and multiparametric MRI for pelvic lymph node staging prior to radical prostatectomy in patients with intermediate to high-risk prostate cancer: a meta-analysis. Front Oncol. 2021;11:737989.
54. Lin M, Ta RT, Kairemo K, Le DB, Ravizzini GC. Prostate-specific membrane antigen-targeted radiopharmaceuticals in diagnosis and T nulcerapy of prostate cancer: current status and future perspectives. Cancer Biother Radiopharm. 2021;36:237–51.

55. Kairemo K, Kangasmäki A, Kappadath SC, Joensuu T, Macapinlac HA. A retrospective comparative study of sodium fluoride $Na^{18}F$-PET/CT and ^{68}Ga-PSMA-11 PET/CT in the bone metastases of prostate cancer using a volumetric 3-D radiomic analysis. Life (Basel). 2022;12:1977.
56. Sonni I, Dal Pra A, O'Connell DP, et al. ^{68}Ga-PSMA PET/CT-based atlas for prostate bed recurrence after radical prostatectomy: clinical implications for salvage radiation therapy contouring guidelines. J Nucl Med. 2023;64:902–9.
57. Gaudreault M, Chang D, Hardcastle N, et al. Feasibility of biology-guided radiotherapy using PSMA-PET to boost to dominant intraprostatic tumour. Clin Transl Radiat Oncol. 2022;35:84–9.
58. Petit C, Delouya G, Taussky D, Barkati M, Lambert C, Beauchemin MC, et al. PSMA-PET/CT-guided intensification of radiation therapy for prostate cancer (PSMAgRT): findings of detection rate, effect on cancer management, and early toxicity from a phase 2 randomized controlled trial. Int J Radiat Oncol Biol Phys. 2023;S0360-3016(23):00006–8.
59. Gunnlaugsson A, Johannesson V, Wieslander E, et al. A prospective phase II study of prostate-specific antigen-guided salvage radiotherapy and ^{68}Ga-PSMA-PET for biochemical relapse after radical prostatectomy—the PROPER 1 trial. Clin Transl Radiat Oncol. 2022;36:77–82.
60. Hölscher T, Baumann M, Kotzerke J, et al. Local control after locally ablative, image-guided radiotherapy of oligometastases identified by gallium-68-PSMA-positron emission tomography in castration-sensitive prostate cancer patients (OLI-P). Cancers (Basel). 2022;14:2073.
61. Treglia G, Annunziata S, Pizzuto DA, Giovanella L, Prior JO, Ceriani L. Detection rate of (^{18}) F-labeled PSMA PET/CT in biochemical recurrent prostate cancer: a systematic review and a meta-analysis. Cancers (Basel). 2019;11(5):710.
62. Huang YT, Tseng NC, Chen YK, et al. The detection performance of ^{18}F-prostate-specific membrane antigen-1007 PET/CT in primary prostate cancer: a systemic review and meta-analysis. Clin Nucl Med. 2022;47:755–62.
63. Liu X, Wang Q, Zhang B, Jiang T, Zeng W. Diagnostic accuracy of (^{18})F-PSMA-1007PET/CT for prostate cancer in primary staging and biochemical recurrence with different serum PSA levels: a systematic review and meta-analysis. Hellenic J Nucl Med. 2022;25:88–102.
64. Kawada T, Yanagisawa T, Rajwa P, et al. Diagnostic performance of prostate-specific membrane antigen positron emission tomography-targeted biopsy for detection of clinically significant prostate cancer: a systematic review and meta-analysis. Eur Urol Oncol. 2022;5:390–400.
65. Rowe L, Harmon S, Horn A, et al. Pattern of failure in prostate cancer previously treated with radical prostatectomy and post-operative radiotherapy: a secondary analysis of two prospective studies using novel molecular imaging techniques. Radiat Oncol. 2021;16:32.
66. Floberg JM, Wells SA, Ojala D, et al. Using ^{18}F-DCFPyL prostate-specific membrane antigen-directed positron emission tomography/magnetic resonance imaging to define intraprostatic boosts for prostate stereotactic body radiation therapy. Adv Radiat Oncol. 2023;8(5):101241.
67. Marinescu IM, Spohn SKB, Kiefer S, et al. Intraindividual comparison between [^{18}F] PSMA-1007 PET/CT and multiparametric MRI for radiotherapy planning in primary prostate cancer patients. Front Oncol. 2022;12:880042.
68. Chen L, Liu M, Bao J, Xia Y, Zhang J, Zhang L, et al. The correlation between apparent diffusion coefficient and tumor cellularity in patients: a meta-analysis. PLoS One. 2013;8:e79008.
69. Decazes P, Hinault P, Veresezan O, Thureau S, Gouel P, Vera P. Trimodality PET/CT/MRI and radiotherapy: a mini-review. Front Oncol. 2021;10:614008.
70. Chapman ER, Nicholls L, Suh YE, et al. Interobserver variation in clinical target volume (CTV) delineation for stereotactic radiotherapy to non-spinal bone metastases in prostate cancer: CT, MRI and PET/CT fusion. Radiother Oncol. 2023;180:109461.
71. Chan TH, Haworth A, Wang A, et al. Detecting localised prostate cancer using radiomic features in PSMA PET and multiparametric MRI for biologically targeted radiation therapy. Eur J Nucl Med Mol Imaging Mol Imaging Res. 2023;13(1):34. https://doi.org/10.1186/s13550-023-00984-5. PMID: 37099047

72. Kairemo K, Rasulova N, Partanen K, Joensuu T. Preliminary clinical experience of trans-1-Amino-3-(18)F-fluorocyclobutanecarboxylic acid (anti-(18)F-FACBC) PET/CT imaging in prostate cancer patients. Biomed Res Int. 2014:305182.
73. Suzuki H, Inoue Y, Fujimoto H, , et al. Diagnostic performance and safety of NMK36 (trans-1-amino-3-[^{18}F]fluorocyclobutanecarboxylic acid)-PET/CT in primary prostate cancer: multicenter Phase IIb clinical trial. Jpn J Clin Oncol 2016;46:152–162.
74. Nanni C, Zanoni L, Pultrone C, et al. (^{18})F-FACBC (anti1-amino-3-(^{18})F-fluorocyclobutane-1-carboxylic acid) versus (^{11})C-choline PET/CT in prostate cancer relapse: results of a prospective trial. Eur J Nucl Med Mol Imaging. 2016;43:1601–10.
75. Pernthaler B, Kulnik R, Gstettner C, Salamon S, Aigner RM, Kvaternik H. A prospective head-to-head comparison of ^{18}F-fluciclovine with ^{68}Ga-PSMA-11 in biochemical recurrence of prostate cancer in PET/CT. Clin Nucl Med. 2019;44:e566–73.
76. Calais J, Ceci F, Eiber M, et al. ^{18}F-fluciclovine PET-CT and 68Ga-PSMA-11 PET-CT in patients with early biochemical recurrence after prostatectomy: a prospective, single-centre, single-arm, comparative imaging trial. Lancet Oncol. 2019;20:1286–94.
77. Lawal IO, Jani AB, Adediran OA, et al. Differences in failure-free survival after salvage radiotherapy guided by conventional imaging versus ^{18}F-fluciclovine PET/CT in postprostatectomy patients: a post hoc substratification analysis of the EMPIRE-1 trial. J Nucl Med. 2023;64:586–91.
78. Pinkawa M, Holy R, Piroth MD, et al. Intensity-modulated radiotherapy for prostate cancer implementing molecular imaging with ^{18}F-choline PET-CT to define a simultaneous integrated boost. Strahlenther Onkol. 2010;186:600–6.
79. Picchio M, Berardi G, Fodor A, et al. (^{11})C-choline PET/CT as a guide toradiation treatment planning of lymph-node relapses in prostate cancer patients. Eur J Nucl Med Mol Imaging. 2014;41:1270–9.
80. Rischke HC, Schultze-Seemann W, Wieser G, et al. Adjuvant radiotherapy after salvage lymph node dissection because of nodal relapse of prostate cancer versus salvage lymph node dissection only. Strahlenther Onkol. 2015;191:310–20. https://doi.org/10.1007/s00066-014-0763-5.
81. Kairemo K, Partanen K, Bützow A, Valle T, Ala-Opas M, Joensuu T. Personalized imaging approach in the clinical diagnosis of prostate cancer with suspicion of liver metastases. Medical case reports. iMedJournals. 2015;10:1.
82. Seppälä J, Seppänen M, Arponen E, Lindholm P, Minn H. Carbon-11 acetate PET/CT based dose escalated IMRT in prostate cancer. Radiother Oncol. 2009;93:234–40.
83. Hodolič M, Fettich J, Kairemo K. Hypoxia PET tracers in EBRT dose planning in head and neck cancer. Curr Radiopharm. 2015;8:32–7.
84. Fox JJ, Gavane SC, Blanc-Autran E, et al. Positron emission tomography/computed tomography-based assessments of androgen receptor expression and glycolytic activity as a prognostic biomarker for metastatic castration-resistant prostate cancer. JAMA Oncol. 2018;4:217–24.
85. Kairemo K, Ravizzini GC, Macapinlac HA, Subbiah V. An assessment of early response to targeted therapy via molecular imaging: a pilot study of 3′-deoxy-3′[(18)F]-fluorothymidine positron emission tomography ^{18}F-FLT PET/CT in prostate adenocarcinoma. Diagnostics (Basel). 2017;7:E20.
86. Kairemo K, Kappadath SC, Joensuu T, Macapinlac HA. A retrospective comparative study of sodium fluoride (NaF-18)-PET/CT and fluorocholine (F-18-CH) PET/CT in the evaluation of skeletal metastases in metastatic prostate cancer using a volumetric 3-D radiomics analysis. Diagnostics (Basel). 2020;11:17.
87. Song C, Kim YS, Hong JH, Kim CS, Ahn H. Treatment failure and clinical progression after salvage therapy in men with biochemical recurrence after radical prostatectomy: radiotherapy vs androgen deprivation. BJU Int. 2010;106:188–93.

Brief Overview of Prostate Cancer Treatment Modalities

12

This chapter describes briefly the landscape of prostate cancer (PCa) treatments beyond radionuclide therapies and external beam radiation therapy which have been discussed elsewhere. Figure 12.1 illustrates the development of prostate cancer from local hormone dependent to metastatic castration-resistant disease together with treatment options. The list is by no means complete, because new therapies are developed continuously.

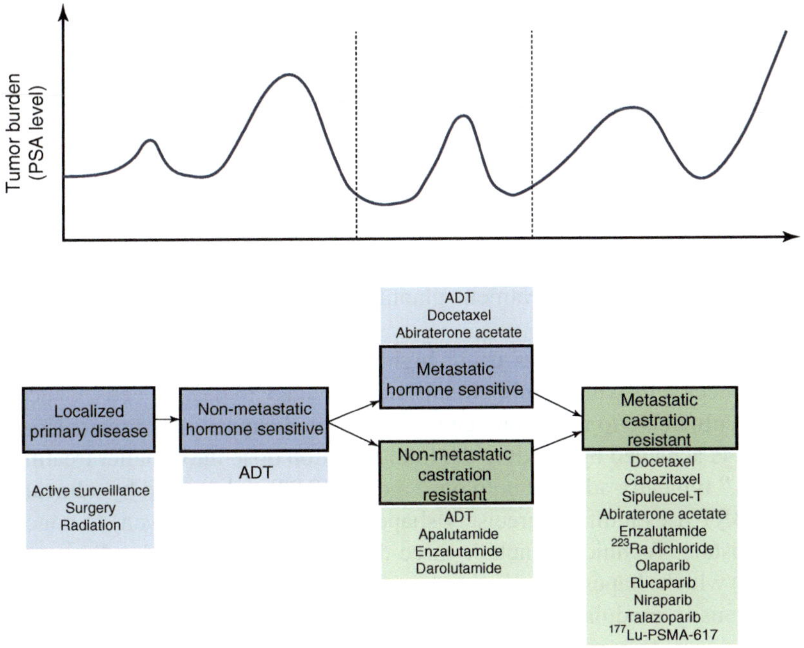

Fig. 12.1 Schematic curve of development (tumor burden/S-PSA) of prostate cancer with presentation of possible treatment options, updated and modified from [1]

K. Kairemo, *Prostate Cancer from a Nuclear Oncology Perspective*,
https://doi.org/10.1007/978-3-031-90337-3_12

Focal Therapies

For the focal therapy, multiple options are available of the localized primary disease—the main options are active surveillance, surgery, and radiation therapy. Patients with localized PCa undergo radical prostatectomy (RP) or external beam radiotherapy (EBRT), brachytherapy, or both or, in selected high-risk patients, RP followed by adjuvant EBRT. Radionuclide methods may play role in the primary staging and planning of the therapy and tentatively in intraoperative guiding of surgery. For PCa patients, initial diagnostics aim to detect the dominant intraprostatic lesion (DIL) while avoiding to detect insignificant intraprostatic lesions. A targeted biopsy is better and safer than a template-based 12-needle biopsy. The PRIMARY study [2] found a combination of PSMA PET and mpMRI (multiparametric magnetic resonance imaging) better detected significant PCa than mpMRI alone. The combination can detect intraprostatic lesions [3]. For most patients, PSA declines after RP to undetectable values, and a quarter of the patients relapse with a rise of PSA (biochemical recurrence or PSA relapse) [3].

In this section, EBRT and brachytherapy are mentioned only briefly, because they have been discussed elsewhere comprehensively, especially in relation to targeted diagnosis using radiopharmaceuticals.

Alternative methods for local therapy, such as high intensity focused ultrasound, cryotherapy, and electroporation, are presented briefly.

EBRT

External beam radiation therapy (EBRT) plays a critical role in managing prostate cancer. PSMA PET, a type of positron-emission tomography (PET) scan, is "almost" recognized as the gold standard for whole-body staging in prostate cancer, surpassing conventional imaging techniques (CT, MRI, bone scan) and older PET tracers in localizing cancer lesions. This precision helps direct radiation therapy, making it a crucial step in modern treatment planning. This has been discussed in Chaps. 10 and 11.

Radiation therapy involves using high-energy X-rays to penetrate tissues and destroy cancer cells while aiming to minimize damage to healthy cells. Cancer cells are more vulnerable to radiation due to their limited capacity for repair. This selective effect is achieved by dividing the total radiation dose into smaller treatments or "fractions," typically administered once a day. EBRT is delivered by a linear accelerator. EBRT uses multiple precisely shaped beams (three to seven) to concentrate on the prostate. Techniques include three-dimensional conformal radiation therapy (3D-CRT) which shapes the radiation beams to conform closely to the prostate's 3D shape; intensity modulated radiation therapy (IMRT) which allows modulation of radiation doses to spare surrounding healthy tissues, increasing cure rates by enabling higher doses on the target area; and volumetric modulated arc therapy (VMAT) which delivers treatment as a single machine rotation, reducing the treatment time to about 1 min.

Brachytherapy involves implanting radioactive pellets (seeds) directly into the prostate. Brachytherapy allows for a high radiation dose in a targeted area but doesn't cover the lymph nodes, which may be necessary for high-risk cancers. It delivers a higher radiation dose to cancer cells, improving the cure rate. Treatment is completed in a single day, significantly reducing patient burden.

Radiation therapy is suitable for prostate cancer at all stages. It is commonly used also for patients with residual cancer after prostatectomy and recurrent cases, except in those with prior high-dose radiation near the prostate or conditions like ulcerative colitis.

PSA levels are regularly monitored posttreatment to check for recurrence: after EBRT, PSA levels typically fall to around 0.5 µg/l within 4 years; brachytherapy patients often reach PSA levels of 0.1 µg/l, with some experiencing a temporary increase 1–3 years posttreatment before stabilizing; a PSA rise above 2 µg/l may indicate cancer recurrence.

High Intensity Focused Ultrasound

High intensity focused ultrasound (HIFU) uses the energy that can be generated by an ultrasound beam to heat tissue, which kills off living cells, including cancers. For PCa, the ultrasound device is similar to that used for a prostate biopsy, but the ultrasound energy is focused to a small spot—a few millimeters. The whole prostate gland will be treated spot by spot, under anesthesia and transrectal ultrasound control over several hours. Two main types of HIFU treatments exist: algorithm-directed HIFU, which relies on preset power and time parameters, and visually directed HIFU, which allows real-time power adjustments based on live tissue feedback, providing potentially more tailored ablation of cancerous tissue [5].

The most detailed reports in the medical-scientific literature currently show that HIFU is not as effective as standard therapies. For men with low-risk prostate cancer, 65% are free of cancer 7 years later, whereas the results with brachytherapy or surgery are around 80–95%. Side effects are about as troublesome as side effects after surgery or radiation therapy. Therefore, HIFU is more often used for salvage therapy, e.g., for biochemical recurrence after high-dose radiation therapies.

Limited evidence from eight observational studies demonstrated that visually directed HIFU for focal treatment of localized prostate cancer was associated with a relatively low risk of complications and acceptable cancer control over medium-term follow-up [5]. This systematic review and meta-analysis aimed to evaluate the outcomes of visually directed HIFU used for the focal treatment of localized prostate cancer. The study specifically analyzed cancer-control efficacy, PSA reduction, biopsy results, salvage treatment requirements, and complication rates associated with this approach. The review followed the PRISMA guidelines and incorporated data from 8 observational studies, involving a total of 1819 patients treated with visually directed focal HIFU [5].

The PSA nadir, a measure of successful treatment, showed an average of 2.2 µg/l (95% CI, 0.9–3.5 µg/l) reached approximately 6 months post-HIFU. Although the reduction in PSA levels varied widely between studies, this nadir indicated effective cancer ablation, comparable with other forms of focal prostate cancer therapy [5]. Rates of clinically significant positive biopsy post-HIFU were observed in 19.8% of patients (95% CI, 12.4–28.3%) [5]. Higher prostate volume was statistically associated with a higher rate of positive biopsy, possibly due to treatment challenges in larger prostates where energy penetration may be inconsistent. 16.2% of patients (95% CI, 9.7–23.8%) required either focal or whole-gland salvage treatment following HIFU. A lower percentage (8.6%) specifically required whole-gland salvage treatment, indicating that the initial HIFU treatment successfully delayed or eliminated the need for more aggressive interventions for many patients [5]. The complication rates for visually directed HIFU were favorable, showing erectile dysfunction in 16.7% of the patients (95% CI, 9.9–24.6%), often decreasing over time for some patients, and urinary complications such as retention (6.2%), infection (3.0%), and incontinence (1.9%) [5].

The real-time power adjustments in visually directed HIFU may help mitigate treatment risks, such as urinary complications and erectile dysfunction. However, the variability in cancer-control outcomes across the studies—attributable to differences in patient demographics, prostate volume, and HIFU protocols—underscores the need for standardized protocols.

Cryotherapy

Cryotherapy uses the opposite approach to that of HIFU—it destroys tissue by freezing it. Cancer cells are particularly susceptible to extremes of temperature, and if the surrounding normal tissues can be protected by being kept warm, then the prostate can be safely treated. The freezing is accomplished by inserting fine tubes into the prostate tissues, which are then frozen using liquid nitrogen; an "ice ball" forms and envelopes the prostate gland. Thawing is then allowed to occur and the freezing is repeated a second time. This can be applied for the whole gland of focally. Most often, this method is used as a salvage treatment for biochemical recurrence [6].

The Cryo On-Line Database (COLD) registry, based on 419 patients, reported biochemical recurrence-free survival (BRFS) rates of 78.3% for patients with PSA < 5 μg/L at 5 years, compared to 52.9% for those with PSA > 5 μg/L [7]. Higher Gleason scores, advanced tumor stages (cT3–4), and PSA values over 10 μg/L were all linked to increased risk of posttreatment recurrence [7].

A study by Spiess et al. [8] reported that whole-gland cryotherapy provided a BRFS rate of 45.5% at 5 years. Key predictors of success included a post-cryoablation PSA nadir of <2.5 μg/L and a pretreatment Gleason score of ≤7. BRFS outcomes are generally lower than whole-gland cryotherapy but vary widely by patient selection. Li et al. [9] observed BRFS rates of 95.3% at 1 year, 72.4% at 3 years, and 46.5% at 5 years in a cohort treated with focal cryotherapy, indicating good medium-term disease control. Another study by Tan et al. [10] noted failure-free survival rates at 100% at 1 year, 80% at 2 years, and 40% at 3 years, suggesting a rapid decline in BRFS over time. In Li et al.'s cohort [9], 28.6% of patients experienced local recurrence posttreatment, highlighting a limitation in focal cryotherapy's ability to fully eradicate cancer when used in a more targeted manner.

Focal cryotherapy has consistently shown lower incontinence rates than whole-gland treatment [6]. For example, Li et al. [9] reported incontinence in only 5.5% of patients over 12 months, while Ismail et al. [11] found a 13% incontinence rate, which was lower than typical whole-gland rates. Erectile dysfunction rates are significantly reduced compared to whole-gland cryotherapy, but still notable. For instance, Ismail et al. reported erectile dysfunction in 86% of patients undergoing focal cryotherapy, while other studies found lower rates, especially when nerve-sparing techniques were used. Li et al. found that 50% of patients retained potency posttreatment [9].

Cryotherapy and HIFU offer similar biochemical control rates, but cryotherapy is generally associated with lower urinary tract complications [6]. However, cryotherapy has higher reported rates of erectile dysfunction.

One potential drawback of HIFU is that if it fails to cure the cancer—it will be impossible to carry out brachytherapy treatment (due to the high risk of incontinence that would result), and surgery may be very challenging or impossible. Focal cryotherapy may benefit patients focused on preserving function, though it may require additional treatments over time. In studies where local cancer-control rate of cryotherapy has been compared with external radiation, cryotherapy had inferior cure rates. Since the results of radiation have substantially improved with modern intensity modulated radiation therapy techniques, which allow higher radiation doses to be given without an increase in side effects, cryotherapy is rarely used. Because diagnostics of PCa is increasing these focal treatments, HIFU and cryotherapy may still have some role in selected patients.

Irreversible Electroporation

Irreversible electroporation (IRE) is a new alternative technology for local treatment of prostate cancer (PCa). It is based on destabilization of the cell membrane, causing the alteration of membrane shape and the formation of nanopores by electric current. The method can precisely target and destroy small prostate tumors that are visible with real-time magnetic resonance imaging (MRI). Generated consecutive electrical pulses between pairs of electrodes which move through tumor cells irreversibly perforate their membranes and eventually lead to cell death while avoiding tissue thermal effect. The excessive permeability of these cells disrupts the osmotic balance, leading to irreversible damage and the process of apoptosis. Because the treatment focuses on just one small area of the prostate rather than the entire organ, the risk of side effects is greatly reduced.

A recent systematic review analyzed 19 studies, with 1452 prostate cancer patients who underwent irreversible electroporation (IRE) treatment. The studies spanned from 2014 to 2023 and primarily focused on low- to intermediate-risk localized prostate cancer, though a few studies included a small percentage of high-risk cases [12]. After IRE treatment, the recurrence rate for clinically significant prostate cancer within the treated area ranged from 0% to 33.3%. For instance, in 4 larger studies with over 100 patients, the rate of in-field clinically significant recurrence was between 1% and 9.9%.

Out-of-field recurrence rates for clinically significant cancer were observed between 0% and 30.8%.

Failure-free survival (FFS) at 3 years was high, ranging from 90% to 96.8%, showing that IRE effectively manages cancer progression in localized cases [12]. A separate study noted FFS rates over 5 years with variations by tumor grade: 95% for Gleason 6 tumors, 85% for Gleason 7 tumors, and 61% for Gleason scores above 7 [13].

Across 12 studies, PSA levels generally decreased significantly within 6–12 months post-IRE, indicating a reduction in cancer activity. Urinary function outcomes were favorable, with a high pad-free rate posttreatment (96.7–100% across studies). Erectile function varied, with some patients experiencing declines, especially noted at 6 months, though some studies reported a gradual recovery over time. Common mild to moderate complications included urinary tract infections and hematuria. Severe complications were rare, with most studies reporting a 0.9–8.5% rate for grade 3 complications, which is notably lower than traditional therapies [12].

IRE for localized prostate cancer shows promising control over cancer progression with minimal adverse effects on urinary and erectile functions, suggesting it as a viable alternative for low- to intermediate-risk patients. However, the recurrences outside the treatment field and the moderate need for re-treatment (8–36.6%) highlight that further refinement in technique and patient selection may be beneficial [12].

IRE for prostate cancer is feasible with minimal functional impact on urinary and sexual function. The high rate of recurrence underscores IRE's limitations as a standalone curative approach; thus, it should not be viewed as equivalent to radical treatments. IRE might benefit patients seeking to delay aggressive treatment without significant added morbidity but must include rigorous follow-up, including early biopsies [14].

Systemic Therapies

Hormone Therapy

Hormonic treatments are discussed here very briefly. Hormone treatment is used for nonmetastatic and metastatic hormone sensitive prostate cancer (PCa) as shown in Fig. 12.1. In the literature, terms androgen deprivation therapy (ADT) or even total androgen blockade (TAB) have been used. Hormone receptor imaging is discussed in Chap. 7.

Testosterone, the primary male hormone, is a significant driver of prostate cancer-cell growth. Cancer cells in the prostate rely on testosterone, produced mainly in the testicles, to survive and multiply. Reducing testosterone, either through surgical removal of the testicles (orchiectomy) or through pharmaceutical means, can suppress cancer progression in up to 95% of cases, making it a standard approach for advanced prostate cancer treatment.

The different types of hormone therapy are listed briefly here:

Surgical hormone therapy (orchiectomy): Orchiectomy involves removing both testicles to permanently lower testosterone. This straightforward surgery requires minimal recovery and is generally well tolerated. Side effects are limited but may include scrotal swelling or minor infection at the incision. Scarring and some shrinkage of the scrotum post-surgery are common.

Drug-based hormone therapies are listed in the following:

Antiandrogens: Antiandrogens block testosterone from binding to prostate cells. Nonsteroidal options (e.g., flutamide, bicalutamide, nilutamide, darolutamide) are commonly used because they don't reduce blood testosterone levels, thus preserving some aspects of sexual function. Nonsteroidal antiandrogens may cause breast enlargement, gastrointestinal issues, and, in rare cases, liver toxicity. Steroidal options are less common due to adverse effects.

LHRH agonists: Drugs like leuprolide, goserelin, and buserelin halt testosterone production by acting on the body's hormone-regulating pathways. LHRH agonists temporarily surge testosterone at treatment initiation, potentially worsening symptoms temporarily; thus, they are often paired with antiandrogens initially. These drugs may cause common menopause-like symptoms including hot flashes and fatigue.

LHRH antagonists: LHRH antagonists, such as degarelix, prevent testosterone production without the initial surge, making them a safer option for some patients. Because these drugs are administered as injections, they may cause mild injection site reactions, including redness and swelling.

Estrogen: While effective, oral estrogen is rarely used due to severe side effects, such as blood clots and cardiovascular complications. Transdermal estrogen patches are under study to offer a safer alternative by potentially lowering side effects like blood clots.

Hormone therapy slows but rarely cures prostate cancer. Some cancer cells adapt to grow without testosterone or produce it locally, leading to castration-resistant prostate cancer. Intermittent therapy, which cycles on and off hormone suppression, can help manage quality of life and maintain therapeutic responsiveness.

Combining hormone therapy with radiation improves treatment outcomes, particularly in high-risk patients, by sensitizing cancer cells to radiation. Hormone therapy, external beam radiation therapy (EBRT), and brachytherapy together show promise for high-risk cases.

Side effects of hormonal treatments are multiple, not discussed in detail here, but they include hot flashes, loss of libido, impotence, fatigue, weight gain, muscle loss, and osteoporosis. Emotional and cognitive changes may occur: Patients also may experience mood swings, anxiety, or cognitive impairment. Due to changes in metabolism, weight gain, higher triglycerides in the blood, and risk of diabetes and heart issues can occur.

Intermittent therapy offers periods of relief from side effects, potentially enhancing quality of life without compromising survival. Weighing of the benefits of hormone therapy against side effects is relevant, especially if prostate cancer progression is slow.

Combining hormone therapy with radiation improves treatment outcomes, particularly in high-risk patients, by sensitizing cancer cells to radiation. Triple therapy includes hormone therapy, external beam radiation therapy (EBRT), and brachytherapy, showing promise for high-risk cases. This triple therapy form is presented in my own history.

Immunotherapy

I have been involved with the article "Immune Checkpoints, Inhibitors, and Radionuclides in Prostate Cancer: Promising Combinatorial Therapy Approach" by Kgatle et al. [15]. We reviewed the current treatment landscape of prostate cancer (PCa), specifically exploring immune checkpoint inhibitors (ICIs) and their potential synergy with radionuclide therapy. Prostate cancer is a highly heterogeneous and often aggressive cancer, especially in advanced stages. Standard treatments like androgen deprivation therapy (ADT), radiation, and chemotherapy offer limited long-term benefits as resistance frequently develops, especially in metastatic castration-resistant prostate cancer (mCRPC). Given this challenge, we suggest that integrating ICIs with other therapies, particularly radionuclides, could provide a new, effective approach.

Unlike other cancers, PCa's immune environment is often "cold," meaning it has a low level of immune cell infiltration, making it less responsive to immunotherapies such as ICIs. Despite their success in cancers like melanoma, ICIs alone have shown limited success in PCa due to its unique immune profile.

The article highlights several immune checkpoints that tumors exploit to evade the immune system, each of which may be targeted in novel treatments [15]:

1. CTLA-4 (Cytotoxic T-Lymphocyte-Associated Protein 4): CTLA-4 inhibits T-cell activation, weakening immune responses. Blocking CTLA-4 can enhance T-cell activity against cancer, although it shows limited benefit alone in PCa. Combining CTLA-4 inhibitors (such as ipilimumab) with other treatments has shown some promise but often results in significant side effects.
2. PD-1/PD-L1 (Programmed Death-1/Programmed Death Ligand-1): PD-1 on immune cells binds with PD-L1 on tumor cells, suppressing T-cell activity and allowing tumors to evade immune detection. PD-1/PD-L1 inhibitors, such as pembrolizumab and nivolumab, have achieved limited success in PCa. However,

some patients with specific genetic mutations (like DNA mismatch repair deficiencies) respond better to these inhibitors.

3. Emerging Checkpoints.

   VISTA (V-domain immunoglobulin suppressor of T-cell activation): Primarily expressed on tumor-infiltrating lymphocytes, VISTA suppresses immune responses, often compensating when other checkpoints are blocked.

   TIM-3 (T-cell Immunoglobulin Domain and Mucin Domain 3) and *LAG-3* (lymphocyte-activation gene 3): These checkpoints regulate immune responses and, when overexpressed in PCa, correlate with aggressive cancer characteristics. Blocking TIM-3 and LAG-3 has shown promise in preclinical models.

   B7-H3 (B7 homolog 3) and *TIGIT* (T-cell immunoreceptor with Ig and ITIM domains): These have roles in immune suppression and are upregulated in PCa. They are currently being explored as novel targets for immunotherapy.

Combination of ICIs with Radionuclide Therapy

We propose a strategy of combining ICIs with radionuclide therapy (alpha-emitters ^{225}Ac and ^{223}Ra, beta-emitter ^{177}Lu), which delivers targeted radiation to tumor cells and can alter the immune environment, potentially making it more responsive to ICIs. This combination approach aims to enhance immune cell infiltration into the tumor; increase antigen release from dying cancer cells, making them more recognizable to the immune system; and potentially improve overall survival and progression-free survival by simultaneously targeting multiple pathways.

Figure 12.2 illustrates schematically the landscape of prostate cancer treatments and how immune checkpoints that can potentially be targeted for therapy and how immunotherapy and chemotherapy, radiotherapy, surgery, and ADT can be combined [15]. We also summarize recent and ongoing clinical trials assessing combination therapies in PCa, especially those integrating ICIs with ADT, chemotherapy, or radionuclides [15]. The CheckMate 650 trial combines nivolumab and ipilimumab in mCRPC patients. Although this combination showed some antitumor activity, it led to significant side effects, indicating a need for careful management of dosage and treatment duration [16].

Enzalutamide (an androgen receptor inhibitor) combined with pembrolizumab showed enhanced responses in patients previously treated with ADT. This dual therapy has resulted in increased T-cell activity in the tumor microenvironment and reduced PSA levels in some patients [17]. Preliminary evidence suggests that bipolar androgen therapy, when combined with anti-PD-1 therapy, could sensitize PCa cells to immune attacks, particularly in genetically distinct patient subgroups [18].

Emerging research demonstrates that co-inhibitory immune checkpoints (ICs) remain the most promising immunotherapy targets in various malignancies [15]. Nonetheless, ICIs have offered insignificant clinical benefits in the treatment of advanced prostate cancer (PCa) especially when they are used as monotherapies.

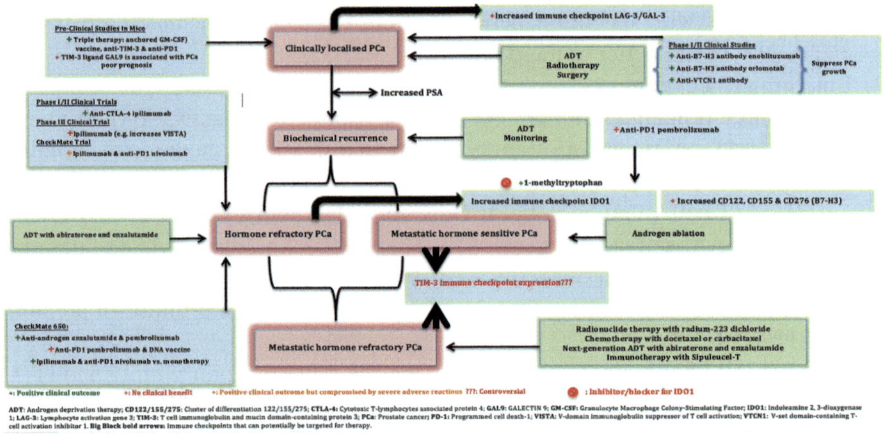

Fig. 12.2 Clinical disease progression, pathophysiology, and current therapeutic interventions of prostate cancer. Most PCa patients usually progress slowly to mCRPC or mHSPC. PCa treatment varies according to stages and pathophysiology of the disease, and these currently include chemotherapy, radiotherapy, surgery, and ADT. Various preclinical and clinical trials have been tested for immunotherapy approaches targeting various immune checkpoints although these have demonstrated minimal clinical benefit in PCa especially when used as monotherapies. **Bold arrows** represent immune checkpoints that can potentially be targeted for therapy. Color codes: pink boxes, clinical disease progression; green boxes, established therapy strategies; blue boxes, novel therapy option. (Presented in [15])

Current existing PCa treatment initially offers an improved clinical outcome and overall survival (OS); however, after a while, the treatment becomes resistant leading to aggressive and uncontrolled disease associated with increased mortality and morbidity.

When the diverse genetic and immunologic profiles of PCa patients have been recognized, more personalized approaches can be recommended, including genetic testing, to identify patients who would benefit most from specific combination therapies. Concurrent combination of the ICIs with radionuclide therapy that has rapidly emerged as safe and effective targeted approach for treating PCa patients may shift the paradigm of PCa treatment. Extensive clinical research is needed to optimize dosing strategies, reduce adverse effects, and validate the efficacy of combination therapies involving ICIs and radionuclides. Ensuring that these new therapies not only extend survival but also improve quality of life will be essential in evaluating their success.

About Combinatory and Personalized Treatment Strategies

The more complex the PCa disease is, the more personalized treatments we need. The operational framework would aim to improve survival rates among patients in different disease stages and comprises multidisciplinary approach, e.g., with the geneticist, urologist (surgeon), nuclear medicine physician, endocrinologist, tumor biologist, pathologist, radiologist, oncologist, and palliative care specialists. Radionuclide therapy is currently a revolutionary theranostics approach for advanced PCa, which is usually difficult to treat. We have earlier shown that immune checkpoint inhibition and targeted radionuclide therapy stand at the forefront of this evolving therapeutic landscape [15].

I personally learned the power of an aggressive combinatory treatment already more than 10 years ago. We combined antiandrogen therapy with radiotherapy in a first-line setting for metastatic prostate cancer aiming to cause maximal cancer-cell death to delay the emergence of castration-resistant disease. We combined antiandrogen therapy with radiotherapy in a first-line setting for metastatic prostate cancer aiming to cause maximal cancer-cell death to delay the emergence of castration-resistant disease [19]. In this nonrandomized retrospective series of 46 patients, the initial median S-PSA was 98.5 μg/l (range: 6.7–15,500 μg/l), with median GS 9, and most men had at least T3N1M1 disease. At PSA nadir, all patients received VMAT radiotherapy of the prostate. Overall survival (OS) at 5 years was 81.3%. The feasibility and safety of aggressive multimodality treatment were good resulting in an excellent median OS of 8.35 years. In conclusion, multimodal primary treatment of metastatic prostate cancer with both androgen deprivation and radiation is demonstrated to be potentially feasible in the patient series reported here. Impressive overall survival data encouraged us to extend this approach into clinical trials.

However, the situation changed in the 2010s, because six new drugs have been found to increase overall survival for patients with metastatic castration-resistant prostate cancer (mCRPC) [20–25]. Patients with symptomatic mCRPC had initially been treated with docetaxel [20]. Cabazitaxel, sipuleucel-T, abiraterone acetate, enzalutamide, and ^{223}radium increase overall survival for patients who had failed treatment with docetaxel [21–25]. The approved treatments both by FDA and EMA have been listed in Table 12.1. There are also the new drugs approved in the 2020s, e.g., olaparib [26] and ^{177}lutetium-PSMA-617 (vipivotide tetraxetan) [27].

However, there were no randomized trials which would have evaluated the drugs for patients with failure in response to second-line treatment following recurrence after docetaxel. Therefore, we conducted a systematic review discussed in Chap. 16. We compared sixteen studies including 1338 patients receiving third-line treatment (cabazitaxel, abiraterone acetate, enzalutamide) with twelve studies including 669 patients treated with ^{177}Lu-PSMA-radioligand therapy (RLT). Overall, 44% of the patients responded (decline of PSA of ≥50%) following treatment with ^{177}Lu-PSMA RLT, whereas 22% of the patients had a best decline of PSA of ≥50% following third-line treatment [28]. We had reliable results before the actual registration trial of ^{177}Lu-PSMA [27]. Meta-analyses and systematic reviews are helpful, if the indications and patient populations are comparable. The overall survivals in the table cannot directly be compared, because the patient populations are not uniform—both inclusion and exclusion criteria in the randomized trials differ even though the disease is similar.

Table 12.1 Approved treatments for metastatic castration-resistant prostate cancer (mCRPC)

Approved by FDA/EMA	Mechanism of action	Patient population	Control group	Benefit in OS (months) [ref]
Docetaxel 2004/2007	Microtubule inhibitor	mCRPC	Mitoxantrone	19.2 vs. 16.3 [20]
Cabazitaxel 2010/2011	Microtubule inhibitor	mCRPC post taxanes	Mitoxantrone	15.1 vs. 12.7 [21]
Sipuleucel-T 2010/2013	Autologous immunotherapy	mCRPC, no or minimal symptoms	Placebo	25.8 vs. 21.7 [22]
Abiraterone acetate 2011/2011	Androgen inhibitor	mCRPC post taxanes	Prednisone	15.8 vs. 11.2 [23]
Enzalutamide 2012/2013	AR inhibitor	mCRPC post taxanes	Placebo	18.4 vs. 13.6 [24]
^{223}Ra-dichloride 2013/2013	Bone targeted alpha therapy	mCRPC with bone mets	Placebo	14.9 vs. 11.3 [25]
Olaparib 2020/2022	PARP inhibitor	mCRPC post enzalutamide or abiratone	Enzalutamide or abiraterone	17.3 vs. 14.0 [26]
^{177}Lu-PSMA-617 2022/2022	Radioligand therapy, PSMA inhibitor	mCRPC post taxanes and ADT	Best supportive care	15.3 vs. 11.3 [27]

Abbreviations: AR androgen receptor, *ADT* androgen deprivation therapy, *EMA* European Medicines Agency, *FDA* Food and Drug Administration, *mCRPC* metastatic castration-resistant prostate cancer, *OS* overall survival, *PARP* poly-ADP-ribose polymerase, *PSMA* prostate specific membrane antigen

The great challenge is to identify the best individual combinations in high-risk cancers. Before they can end up with official treatment recommendations, the right dosing order and the right drug combinations need to be studied by randomization. Anyway, we have already learned that never is too late. But on the one hand, we know that not all patients will respond.

References

1. Abou D, Benabdallah N, Jiang W, et al. Prostate cancer theranostics—an overview. Front Oncol. 2020;10:884.
2. Emmett L, Buteau J, Papa N, et al. The additive diagnostic value of prostate-specific membrane antigen positron emission tomography computed tomography to multiparametric magnetic resonance imaging triage in the diagnosis of prostate cancer (PRIMARY): a prospective multicentre study. Eur Urol. 2021;80:682–9.
3. Prive BM, Israel B, Schilham MGM, et al. Evaluating F-18-PSMA-1007-PET in primary prostate cancer and comparing it to multi-parametric MRI and histopathology. Prostate Cancer Prostatic Dis. 2021;24:423–30.
4. von Eyben FE, Kairemo K, Kapp DS. Prostate-specific antigen as an ultrasensitive biomarker for patients with early recurrent prostate cancer: how low shall we go? A systematic review. Biomedicine. 2024;12:822.

5. Peretsman SJ, Emberton M, Fleshner N, Shoji S, Bahler CD, Miller LE. High-intensity focused ultrasound with visually directed power adjustment for focal treatment of localized prostate cancer: systematic review and meta-analysis. World J Urol. 2024;42:175.
6. Pio F, Murdock A, Fuller RE, Whalen MJ. The role of whole-gland and focal cryotherapy in recurrent prostate cancer. Cancers (Basel). 2024;16:3225.
7. Campbell SP, Deivasigamani S, Arcot R, et al. Salvage cryoablation for recurrent prostate cancer following primary external beam radiotherapy or primary cryotherapy: a propensity score matched analysis of mid-term oncologic and functional outcomes. Clin Genitourin Cancer. 2023;21:555–62.
8. Spiess PE, Levy DA, Pisters LL, Mouraviev V, Jones JS. Outcomes of salvage prostate cryotherapy stratified by pre-treatment PSA: update from the COLD registry. World J Urol. 2013;31:1321–5.
9. Tan WP, Kotamarti S, Ayala A, et al. Oncological and functional outcomes for men undergoing salvage whole-gland cryoablation for radiation-resistant prostate cancer. Eur Urol Oncol. 2023;6:289–94.
10. Li YH, Elshafei A, Agarwal G, Ruckle H, Powsang J, Jones JS. Salvage focal prostate cryoablation for locally recurrent prostate cancer after radiotherapy: initial results from the cryo on-line data registry. Prostate. 2015;75:1–7.
11. Ismail M, Ahmed S, Kastner C, Davies J. Salvage cryotherapy for recurrent prostate cancer after radiation failure: a prospective case series of the first 100 patients. BJU Int. 2007;100:760–4.
12. Zhang K, Teoh J, Zhu G, Ng CF, Suberville M, Laguna P, de la Rosette J. Irreversible electroporation for the focal treatment of prostate cancer: a systematic review. World J Mens Health. 2024; https://doi.org/10.5534/wjmh.240012. Epub ahead of print. PMID: 39028129
13. Guenther E, Klein N, Zapf S, et al. Prostate cancer treatment with irreversible electroporation (IRE): safety, efficacy and clinical experience in 471 treatments. PLoS One. 2019;14:e0215093.
14. Popeneciu IV, Mohr MN, Strauß A, Leitsmann C, Trojan L, Reichert M. Personalized treatment strategy in "low-risk prostate cancer active surveillance candidates" using irreversible electroporation: prospective evaluation of feasibility, morbidity, functional and oncological outcomes. World J Mens Health. 2024;42:821–9.
15. Kgatle MM, Boshomane TMG, Lawal IO, et al. Immune checkpoints, inhibitors and radionuclides in prostate cancer: promising combinatorial therapy approach. Int J Mol Sci. 2021;22:4109.
16. Sharma P, Pachynski RK, Narayan V, et al. Nivolumab plus ipilimumab for metastatic castration-resistant prostate cancer: preliminary analysis of patients in the CheckMate 650 trial. Cancer Cell. 2020;38:489–499.e3.
17. Graff JN, Beer TM, Alumkal JJ, et al. A phase II single-arm study of pembrolizumab with enzalutamide in men with metastatic castration-resistant prostate cancer progressing on enzalutamide alone. J Immunother Cancer. 2020;8:e000642.
18. Markowski MC, Shenderov E, Eisenberger MA, et al. Extreme responses to immune checkpoint blockade following bipolar androgen therapy and enzalutamide in patients with metastatic castration resistant prostate cancer. Prostate. 2020;80:407–11.
19. Joensuu T, Joensuu G, Kairemo K, et al. Multimodal primary treatment of metastatic prostate cancer with androgen deprivation and radiation. Anticancer Res. 2016;36:6439–47.
20. Tannock IF, de Wit R, Berry WR, et al. Docetaxel plus prednisone or mitoxantrone plus prednisone for advanced prostate cancer. N Engl J Med. 2004;351:1502–12.
21. Kantoff PW, Higano CS, Shore ND, et al. Sipuleucel-T immunotherapy for castration-resistant prostate cancer. N Engl J Med. 2010;363:411–22.
22. de Bono JS, Oudard S, Ozguroglu M, et al. Prednisone plus cabazitaxel or mitoxantrone for metastatic castration-resistant prostate cancer progressing after docetaxel treatment: a randomised open-label trial. Lancet. 2010;376:1147–54.
23. de Bono JS, Logothetis CJ, Molina A, et al. Abiraterone and increased survival in metastatic prostate cancer. N Engl J Med. 2011;364:1995–2005.
24. Scher HI, Fizazi K, Saad F, et al. Increased survival with enzalutamide in prostate cancer after chemotherapy. N Engl J Med. 2012;367:1187–97.

25. Parker C, Nilsson S, Heinrich D, et al. Alpha emitter radium-223 and survival in metastatic prostate cancer. N Engl J Med. 2013;369:213–23.
26. Hussain M, Mateo J, Fizazi K, et al. Survival with Olaparib in metastatic castration-resistant prostate cancer. N Engl J Med. 2020;383:2345–57.
27. Sartor O, de Bono J, Chi KN, et al. Lutetium-177-PSMA-617 for metastatic castration-resistant prostate cancer. N Engl J Med. 2021;385:1091–103.
28. von Eyben FE, Roviello G, Kiljunen T, et al. Third-line treatment and ^{177}Lu-PSMA radioligand therapy of metastatic castration-resistant prostate cancer: a systematic review. Eur J Nucl Med Mol Imaging. 2018;45:496–508.

Part III

Targeted Therapy (Radionuclides)

Radium-223 Dichloride (Ra-223) for the Treatment of Metastatic Castration-Resistant Prostate Cancer

13

Radium-223 is a targeted alpha-emitting radiopharmaceutical approved for mCRPC with symptomatic bone metastases. It selectively binds to areas of increased bone turnover in metastases, delivering highly localized radiation that causes double-stranded DNA breaks in cancer cells, sparing surrounding healthy tissue. It was particularly effective for bone metastases, which are common in mCRPC patients, affecting around 90% of cases. In the ALSYMPCA clinical trial [1], radium-223 was shown to prolong overall survival (14.9 months vs. 11.3 months with placebo), delay skeletal-related events (SREs), and improve the quality of life in patients. In this registration trial, it was found out that Ra-223 significantly delayed the time to the first symptomatic skeletal-related event (SRE) (15.6 months vs. 9.8 months with placebo), reducing the risk of complications such as pathological fractures and spinal cord compression [1].

The study also found that Ra-223 delays increased in prostate-specific antigen (PSA) and alkaline phosphatase (ALP) levels, the latter being a key biomarker for bone activity and metastatic progression. Radium-223 dichloride (Xofigo®) was the alpha-emitting radiopharmaceutical to get marketing authorization in 2013. This chapter reviews the use of radium-223 in treating metastatic castration-resistant prostate cancer (mCRPC) and provides guidance on optimizing clinical practices.

Clinical Practice

My own first contact with Ra-223 was in the early 2000s in Uppsala University Hospital in Sweden. Actually, I invited Roy Larsen (one of the Ra-223 patent holders) from Oslo to give the presentation "Treatment of Skeletal Metastases with Alpha-Emitters" at the Inauguration Symposium of the new Nuclear Medicine Clinic in March 2002. Later I learned this was the very first lecture about this topic in the world.

Ra-223 was approved for mCRPC patients with symptomatic bone metastases but no visceral metastases in 2013. It is often used in patients either before or after

K. Kairemo, *Prostate Cancer from a Nuclear Oncology Perspective*,
https://doi.org/10.1007/978-3-031-90337-3_13

chemotherapy and can be combined with other treatments like abiraterone and enzalutamide. The recommendation in the European consensus was to start Ra-223 in patients with early symptoms to maximize the likelihood of completing the full treatment course, i.e., six cycles, thus improving clinical outcomes [2].

Treatment requires collaboration between nuclear medicine specialists, oncologists, urologists, and other healthcare professionals to ensure proper patient selection, treatment administration, and follow-up care [2]. This is because the use of alpha-emitters in the clinic was a new concept. Additionally, monitoring during treatment included regular blood counts to check for bone marrow suppression [2].

Radium-223 has a favorable safety profile, with fewer adverse events than placebo. The most common side effects include mild bone pain, nausea, diarrhea, and mild hematologic effects like thrombocytopenia (6% of patients) [1, 2]. Long-term follow-up data have shown no significant increase in the risk of serious conditions like acute myelogenous leukemia or primary bone cancers, suggesting the long-term safety of Ra-223 [2]. One of the significant advantages of Ra-223 compared to traditional radiopharmaceuticals and chemotherapy agents like docetaxel is its low rate of myelosuppression. Myelosuppression is a reduction in bone marrow activity, leading to lower levels of red and white blood cells and platelets. This condition can lead to anemia, infections, and bleeding [2]. The ALSYMPCA trial showed low incidences of severe hematologic toxicities: Grade 3/4 thrombocytopenia (low platelet count) occurred in only 6% of patients treated with Ra-223, compared to 2% in the placebo group; Grade 3/4 neutropenia (low neutrophil count) was seen in just 3% of Ra-223 patients, compared to 1% of those on placebo [1].

Common gastrointestinal side effects include nausea (36%), diarrhea (25%), and vomiting (18%). These side effects were mostly mild and manageable in clinical practice. Diarrhea and nausea are thought to arise from the systemic distribution of radium-223, with small amounts being excreted through the intestines [1].

Bone pain was the most frequent non-hematologic adverse event, occurring in 50% of Ra-223 patients. However, this was actually less common than in the placebo group (62%), suggesting that Ra-223 can have a pain-relieving effect in many patients, which aligns with its role in targeting bone metastases [2].

The overall discontinuation rate due to adverse events was relatively low, with 16% of patients stopping treatment due to side effects, compared to 21% in the placebo group [1]. The tolerability of Ra-223 makes it particularly well-suited for patients who are frail or have limited bone marrow reserve, often allowing them to complete the full six-cycle course. Ra-223's alpha radiation has a very short range (less than 100 micrometers), limiting exposure to surrounding healthy tissues [2]. This makes it safer for patients and their caregivers in terms of radiation exposure.

Patients are instructed to follow basic hygiene practices, such as avoiding direct contact with bodily fluids for a week posttreatment to minimize exposure risks. There is no need for prolonged isolation, and restrictions on contact with family members, including children, are minimal [2].

Selecting the right patients for Ra-223 treatment is essential to maximize benefits and minimize risks. Because Ra-223 was approved for use in mCRPC patients with symptomatic bone metastases and no known visceral metastases, the main criteria and considerations for patient selection are as follows [2]:

1. Bone metastases detectable by imaging: Ra-223 candidates must have at least two bone metastases, which are typically confirmed via imaging modalities like a ^{99m}Tc-phosphonate bone scan or an ^{18}F-NaF PET/CT scan.
2. Adequate bone marrow function: Since Ra-223 can affect the bone marrow, patients must have adequate baseline bone marrow function, measured by hemoglobin levels >100 g/l; absolute neutrophil count (ANC) $\geq 1.5 \times 10^9$/l; and platelet count $\geq 100 \times 10^9$/l.

Unsuitable candidates are patients with visceral metastases, e.g., patients with metastases to organs like the liver, lungs, or brain should be excluded. Similarly, patients with an active intestinal disease are not suitable: patients with conditions such as Crohn's disease or ulcerative colitis are excluded due to the risk of exacerbation from radiation, as Ra-223 is partially excreted through the intestines. Patients with an expected survival of less than 3 months are generally not considered, as they may not have enough time to benefit from the treatment [2].

Biomarkers for Ra-223 Treatment

Alkaline Phosphatase (ALP) A reduction in ALP is commonly observed and is indicative of a positive response to Ra-223 treatment [3, 4]. While this decrease correlates with treatment success, the role of ALP as a definitive marker is described later.

Prostate-Specific Antigen (PSA) PSA is not a reliable marker for response to Ra-223, as bone-targeting therapies may not always lead to a reduction in PSA levels, unlike other treatments (e.g., chemotherapy). PSA is a protein produced by both normal and malignant prostate cells. It is widely used as a biomarker in prostate cancer to monitor disease progression and response to treatment. However, PSA responses are not reliable in patients treated with Ra-223 [3, 4]. Unlike other therapies (e.g., chemotherapy or androgen receptor-targeted agents), where a PSA decline is indicative of treatment efficacy, Ra-223's primary action is on bone metastases, not directly on prostate cancer cells. Thus, PSA levels often do not decrease during Ra-223 treatment. In some studies, PSA responses (defined as a decline of 30% or more) were observed in only a small subset of Ra-223-treated patients (6.3%), suggesting that PSA is not a suitable predictive biomarker for Ra-223 therapy [5]. PSA remains an important marker for other treatments but should not be relied upon for assessing Ra-223 efficacy. However, rising PSA during Ra-223 treatment might indicate the development of soft-tissue metastases not targeted by Ra-223.

Many patients experience significant pain relief during treatment, although it is not a universal indicator of response.

Because PSA are not predictive of response to Ra-223, there is a need for new biomarkers. Some of these are reviewed briefly here, such as markers of bone metabolism, circulating tumor DNA (ctDNA), and imaging techniques, to predict patient response and stratify treatment. Two patient examples are shown, where there is a PSA response (Fig. 13.1) and no PSA response (Fig. 13.2) related to Ra-223 treatment [6]. The response is better seen with ALP (as indicated with AFOS in Figs. 13.1 and 13.2).

Bone-Specific Alkaline Phosphatase (b-ALP) Bone-specific alkaline phosphatase (b-ALP) and collagen degradation products (e.g., CTx, NTx) are highlighted as promising biomarkers that might correlate with treatment outcomes, although more research is needed [7, 8]. b-ALP is an enzyme produced by osteoblasts, the bone-forming cells. It is a marker of bone formation and is often elevated in patients with bone metastases due to the increased osteoblastic activity induced by prostate cancer cells. In mCRPC, bone metastases are predominantly osteoblastic, leading to the overproduction of bone matrix. b-ALP reflects this abnormal bone turnover and is considered a key biomarker for bone metastasis activity. Elevated baseline levels of

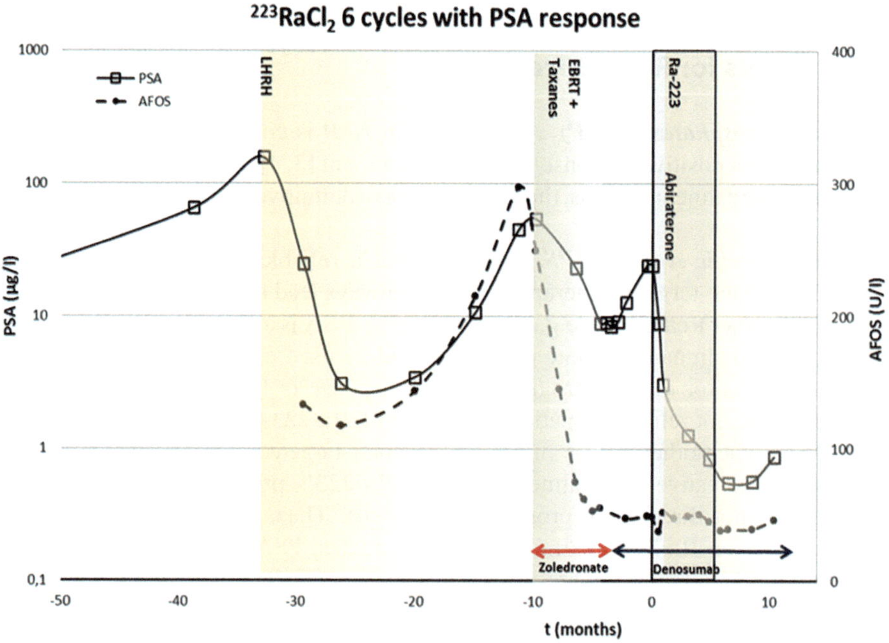

Fig. 13.1 The timing of various treatments of 64-year-old male with prostate cancer (Gleason score 8 (4 + 4)) and $^{223}RaCl_2$ therapeutic dosing schedule. S-PSA and S-AFOS concentrations are presented as well. This patient demonstrated a S-PSA response due to $^{223}RaCl_2$ treatment. (From Kairemo et al. [6])

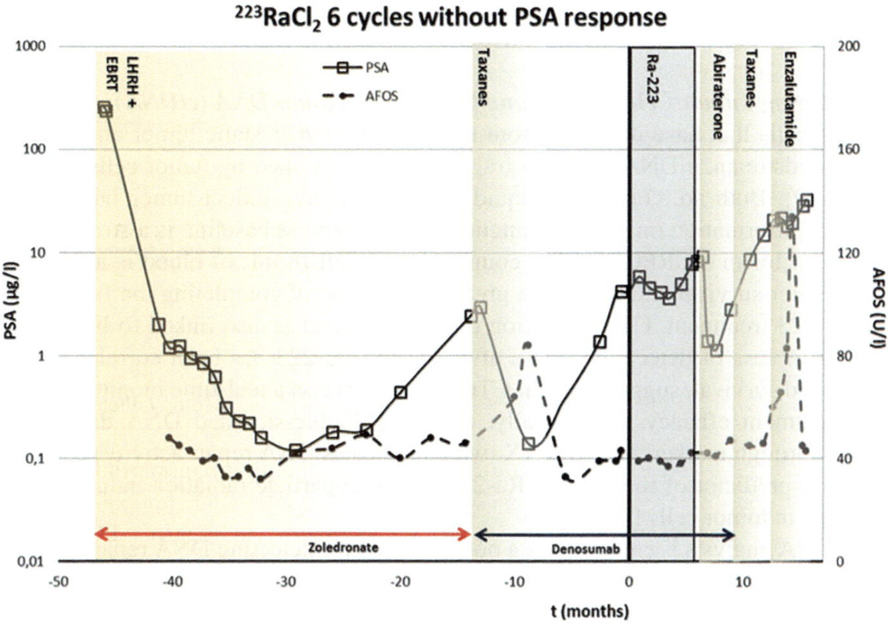

Fig. 13.2 The timing of various treatments of 61-year-old male with prostate cancer (Gleason score 7 (4 + 3)) and $^{223}RaCl_2$ therapeutic dosing schedule. S-PSA and S-AFOS concentrations are presented as well. This patient demonstrated only a change in S-PSA velocity due to $^{223}RaCl_2$ treatment. (From Kairemo et al. 2015 [6])

b-ALP are associated with a higher tumor burden and increased bone turnover, which correlates with shorter overall survival (OS). A decrease in b-ALP during Ra-223 therapy suggests a positive response to treatment.

Bone Metabolism Markers (CTx, NTx, P1NP) These markers are by-products of bone collagen turnover. C-telopeptide (CTx) and N-telopeptide (NTx) are released during bone resorption, while P1NP is a marker of bone formation. In patients treated with Ra-223, decreases in these markers (particularly NTx and P1NP) are associated with improved radiographic responses and longer progression-free survival [7, 8]. These markers reflect changes in bone metabolism due to the therapeutic effects of Ra-223 on bone metastases. However, not all studies have confirmed their predictive value consistently, and their use in clinical practice is still evolving.

Lactate Dehydrogenase (LDH) LDH is an enzyme involved in cellular energy production and is elevated in many cancers due to increased tumor glycolysis (the Warburg effect). High LDH levels reflect an aggressive tumor phenotype and correlate with higher tumor burden. LDH has been identified as a prognostic marker in mCRPC, where higher LDH levels at baseline are associated with worse outcomes. Patients with elevated LDH tend to have shorter survival irrespective of treatment. In Ra-223-treated patients, elevated LDH at baseline predicts a poor prognosis [3,

5]. Although LDH does not serve as a direct indicator of Ra-223 response, its levels provide insight into the overall aggressiveness of the disease.

Circulating Tumor Cells (CTCs) and Circulating Tumor DNA (ctDNA) CTCs are cancer cells that have detached from the primary or metastatic tumor and entered the bloodstream. ctDNA refers to fragments of DNA shed by tumor cells into the blood [9]. Both are considered liquid biopsy tools that reflect tumor burden and provide information on genetic mutations. CTC count at baseline is a strong prognostic factor in mCRPC. A CTC count below 5 cells/8 mL of blood is associated with better survival and predicts a greater likelihood of completing the full course of Ra-223 treatment. CTC reduction during treatment is also linked to better outcomes. A loss of detectable CTCs after starting Ra-223 has been correlated with improved survival, suggesting that CTCs could serve as a real-time monitoring tool for treatment efficacy. Additionally, detecting double-stranded DNA damage in CTCs through markers like γH2AX (which indicates DNA repair activity) could be an early predictor of response to Ra-223, as alpha-particle radiation induces DNA damage in tumor cells [9].

ctDNA analysis is emerging as a powerful tool for detecting DNA repair defects, such as homologous recombination deficiency (HRD), which is discussed below [9, 10]. This allows for patient selection based on molecular profiling, but specific studies on Ra-223 and ctDNA are still lacking.

Homologous Recombination Deficiency (HRD) HRD is caused by mutations in genes like BRCA1, BRCA2, and ATM, which are involved in DNA repair [10]. Cells with HRD are more susceptible to therapies that induce DNA damage, such as Ra-223, which works by causing double-stranded breaks in cancer cell DNA. Patients with HRD, especially BRCA2 mutations, may respond better to Ra-223 because their tumors are less capable of repairing the damage caused by alpha particles. Several studies reported that patients with HR gene mutations had better outcomes, including longer survival and better biomarker responses (e.g., ALP declines). Ongoing clinical trials are exploring the combination of Ra-223 with PARP inhibitors (which target DNA repair defects), particularly in patients with HRD. This suggests that HRD could serve as both a predictive biomarker for Ra-223 and a basis for combination therapies.

Imaging Biomarkers

Conventional imaging, such as bone scans and CT scans, are limited in their ability to assess response to Ra-223. Advanced PET techniques, particularly with radiotracers like [^{18}F]NaF or PSMA, offer more precise evaluation of bone metastasis response and may improve patient monitoring during Ra-223 treatment. The capability of the various PET tracers has been discussed in their own chapters. However, simultaneous use of the^{18}F-fluorocholine and Na^{18}F and Ga-PSMA-11 PET has been analyzed in two studies [11, 12], briefly described in Chap. 3. Additional examples are shown here. Ra-223 itself is not good for patient imaging, because it only produces 1.1% gamma emission, which could provide dosimetric estimates. To create the Ra-223-image as shown in Fig. 13.3, the acquisition took more than 60 min, meaning that it is impossible to apply this method for routine imaging [6].

Bone scintigraphy may still be useful for assessing response, if used quantitatively. For example, bone scintigraphy index (BSI) quantifies the extent of skeletal tumor burden and showed earlier promise as a prognostic biomarker [14]. A lower BSI at baseline correlates with better outcomes. However, $Na^{18}F$ turned out to be much more sensitive, and a few methods were developed to standardize its use. We used criteria for regional samples [13], and several methods for total fluoride burden (TLF) were developed [15, 16]. These methods used different cutoff values for response assessment. I used the SUVvalue SUV > 10 both in Texas (MD Anderson Cancer Center) [15] and Helsinki (Docrates Cancer Center) [13]. Figures 13.4 and 13.5 demonstrate patients who had quantitative minor response based on $Na^{18}F$-PET imaging. The patient in Fig. 13.4 has extensive disease which is not possible to evaluate visually—here quantification helps [13]. The patient in Fig. 13.5 is a young patient with an aggressive disease treated previously with multiple regimens. Therefore, it is crucial to identify a skeletal response, even minor, because most of

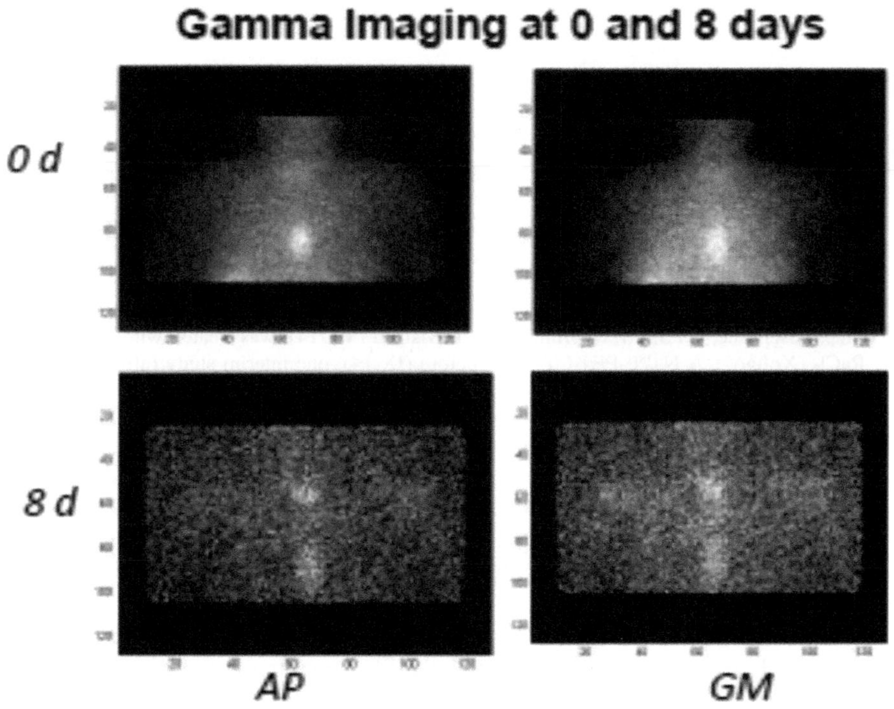

Fig. 13.3 Gamma imaging at 0 and 8 days after $^{223}RaCl_2$ therapeutic dose using gamma camera, AP views on the left and geometric mean (GM) images on the right. This patient has a lesion in the sternum and in the thoracic vertebra. (From [6])

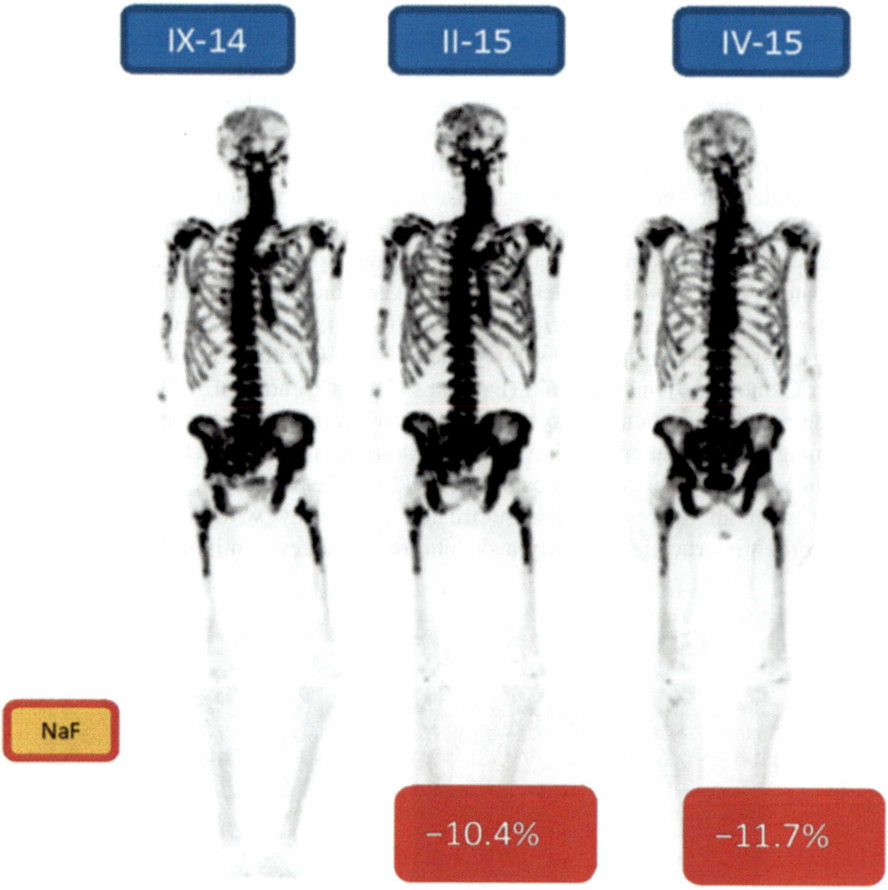

Fig. 13.4 A 69-year-old male, Gleason score 8 (diagnosed in 2012), treated earlier with bicalutamide, gosereline, S-PSA 671 ng/mL at initial visit in (VII/14), was treated with six cycles of $^{223}RaCl_2$ (Xofigo®). A Na^{18}F-PET-CT study before (IX-14), one interim study (after two cycles, II-15), and one study (IV-15) after the six cycles are shown. There is a quantitative response (−10.4% and −11.7%) in both the interim and post therapy Na^{18}F-PET-MIP (maximum intensity projection) images. There is a quantitative response which cannot be seen visually. (From [13])

the prostate cancer patients die because of skeletal metastases or SREs. We reported early in Helsinki that interim analysis does help to predict the outcome [13]. We got the same result later in Texas in analysis of 161 men with mCRPC and a total of 773 ^{223}Ra therapy cycles [17].

At MDACC, the median overall survival (95% CI) was 12.4 (9.1, 16.1) months in the whole patient population [17]. Na^{18}F-PET imaging at baseline, after three cycles (n = 14) and after six cycles, and TLF_{10} (skeletal disease burden at SUV values >10 on Na^{18}F-PET) were calculated in all these PET studies. From these results, we found that interim imaging did not help in assessing the final outcome

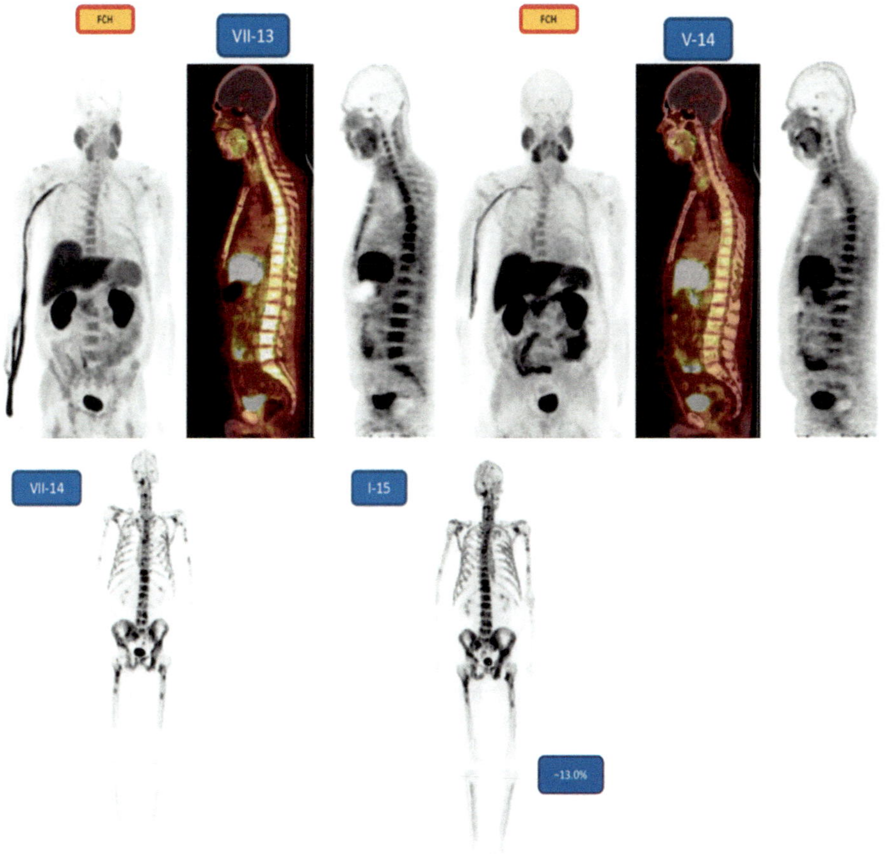

Fig. 13.5 The images demonstrate a young patient (49 years) with GS 9, treated earlier with cyproterone, degarelix, bicalutamide, zoledronate, docetaxel, Sm-153-EDTMP, mitoxantrone, EBRT (P), docetaxel, abiraterone. A response to the treatments is seen on FCH-PET in 10 months, especially in the bone marrow disease—MIP image, sagittal fusion FCH-PET on CT, and sagittal FCH-PET figures are shown in July 2013 (VII-13) and corresponding data in May 2014 (V-14). NaF-PET 6 weeks (VII-14) later in July 2014 demonstrated a widespread active cortical bone disease. He responded to the Ra-223 treatment, because after six cycles, a response was seen in January 2015 (−13.0% change, I-15). (From [13])

of ^{223}Ra therapy. The survival benefit of ^{223}Ra therapy alone is more than a year in a high-risk group of advanced prostate cancer [17]. A patient example is shown in Fig. 13.6.

Thousands of patients have been treated with ^{223}Ra therapy. A recent real-world evidence of 48 patients (25 docetaxel-naïve, 23 post-docetaxel) who were followed for 12.4 months (accidentally) showed a significantly lower all-cause mortality rate versus the post-docetaxel group (40.0% vs. 78.3%, $P = .02$), as well as a significantly higher treatment completion rate (72.0% vs. 26.1%, $P < .01$) [18]. There were no significant differences in pain control, change in biochemical parameters,

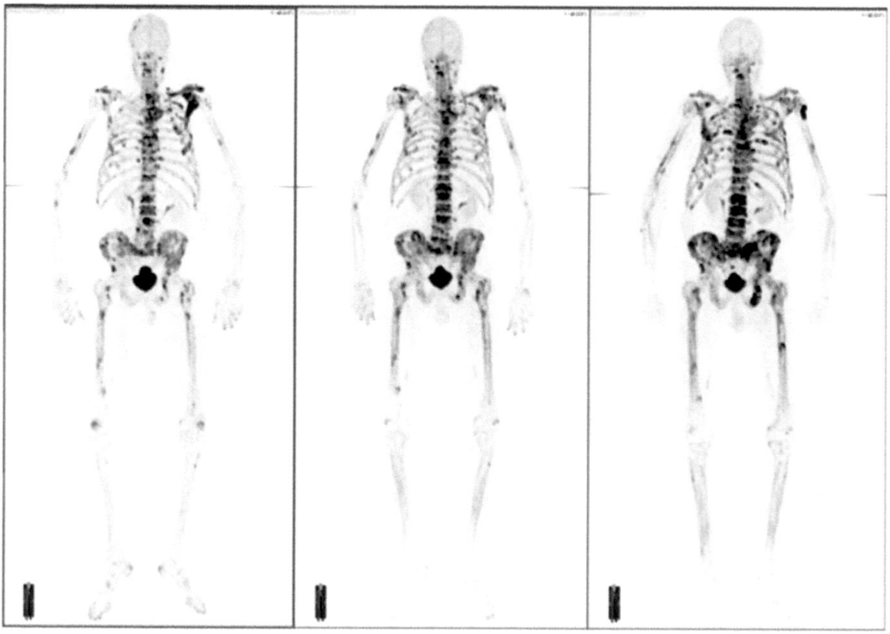

Fig. 13.6 The images demonstrate 1 case out of 161 men with mCRPC who received a total of 773 ^{223}Ra therapies; their median overall survival was 12.4 months. Na^{18}F-PET in 14 patients at baseline, after 3 cycles and after 6 cycles (1 patient shown), demonstrated no significant association between change in total Na^{18}F burden (TLF10) after 3 and 6 cycles. (Presented in [17])

biochemical response, or hematologic treatment-emergent adverse events between the two groups.

Docetaxel-naïve group had a numerically higher pain control rate, numerically greater improvements in ALP and PSA, and numerically lower rates of grade ≥3 neutropenia and grade ≥3 thrombocytopenia than the post-docetaxel group [18]. This supports earlier real-world evidence [2] that Ra-223 may be used safely and effectively in earlier lines of treatment for bone-predominant mCRPC.

There is a rather new network meta-analysis consisting of 5 trials with 3862 patients comparing 4 treatments (abiraterone, enzalutamide, cabazitaxel, and radium-223) [19]. All the four treatments were associated with improved overall survival (OS) and biochemical progression-free survival relative to best supportive care. Among them, enzalutamide (hazard ratio [HR] = 0.58, 95% confidence interval [CI]: 0.49–0.69) had the highest probability of ranking first in terms of OS, followed by cabazitaxel (HR = 0.70, 95% CI: 0.59–0.83), radium-223 (HR = 0.71, 95% Cl: 0.56–0.90), and abiraterone (HR = 0.73, 95% CI: 0.63–0.84) [19]. In terms of safety, treatments ranked from the safest to the least safe were radium-223 (OR = 0.58, 95% CI: 0.20–1.68), enzalutamide (OR = 0.80, 95% CI: 0.28–2.29), abiraterone (OR = 0.94, 95% CI: 0.39–2.27), and cabazitaxel (OR = 2.50, 95% CI:

0.84–7.44) [19]. Although this network meta-analysis provided indirect comparisons and ranking probabilities, the results should be treated with caution because they cannot replace randomized direct comparison. According to this, for patients with mCRPC who progressed after docetaxel, enzalutamide may offer the most significant survival benefits, but Ra-223 is safest.

Conclusive Remarks

Radium-223 offers a well-tolerated and effective treatment option for patients with mCRPC and symptomatic bone metastases. Its low toxicity and favorable safety profile make it particularly suitable for patients who are unable to tolerate chemotherapy or who have limited bone marrow reserve. Careful patient selection is crucial, focusing on those with bone-only metastases and early symptoms, while avoiding patients with visceral metastases or advanced intestinal disease. Combination strategies with other therapies are not discussed here, because they continue to be explored to further enhance the clinical outcomes of Ra-223 treatment.

This chapter is a review focused on understanding the use of radium-223 dichloride (Ra-223) for treating metastatic castration-resistant prostate cancer (mCRPC) with bone metastases. Radium-223 is a crucial treatment option for mCRPC with bone metastases, offering survival benefits, quality-of-life improvements, and reduced skeletal complications. Its integration into clinical practice marks a shift toward nuclear medicine as a frontline treatment. To optimize patient outcomes, multidisciplinary teams are essential, and further research is ongoing to explore combinations and biomarkers to enhance Ra-223's efficacy.

Among the biomarkers explored for Ra-223 treatment, b-ALP and HRD stand out as promising tools for predicting response and guiding patient selection. Other markers, such as CTCs, bone metabolism markers, and imaging modalities, especially quantitative $Na^{18}F$ show potential but need further validation. PSA, while useful in other treatments, is largely ineffective in assessing Ra-223 outcomes, highlighting the need for novel, reliable biomarkers in mCRPC management.

While Ra-223 is effective in treating mCRPC with bone metastases, there is a need for reliable biomarkers to better stratify patients and monitor responses. Current biomarkers like PSA are insufficient, and future research is focusing on bone metabolic markers, genetic defects, and advanced imaging techniques to fill this gap.

Patients must be well-informed about the goals of Ra-223 therapy, which include symptom improvement, prolongation of overall survival, and reduction in skeletal-related events (SREs)**. It is important to emphasize that Ra-223 is not curative but can significantly enhance quality of life and delay disease progression. Patients should also be aware of potential side effects and the importance of completing the "official" six treatment cycles to maximize the benefits.

References

1. Parker C, Nilsson S, Heinrich D, et al. Alpha emitter radium-223 and survival in metastatic prostate cancer. N Engl J Med. 2013;369:213–23.
2. Oyen W, Sundram F, Haug AR, et al. Radium-223 dichloride (Ra-223) for the treatment of metastatic castration-resistant prostate cancer: optimizing clinical practice in nuclear medicine centers. J OncoPathol. 2015;3:1–25.
3. van der Zande K, Oyen WJG, Zwart W, Bergman AM. Radium-223 treatment of patients with metastatic castration resistant prostate cancer: biomarkers for stratification and response evaluation. Cancer. 2021;13:4346.
4. Agarwal N, Nussenzveig R, Hahn AW, et al. Prospective evaluation of bone metabolic markers as surrogate markers of response to Radium-223 therapy in metastatic castration-resistant prostate cancer. Clin Cancer Res. 2020;26:2104–10.
5. Badrising SK, Louhanepessy RD, van der Noort V, et al. A prospective observational registry evaluating clinical outcomes of Radium-223 treatment in a nonstudy population. Int J Cancer. 2020;147:1143–51.
6. Kairemo K, Joensuu T, Rasulova N, Kiljunen T, Kangasmäki A. Evaluation of alpha-therapy with Radium-223-dichloride in castration resistant metastatic prostate cancer-the role of gamma scintigraphy in dosimetry and pharmacokinetics. Diagnostics (Basel). 2015;5:358–68.
7. Armstrong AJ, Eisenberger MA, Halabi S, et al. Biomarkers in the management and treatment of men with metastatic castration-resistant prostate cancer. Eur Urol. 2012;61:549–59.
8. Frantellizzi V, Monari F, Mascia M, et al. Validation of the 3-variable prognostic score (3-PS) in mCRPC patients treated with ^{223}Radium-dichloride: a national multicenter study. Ann Nucl Med. 2020;34:772–80.
9. Wyatt AW, Annala M, Aggarwal R, et al. Concordance of circulating tumor DNA and matched metastatic tissue biopsy in prostate cancer. J Natl Cancer Inst. 2017;109:djx118.
10. Mateo J, Seed G, Bertan C, et al. Genomics of lethal prostate cancer at diagnosis and castration resistance. J Clin Invest. 2020;130:1743–51.
11. Kairemo K, Kangasmäki A, Kappadath SC, Joensuu T, Macapinlac HA. A retrospective comparative study of sodium fluoride Na^{18}F-PET/CT and ^{68}Ga-PSMA-11 PET/CT in the bone metastases of prostate cancer using a volumetric 3-D radiomic analysis. Life (Basel). 2022;12:1977.
12. Kairemo K, Kappadath SC, Joensuu T, Macapinlac HA. A retrospective comparative study of sodium fluoride (NaF-18)-PET/CT and fluorocholine (F-18-CH) PET/CT in the evaluation of skeletal metastases in metastatic prostate cancer using a volumetric 3-D radiomics analysis. Diagnostics (Basel). 2020;11:17.
13. Kairemo K, Joensuu T. Radium-223-dichloride in castration resistant metastatic prostate cancer-preliminary results of the response evaluation using F-18-fluoride PET/CT. Diagnostics (Basel). 2015;5:413–27.
14. Sabbatini P, Larson SM, Kremer A, et al. Prognostic significance of extent of disease in bone in patients with androgen-independent prostate cancer. J Clin Oncol. 1999;17(3):948–57.
15. Rohren EM, Etchebehere EC, Araujo JC, et al. Determination of skeletal tumor burden on 18F-fluoride PET/CT. J Nucl Med. 2015;56(10):1507–12.
16. Harmon SA, Perk T, Lin C, et al. Quantitative assessment of early [^{18}F] sodium fluoride positron emission tomography/computed tomography response to treatment in men with metastatic prostate cancer to bone. J Clin Oncol. 2017;35:2829–37.
17. Kairemo K, Milton DR, Etchebehere E, Rohren EM, Macapinlac HA. Final outcome of ^{223}Ra-therapy and the role of 18F-fluoride-PET in response evaluation in metastatic castration-resistant prostate cancer—a single institution experience. Curr Radiopharm. 2018;11:147–52.

18. Chiang PC, Chiang PH, Chen IA, et al. Treatment outcomes with radium-223 in docetaxel-naïve versus docetaxel-treated metastatic castration-resistant prostate cancer patients: real-world evidence from Taiwan. Medicine (Baltimore). 2023;102(5):e32671.
19. Chen J, Zhang Y, Zhang X, et al. Comparison of systemic treatments for metastatic castration-resistant prostate cancer after docetaxel failure: a systematic review and network meta-analysis. Front Pharmacol. 2022;12:789319.

Lu-177-PSMA Treatment in Prostate Cancer

14

Introduction

Prostate cancer radioligand therapy (PRLT) with ^{177}Lu-PSMA is still considered as an investigational treatment, even though Pluvicto® got marketing approval by the FDA in December 2022. PRLT in this context involves the systemic intravenous administration of a specific radiopharmaceutical composed of a β-emitting radionuclide chelated to a small molecule for the purpose of delivering cytotoxic radiation to cancer cells. The decision to perform PRLT should be taken by a multidisciplinary team, including all of the specialists involved in the care of patients with metastatic castrate resistant prostate cancer (mCRPC) which is the indication of the approved therapy. CRPC is defined as castrate serum testosterone <50 μg/l or 1.7 nmol/l plus one of the following types of progression [1]. The treatment should take place in an approved nuclear medicine department and must be performed by an experienced nuclear medicine specialist. The nuclear medicine team must have qualified personnel, appropriate radiation safety equipment, and procedures for waste management and handling accidental contamination of the site or personnel. Isolation of patients in nuclear medicine department should be performed according to local radiation regulations for patient release after radionuclide.

Prostate-specific membrane antigen (PSMA), also known as folate hydrolase I or glutamate carboxypeptidase II, is a type II transmembrane protein, which is anchored in the cell membrane of prostate epithelial cells. PSMA is highly expressed on prostate epithelial cells and strongly upregulated in prostate cancer. The PSMA expression levels are directly correlated to androgen independence, metastasis, and prostate cancer progression [2]. Thus, PSMA is a promising molecular target for diagnosis and therapy of metastatic prostate cancer at present [3].

^{177}Lu is a β- and γ-emitting radionuclide with a physical half-life of 6.7 days. It has a maximum and mean β-particle energy of 0.498 MeV and 0.133 MeV, respectively. The maximum and mean soft-tissue penetration depth of ^{177}Lu is 1.7 mm and 0.23 mm, respectively. It has two main gamma emission lines: 113 keV (6% relative abundance) and 208 keV (11% relative abundance).

K. Kairemo, *Prostate Cancer from a Nuclear Oncology Perspective*,
https://doi.org/10.1007/978-3-031-90337-3_14

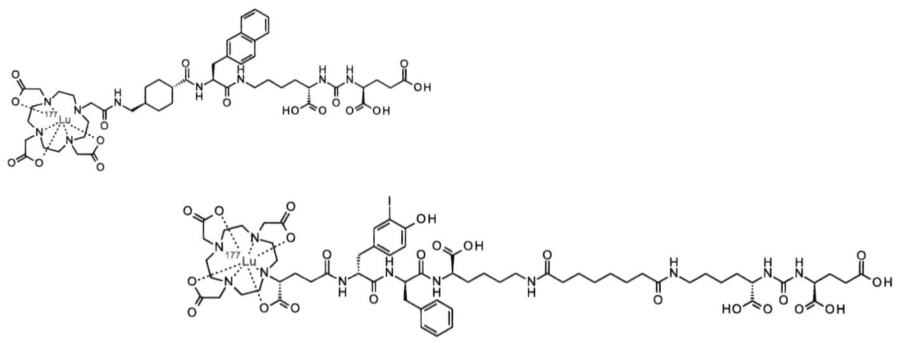

Fig. 14.1 Structure of ^{177}Lu-PSMA-617 (left) and ^{177}Lu-PSMA-I&T (right)

^{177}Lu-PSMA-617, a DOTA derivative of the Glu-urea-Lys motif, has been developed in the German Cancer Research Center (DKFZ), Heidelberg, Germany, for the treatment of patients with metastatic prostate cancer [4]. ^{177}Lu-PSMA for imaging and therapy (I&T) is a third-generation derivative of ^{177}Lu-PSMA compounds which has been used in PRLT as well [5]. The structures of these compounds are shown in Fig. 14.1.

This chapter reviews the use of Lu-177-PSMA with practical patient examples.

Literature Review (Brief History)

Metastatic castration-resistant prostate cancer (mCRPC) remains one of the leading causes of cancer-related deaths globally, and therapeutic options are limited. Traditional treatments such as chemotherapy and hormonal therapies are generally ineffective in completely controlling the disease. Prostate-specific membrane antigen (PSMA) is a promising target for both diagnosis and treatment as discussed in chapters dealing with prostate cancer (PCa) diagnostics. Because PSMA is overexpressed on prostate cancer cells and the use of radiolabeled ligands, particularly ^{177}Lu-PSMA-617 and ^{177}Lu-PSMA-I&T, has emerged as a novel treatment modality, these radiopharmaceuticals deliver beta radiation directly to cancer cells, allowing localized tumor destruction while minimizing damage to surrounding healthy tissues.

In PCa, after unsuccessful therapy with ^{90}Y-CYT-356 monoclonal antibody (MAb), which binds to the intracellular domain of PSMA [6], phase I and II clinical trials utilizing the PSMA MAb J591, radiolabeled with ^{177}Lu or ^{90}Y, showed promising results [7]; however, there were higher rates of hematological toxicity. In 47 patients treated with ^{177}Lu-PSMA MAb J591, grade 4 thrombocytopenia in 46.8% (29.8% received platelet transfusions) and grade 4 neutropenia in 25.5% of the patients were reported [7]. Monoclonal antibodies are large molecules and therefore show poor permeability in solid tumors. This characteristic along with slow clearance from the circulation is the probable cause of grade 4 hematotoxicity. Small molecule inhibitors of PSMA were introduced instead of MAb [8]. First clinical experiences with PSMA-based radionuclide treatment using Iodine-131-labeled PSMA showed promising results with mild hematotoxicity and a PSA decrease >50% in 60% of all treated prostate cancer patients [9]. ^{177}Lu has a half-life of 6.7 days and a lower beta-particle emission energy than I-131, indicating higher probability for less side effects [10].

The early two multicenter retrospective studies with Lu-177-labeled small molecule inhibitors of PSMA, which had a low hematotoxicity and nephrotoxicity profile, showed an efficacy of this therapy with a PSA decline of more than 50% in up to 45% of patients [11, 12]. Rahbar et al. showed in a multicenter analysis of 145 patients that the presence of visceral metastases and an alkaline phosphatase (ALP) >220 U/L were negative predictors of therapy response [11]. The studies by Ahmadzadehfar et al. evaluated the hematotoxicity and nephrotoxicity in patients who received at least three cycles of RLT [13, 14]. They studied 49 patients who were treated with 3 cycles of ^{177}Lu-PSMA-617 and reported anemia, thrombocytopenia, and leukopenia (common toxicity criteria; CTC grade 3°) during the observation period after the third cycle in only 4 (8.2%), 3 (6.1%), and 0 patients, respectively. No CTC grade 4° hematotoxicity was observed in the entire study population. More than 60% of patients did not show any hematotoxicity [14]. In this study, 20 patients (40.8%) received a median of six cycles of radionuclide therapy with ^{223}Ra prior to ^{177}Lu-PSMA-617 therapy. There were no significant differences between the patients with a history of therapy with ^{223}Ra and those without regarding leukopenia and thrombocytopenia. These results confirmed that performing repeated cycles of ^{177}Lu-PSMA-617 after radionuclide therapy using ^{223}Ra seems to be safe with a very small probability of hematotoxicity [14]. The 55 patients who received at least 3 cycles of RLT with ^{177}Lu-PSMA-617 did not show any grade 3 or 4 nephrotoxicity [13]. A significant negative effect on renal function was found for age (>65 years) ($p = 0.049$), hypertension ($p = 0.001$), and preexisting kidney disease ($p = 0.001$).

Rahbar et al. reported the overall survival benefit of RLT in comparison with a historical cohort: the estimated median survival was 29.4 weeks, which was significantly longer than the 19.7 weeks of the historical controls (HR: 0.44 (95% CI 0.20–0.95); $P = 0.031$) [15]. According to Ahmadzadehfar et al. [16], the patients with a favorable response and repeated therapies with ^{177}Lu-PSMA-617 have a significantly longer overall survival in comparison with patients who showed no response to RLT according to PSA changes. According to Braeuer et al., an initial ALP level <220 U/L and a PSA decline measured 2 months after the first cycle were associated with a longer overall survival [17].

Delker et al. reported their dosimetry results with ^{177}Lu-PSMA-617 and calculated a mean absorbed dose/per cycle to the bone marrow, kidneys, liver, spleen, and salivary glands of 0.012 Gy/GBq, 0.6 Gy/GBq, 0.1 Gy/GBq, 0.1 Gy/GBq, and 1.4 Gy/GBq, respectively [18].

Regarding these different promising results, ^{177}Lu-PSMA-617 was found to be a promising therapy option for patients with mCRPC, and it should therefore mostly be offered to patients as a salvage therapy.

^{177}Lu-PSMA RLT was mainly used as a compassionate treatment of patients with end-stage mCRPC [19]. It also could treat lymph node metastatic CRPC. ^{177}Lu-PSMA-617 RLT reduced PSA more than salvage radiotherapy and abiraterone [20].

I was involved with a systematic review (PROSPERO database; reg. no.: CRD42017067743) to compare the two types of treatment [21]: the null hypothesis was that ^{177}Lu-PSMA RLT and third-line treatment of mCRPC have similar effects. The meta-analysis consisted of 12 studies including 669 patients reporting ^{177}Lu-PSMA RLT results and 16 studies including 1338 patients reporting third-line treatment results [21]. Overall, 44% of the patients had a maximum decline of PSA of ≥50% following treatment with ^{177}Lu-PSMA RLT, and PSA decline ≥50% was 22% in third-line treatment (mean 44% versus 22%, $p = 0.0002$, t-test) [21]. This has been discussed in Chap. 16 dealing with own meta-analyses.

Very soon after this meta-analysis, two new randomized clinical trials (RCTs) were published, TheraP and VISION [22, 23]. After these trials, ^{177}Lu-PSMA-617 got marketing authorization.

There was an updated meta-analysis inspired by the increasing clinical use of PRLT and the release of two new randomized clinical trials (RCTs) that add significant weight to the evaluation of PRLT's efficacy [24]. This meta-analysis initially screened 472 paper studies involving human subjects with mCRPC treated with ^{177}Lu-labeled small molecule PRLT ligands—69 studies were ultimately included, covering a total of 4157 patients. Of these, 56 studies focused on ^{177}Lu-PSMA-617 (3365 patients), 7 studies evaluated ^{177}Lu-PSMA-I&T (316 patients), and 2 studies compared both agents without separating results. Notably, only two randomized controlled trials were included, a significant limitation but also a key strength of this updated analysis, as these RCTs provided much-needed controlled data. Forty-four percent of patients showed a ≥50% reduction in PSA levels after receiving ^{177}Lu-PSMA therapy (95% CI 41–48%). The treatment was significantly more effective than controls (OR = 5.33, 95% CI 1.24–22.90), based on two RCTs [24]. This finding is critical as a ≥50% reduction in PSA is strongly associated with better clinical outcomes. When considering any PSA decline, 68% of patients exhibited some level of response (95% CI 64–71%), though heterogeneity in results was noted ($\chi^2 = 63\%$). This suggests that, while most patients derive some benefit, the degree of response varies widely based on factors like tumor burden, prior treatments, and patient health [24]. No statistically significant difference was observed in PSA response rates between ^{177}Lu-PSMA-617 and ^{177}Lu-PSMA-I&T, suggesting both radioligands are equally effective. This is important for clinicians, as it provides flexibility in selecting between the two agents without compromising efficacy [24].

The meta-analysis solidified that ^{177}Lu-PSMA radioligand therapy is an effective treatment for mCRPC, offering both significant PSA responses and survival benefits. The findings supported broader adoption of PRLT, though more randomized controlled trials are necessary to refine its use and ensure optimal patient outcomes. Given the high heterogeneity in treatment protocols, future research should aim to standardize dosages and identify patient subgroups most likely to benefit.

In the following, the current indications and contraindications are presented.

Indications

RLT with ^{177}Lu-PSMA-I &T is indicated for the treatment of patients with mCRPC, who do not have any other approved therapy option planned by a multidisciplinary team. Candidate patients for RLT using ^{177}Lu-PSMA-I &T should fulfill the following criteria:

1. mCRPC with PSMA-positive metastatic disease based upon PSMA-PET or SPECT imaging,
   - There are no limitations regarding the number or site of metastases, i.e., bone or soft-tissue metastases. Caution should be given to patients, e.g., with diffuse bone marrow, perineural, and brain metastases.
2. After initial hormone therapy (LHRH agonists/antagonists).

   Progressive disease, i.e. biochemical and/or radiologic progression, despite newly developed hormone therapies (Abiraterone/Enzalutamide) or these medications were not suitable for the patient.

   Progressive disease despite chemotherapy (Docetaxel and Cabazitaxel) or the patient being unfit for chemotherapy.
3. Not suitable for ^{153}Sm-EDTMP or ^{223}Radium dichloride or other locally available radiopharmaceuticals for bone-targeted therapies due to extra-osseous metastases or diffuse bone marrow metastases or patient avoidance.

   In patients without adequate response to bone-targeted therapies for pain palliation or exacerbation of pain even by such therapy, an RLT with ^{177}Lu-PSMA-I & T can be evaluated.
4. Life expectancy longer than 4–6 months.
5. Decision for salvage therapy at the institutional interdisciplinary tumor board.

In summary, mCRPC patients should undergo hormone therapy and chemotherapy as well as bone-targeted therapy, if indicated. In the case of any contraindication for one of these therapies, it should be discussed and documented in an interdisciplinary tumor board.

Contraindications

1. White blood cell count $\leq 1 \times 10^9$/l.
2. Hemoglobin $\leq$80 g/l.

   In the case of symptomatic anemia, a red blood cell transfusion should precede the therapy. RLT with ^{177}Lu-PSMA may have a positive effect on bone marrow depression, causing the need for less blood to be transfused due to tumor regression in bone marrow. It should be noted that pure anemia without thrombocytopenia and leucopenia is not a contraindication for RLT.

3. Platelets $\leq 70 \times 10^9$/l.
4. Creatinine >1.5 upper normal limit; kidney failure with creatinine clearance <30 mL/min.
5. Renal outflow obstruction.
6. Previous chemotherapy or bone-targeted radionuclide therapy and extended external beam irradiation fields to the bone marrow (pelvis, spine), if performed during 4 weeks preceding the RLT.
7. ECOG performance status >2.
8. Hypersensitivity to the active substance or to any of the excipients.

Side Effects

Acute Side Effects According to the results of different published data, no severe adverse events immediately after injection have been reported to date [11, 15, 25–27]. The most common side effect in the first 48 h after injection is mild nausea and vomiting (in up to 20% of patients) [11, 26, 27], which can be easily treated with antiemetics. Fatigue is the most common complaint in patients after therapy, especially in the first 4 weeks (in up to 25%) [11, 26, 27].

Delayed Side Effects Dry mouth was reported in up to 20% of cases and is transient and tolerable in the majority of patients [11, 15, 28].

Renal Toxicity Dosimetry studies have shown that the most critical organs are the kidneys, with a maximum kidney radiation dose of 0.88 Gy/GBq for ^{177}Lu-PSMA-617 and 0.93 Gy/GBq for ^{177}Lu-PSMA-I&T [27]. None of the early studies reported any high grade nephrotoxicity (CTC grade 3, 4, or 5) [11, 15, 26]. In a study by Yordanova et al., the authors reported renal toxicity in 55 mCRPC patients who received at least three cycles of ^{177}Lu-PSMA-617. They observed increased creatinine levels of CTC 1° or 2° in 14 patients (25%) and increased GFR (grade 1/2) in 16 cases. None of the 55 patients experienced severe nephrotoxicity (grade 3/4) [13].

Bone Marrow Toxicity Severe (grade 3 and 4) bone marrow toxicity is observed in less than 10% of patients in various publications [15, 26–28].

Dosimetry

It has been shown that there is no major difference in absorbed dose estimates between Lu-177-PSMA I &T and Lu-177-PSMA-617—here the specific known dosimetry for Lu-177-PSMA I&T is presented [29].

Dosimetry for Normal Organs The mean whole-body effective dose for four cycles was 0.41 ± 0.18 Sv (0.06 Sv/GBq). The mean absorbed organ doses were 5.3 ± 1.6 Gy (0.72 Gy/GBq) for the kidneys; 0.89 ± 0.42 Gy (0.12 Gy/GBq) for the liver; and 4.0 ± 1.1 Gy (0.55 Gy/GBq) for the parotid, 4.8 ± 2.8 Gy (0.64 Gy/GBq) for the submandibular, and 27 ± 10 Gy (3.8 Gy/GBq) for the lacrimal glands [29].

Dosimetry for Tumor Lesions In total, all lesions received a mean dose per cycle of 23 ± 20 Gy (3.3 Gy/GBq). Mean absorbed dose for bone, lymph node, liver, and lung metastases were 26 ± 20 Gy (3.4 Gy/GBq), 24 ± 16 Gy (3.2 Gy/GBq), 8.5 ± 4.7 Gy (1.28 Gy/GBq), and 13 ± 7.4 Gy (1.7 Gy/GBq).

There is a clear trend toward a lower absorbed dose with an increasing number of the cycle. Mean absorbed dose per lesion was 26 ± 21 Gy (3.5 Gy/GBq) for the first, 24 ± 19 Gy (3.3 Gy/GBq) for the second, 20 ± 18 Gy (2.7 Gy/GBq) for the third, and 18 ± 17 Gy (2.4 Gy/GBq) for the fourth cycle. A similar trend can be seen for the subgroup of bone metastases. No reliable comparison is possible for lymph node, liver, and lung metastases because of a low sample number. One example of this behavior is shown in Fig. 14.2, where the first cycle gives the highest dose in three different bone metastases [30].

Blood sampling was performed in six patients to estimate the mean absorbed dose to the red marrow. The mean absorbed dose to the red marrow in six patients varied from 0.01 to 0.04 mGy/MBq [29]. The effective half-life in tumor lesions was higher than those in the whole body, kidneys, and parotid glands, resulting in the delivery of higher mean absorbed doses to tumors [29]. The maximum absorbed dose delivered to a paraaortic lymph node metastasis that exhibited the highest SUVmax (187.5) before therapy was 468 Gy [29]. In 56 patients, treated with Lu-177-PSMA I&T, during a follow-up period of 28 months, 12 patients died (21.4%). The median overall survival (last assessed 15.5 months after PSMA RLT) was not reached. Survival after 28 months was 78.6%. The median progression-free survival was 13.7 months [29].

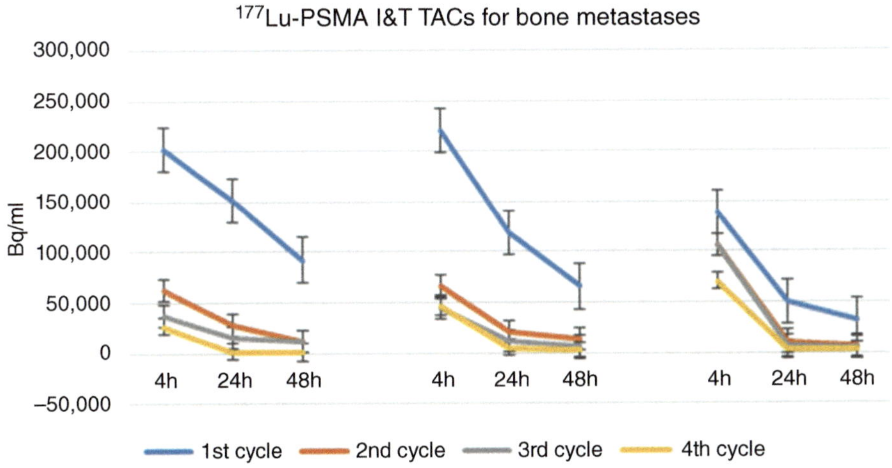

Fig. 14.2 ^{177}Lu time-activity curves (TAC) in three metastatic sites in the skeleton during four cycles of ^{177}Lu-PSMA-I&T RLT. The ^{177}Lu activity concentration decreases toward later time point and toward later cycles. (Presented in [30])

Case Examples

In the following, I present a few challenging different types of patients who have been treated with a major response.

Patient 1

A 63-year-old man was diagnosed with prostate cancer—on biopsies, the grade was Gleason score (GS) 6, but prostatectomy revealed GS 7 disease. Staging appeared to be T3bN0M0, staging based on bone scintigraphy and abdominal ultrasonography. Retropubic radical prostatectomy was done as the primary operation without lymphadenectomy. Adjuvant radiotherapy, bicalutamide, and later on also an LHRH agonist were started. A castration-resistant phase emerged 7 years later when PSA increased from 30 to 75 μg/l during hormonal treatment. PSA continued to increase up to 108 μg/l. Lymph node metastases and two liver metastases (diameters 4.5 cm and 6 cm) were found in CT. Skeletal metastases were detected subsequently. Enzalutamide was started after docetaxel and was given for almost a year, but abiraterone following enzalutamide appeared to be totally ineffective. Biweekly docetaxel was started for castration-resistant bone and liver metastatic disease. When abiraterone was finished, cabazitaxel was started, and it gave the best response—S-PSA was 145 μg/l. ^{177}Lu-PSMA-617 RLT was considered, and the patient came to my institution. ^{68}Ga-PSMA-PET-CT revealed large lymph node metastases were observed, the volume being >70 cm^3. In the liver, there were two inhomogeneous uniform metastases with high uptake of PSMA, the volume in the liver being >500 cm^3 (Fig. 14.3). Seven ^{177}Lu-PSMA-617 RLT treatments were given within seven months, and S-PSA decreased from 145 to 1.2 μg/l, meaning major response and almost a complete biochemical response, 99.2% S-PSA decline (Fig. 14.3).

Patient 2

He had myocardial infarction and coronary angioplasty 8 months before prostate cancer diagnosis. He had primarily urinary retention. Initial S-PSA was only 3.5 μg/l, but aggressive GS 9 (5 + 4) cancer was growing also outside the prostate. Staging was T4N0M0, and the tumor was infiltrating to the pelvic wall, seminal vesicles, and bladder wall, but without distant metastases in fluorocholine-PET-CT.

He was treated with transurethral resection of the prostate and short course of hormone therapy—the radiotherapy was given up to 72 Gy to the prostate and 50 Gy, but not the seminal vesicle region nor the pelvic lymph nodes. The disease remained stable over 3 years. When S-PSA started to increase, the addition of bicalutamide and LHRH agonists was ineffective. When PSA was 46 μg/l, the CT

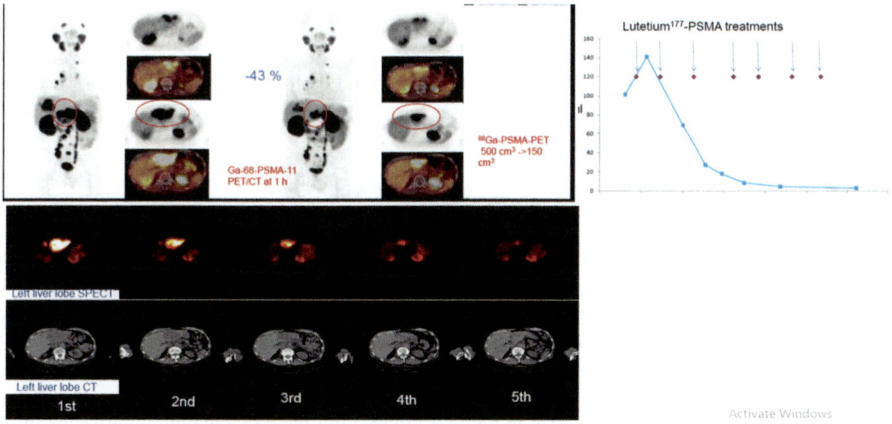

Fig. 14.3 In baseline PET imaging, an extensive liver disease can be seen in the MIP image (red circle, upper panel, left) and also in pelvic liver fusion images (PET on CT) (upper panel, left). This patient had also extensive lymph node disease, e.g., in the retroperitoneum and mediastinum. Normal organs, i.e., salivary and lacrimal glands, liver, spleen, visualize in the MIP images (upper panel). After four cycles, the metabolic liver metastasis volume had decreased from 500 to 150 cm^3. In the control study, the liver disease dramatically decreased in size in the MIP image (red circle) and also in fusion images (PET on CT) (upper panel). SPECT/CT images of the five first ^{177}Lu-PSMA are shown separately at the level of the largest liver metastasis in the left liver lobe (lower left panel), showing how the tumor gets smaller cycle by cycle. The serum PSA (μg/l) curve of the patient who received a total of seven ^{177}Lu-PSMA treatments is shown in the upper right panel. The serum PSA decreased from 145 to 1.2 ng/ml

revealed the tumor being in close contact with sigmoid bowel. Relapses were seen also in the pelvic wall, in lymph nodes, and in the bladder wall. Hydronephrosis was evident on the right side related to the tumor mass. Patient had severe difficulties with defecation, but no tumors were found in colonoscopy. The tumor mass appeared to compress the bowel from outside only, and therefore patient had no stools in many days causing severe abdominal pain. Do not resuscitate (DNR) decision was made and palliative therapy was recommended. Despite the rapid progression and highly symptomatic disease with DNR decision, patient asked second opinion at our institution. ^{68}Ga PSMA-PET-CT showed the tumor mass being strongly PSMA avid and the total disease volume was up to 700 cm^3 (Fig. 14.4). Patient had also metastases in the liver and in adrenals. However, the bones were free of metastases. The big abdominal resistance was also easily observable by palpation. We discussed thoroughly about all risk factors, even death, regarding the high volume of the intraperitoneal disease, as possible severe side effects. We told also that serious bowel irritation might be probable due to the big volume of the disease. Immediately after the first Lutetium^{177}-PSMA therapy, patient had no side effects, but risks were realized when he was hospitalized only 1 week later for 6 days having acute pancreatitis. This pancreatitis was most probably related to the large lymph node next to the pancreas accumulating quite high

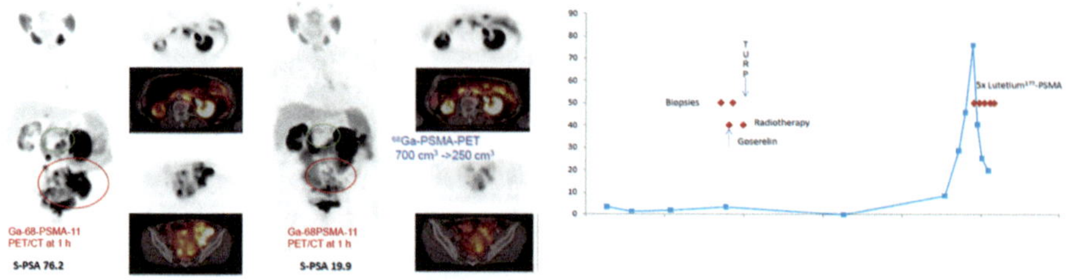

Fig. 14.4 The serum PSA (μg/l) curve of the patient who received five ^{177}Lu-PSMA treatments for his first relapse (upper panel). The Ga-68-PSMA-PET/CT study performed before ^{177}Lu-PSMA therapies shows an extensive pelvic and lower abdominal disease (bladder, pelvic wall, sigmoid bowel, para-aortal, retroperitoneal, retrocrural, left mediastinum, and supraclavicular (red circle), which can also be seen in the MIP image (lower panel, left)). Normal organs, i.e., salivary and lacrimal glands, liver, spleen, visualize in the MIP images (all panels). One month after the third cycle of ^{177}Lu-PSMA treatments, most of the pathologic pelvic and lower abdominal disease (red circle) had disappeared including retroperitoneal, adrenal, and liver regions (lower panel, right). The disease volume decreased from 700 to 250 cm^3 and serum PSA from 76.2 to 19.9 ng/ml. The patient is free from constipation and other quality of life disturbing urinary problems

dose of ^{177}Lu. But he recovered well and was motivated to continue the therapy. Lutetium^{177}-PSMA was given five cycles all together. He received very good response both in S-PSA and in PET-CT scanning (Fig. 14.4)—biochemically there was a 73.9% S-PSA decline. Due to the signs of S-PSA stabilization without further decrease, we decided to continue the follow-up after five treatments with ^{177}Lu-PSMA-RLT. After the treatments, he was 86 years old and completely free from urinary retention and defecation problems.

Patient 3

A 59-year-old man was diagnosed with aggressive GS 9 (4 + 5 in biopsies) prostate cancer, when S-PSA was 28 μg/l. Based on metastatic disease staged by CT and bone scan, the man was told that the given therapies according to national and international guidelines are not curative. Therefore, he looked second opinion from my institution.

Multiparametric prostate MRI together with Na^{18}F- and ^{68}Ga-PSMA-PET/CT confirmed the T4N1M1 disease. Multiple pathologic lymph nodes can seen: Locoregionally, a 9 × 23 mm lymph node chain and a separate 7 mm node in the mesorectum on the left side, a 3 and a 5 mm suspicious node on the right side, and more cranially in the mesorectum at least two 7 mm nodes, a 9 mm obturator and a 9 mm external iliac node on the left and a 7 mm external iliac node, on the right metastatic (M1a) 10 mm right common iliac node. In ^{68}Ga-PSMA-PET-CT, active and aggressive prostate malignancy was observed mainly in the left lobe with local extension and extensive lymph node disease in the pelvic spaces, with the lymph node disease located predominantly on the left with a total volume of 75 cm^3, and it was very active with SUVmax ad 47. There were lymph node lesions in obturator, perirectal, parailiac (ext/int), common iliac, and presacral nodes. Widespread skeletal disease with a low volume (25 cm^3) was observed, but with high uptakes, e.g., in lower spine (SUVmax > 30); solitary metastases in the skull, spine, thorax, and left proximal femur. Since the disease was shown to be aggressive, man was young and otherwise very healthy, and the cancer cells appeared to be extremely avid to PSMA, we decided to start in good agreement with the patient the therapy using Lutetium^{177}-PSMA together with more traditional hormone treatment. Patient decided to stop smoking. In the first early response evaluation, PSA went down from 37.8 to 0.16 μ/l, and the response was confirmed also by ^{68}Ga-PSMA-PET-CT scanning, demonstrating practically complete response by imaging (Fig. 14.5). Earlier active and aggressive prostate malignancy was not anymore active (SUVmax < 2.7). The local extension and extensive and active lymph node disease in the pelvic and retroperitoneal spaces (obturator, perirectal, parailiac (ext/int), common iliac, presacral nodes) had completely vanished. Similarly, the widespread skeletal disease (skull, spine, thorax, and left proximal femur) had fully disappeared (Fig. 14.5). The PSMA-positive disease (skeletal 25 cm^3 + lymph nodes 75 cm^3) demonstrated a visual metabolic complete response. Quantitative "PERCIST" response turned out to be −93%. The biochemical response was excellent, S-PSA decline was 95.8% (Fig. 14.5).

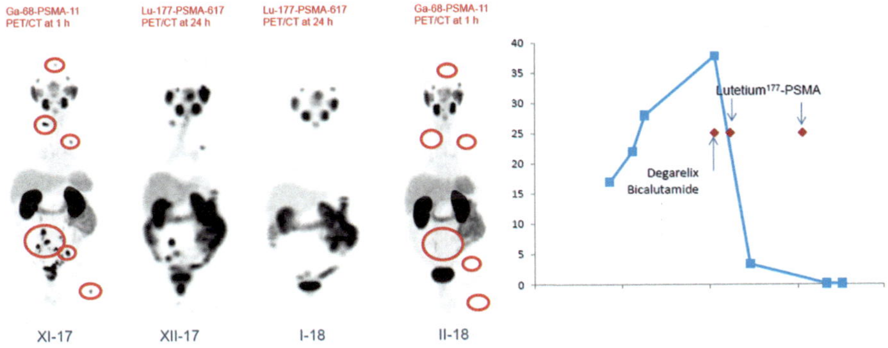

Fig. 14.5 The serum PSA (ng/ml) curve of the patient who received two ^{177}Lu-PSMA treatments as first-line therapy (right panel). Ga-68-PSMA-PET/CT studies performed before and 6 weeks after the ^{177}Lu-PSMA treatments (left panel). In the first Ga-68-PSMA-PET/CT study, i.e., before ^{177}Lu-PSMA therapies, multiple lymph node (obturator, perirectal, parailiac (ext/int), common iliac, presacral nodes) and skeletal metastases (skull, spine, thorax and left proximal femur) are seen, shown by red circles (left panel, most left). Normal organs, i.e., salivary and lacrimal glands, liver, spleen, visualize in the MIP images (all panels). The second Ga-68-PSMA-PET/CT study demonstrates that all metastases have disappeared (red circles, left panel, most right). The serum PSA decreased from 37.8 to 0.16 μg/l

Concluding Remarks

Here I describe three PCa patients who got major response with ^{177}Lu-PSMA-RLT: one patient with extensive metastatic disease in liver and lymph nodes after multiple therapies, one patient with extensive local invasive multiorgan disease, and one patient with metastatic disease where ^{177}Lu-PSMA was used as first-line treatment. The patient with large liver metastases had radical prostatectomy combined with chemical castration and radiation therapy and then anti-androgen and chemotherapies tens of cycles, including the newest third-line treatments, enzalutamide, abiraterone, and cabazitaxel. After all these therapies, he got almost a complete response after seven cycles of ^{177}Lu-PSMA-RLT (Fig. 14.4). The patient extensive local invasive multiorgan disease (the bladder, peritoneum, bowel walls, lymph node, and pelvic wall had no hope and severe life-limiting symptoms including urinary/defecation problems) got his life fully back and a major response after five cycles of ^{177}Lu-PSMA-RLT (Fig. 14.5). The third patient who got ^{177}Lu-PSMA as first-line treatment for aggressive (GS9) metastatic disease had almost a complete response after two cycles of ^{177}Lu-PSMA-RLT (Fig. 14.6). This is not always the case, but this is a possibility which can revolutionize the whole management of prostate cancer, if the patient selection is done properly. We know from our own meta-analysis that it is quite possible that ^{177}Lu could be even more effective than chemotherapies [21], which opinion is supported also by my own experience of several hundreds of treatments so far. Randomized studies comparing head-to-head chemotherapies with ^{177}Lu-PSMA treatment, such as [22], are needed—these treatments are here to stay. It seems also that progression-free survival might be markedly longer after ^{177}Lu than following more traditional chemotherapies. However, possible late side effects are not known yet, although not reported in a great extent. For the side-effect control, we developed a remote patient-reporting system for Lu-177-PSMA side effects. From this, it was easy to analyze if patient was responding: the more side effects, the less tumor burden. The principle is shown in Fig. 14.6. I presented this for the first time in Vienna in 2017 in the WARMTH Conference.

Our example really suggests that it might be worth to test and analyze Lutetium^{177}-PSMA as first-line therapy in randomized clinical setting. In one of our case, the lung metastases were only suspected due to the faint uptake of PSMA [31]. The metastases became much more visible during first ^{177}Lu therapy (the accumulation times are very different, because the ^{177}Lu-PSMA-SPECT was performed at 24 h, whereas the ^{68}Ga-PSMA-PET at 1 h). We found the same phenomenon in eye metastases, where we could visualize the metastasis with ^{177}Lu-PSMA-SPECT (at 24 h) but not with ^{18}F-PSMA-PET (at 1 h) [32]. This therapy works also in patients with multiclonal disease, e.g., we could treat one patient to almost a complete response after fifth recurrence during more than a 15-year follow-up [31].

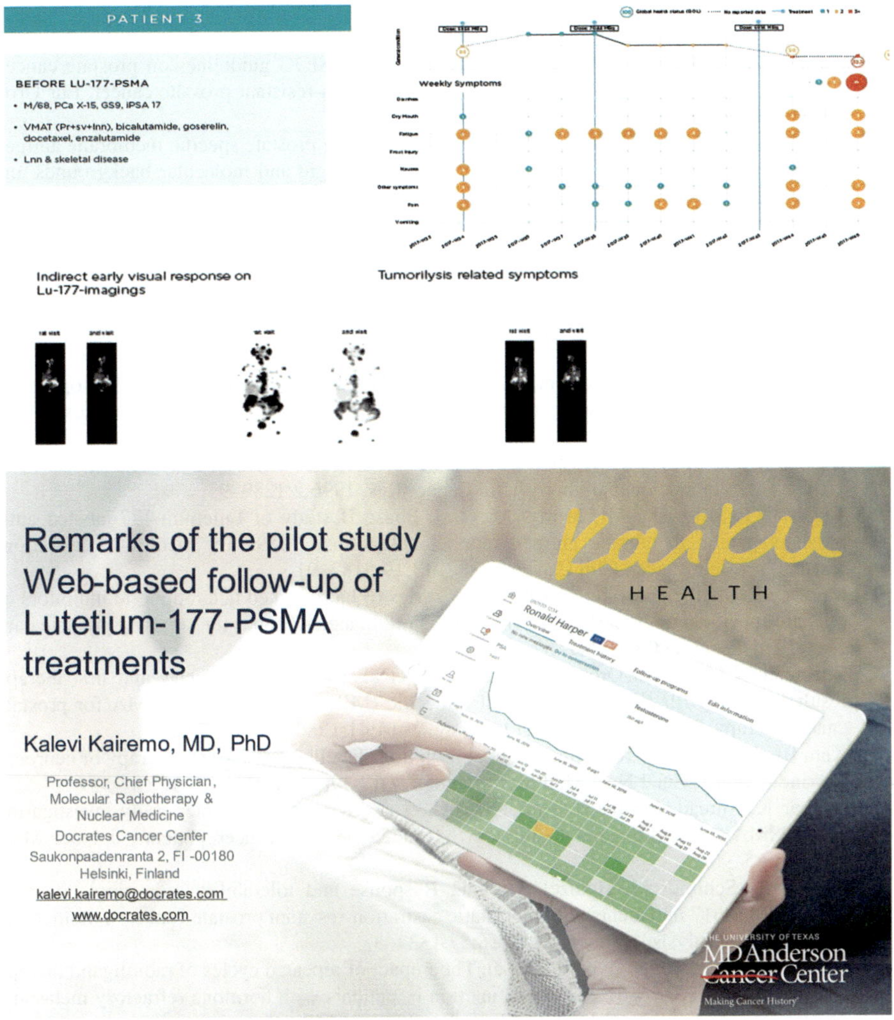

Fig. 14.6 Summary of the patient-reported symptoms of ^{177}Lu-PSMA-617 treatments. On the left, the summary of symptoms after three therapy cycles. The images below demonstrate the actual response—from it, it can be seen that symptoms increase in the summary table (left). On the right is my cover slide from the first presentation in Vienna in 2017 (WARMTH Conference)

In conclusion, my small series show that ^{177}Lu-PSMA therapy can be effective in the prostate, lymph nodes, bones, lungs, and liver. We propose that ^{177}Lu-PSMA should be studied as a new potential treatment of incurable metastatic prostate cancer instead of chemotherapy, besides the chemotherapy and not only in castration/hormone resistant phase but also as first-line therapy. Most importantly, those patients who would likely not to respond should be identified when experience accumulates.

References

1. Cornford P, Bellmunt J, Bolla M, et al. EAU-ESTRO-SIOG guidelines on prostate cancer. Part II: treatment of relapsing, metastatic, and castration-resistant prostate cancer. Eur Urol. 2017;71:630–42.
2. Santoni M, Scarpelli M, Mazzucchelli R, et al. Targeting prostate specific membrane antigen for personalized therapies in prostate cancer: morphologic and molecular backgrounds and future promises. J Biol Regul Homeost Agents. 2014;28:555–63.
3. Haberkorn U, Eder M, Kopka K, Babich JW, Eisenhut M. New strategies in prostate cancer: prostate-specific membrane antigen (PSMA) ligands for diagnosis and therapy. Clin Cancer Res. 2016;22:9–15.
4. Kratochwil C, Giesel FL, Eder M, et al. [^{177}Lu]Lutetium-labelled PSMA ligand-induced remission in a patient with metastatic prostate cancer. Eur J Nucl Med Mol Imaging. 2015;42(6):987–8.
5. Weineisen M, Schottelius M, Simeček J, et al. ^{68}Ga- and ^{177}Lu-labeled PSMA I&T: optimization of a PSMA-targeted theranostic concept and first proof-of-concept human studies. J Nucl Med. 2015;56:1169–76.
6. Deb N, Goris M, Trisler K, et al. Treatment of hormone-refractory prostate cancer with ^{90}Y-CYT-356 monoclonal antibody. Clin Cancer Res. 1996;2:1289–97.
7. Tagawa ST, Milowsky MI, Morris M, et al. Phase II study of Lutetium-177-labeled anti-prostate-specific membrane antigen monoclonal antibody J591 for metastatic castration-resistant prostate cancer. Clin Cancer Res. 2013;19:5182–91.
8. Maresca KP, Hillier SM, Femia FJ, et al. A series of halogenated heterodimeric inhibitors of prostate specific membrane antigen (PSMA) as radiolabeled probes for targeting prostate cancer. J Med Chem. 2009;52:347–57.
9. Zechmann CM, Afshar-Oromieh A, Armor T, et al. Radiation dosimetry and first therapy results with a (^{124})I/ (^{131})I-labeled small molecule (MIP-1095) targeting PSMA for prostate cancer therapy. Eur J Nucl Med Mol Imaging. 2014;41:1280–92.
10. Kam BL, Teunissen JJ, Krenning EP, et al. Lutetium-labelled peptides for therapy of neuroendocrine tumours. Eur J Nucl Med Mol Imaging. 2012;39(Suppl 1):S103–12.
11. Rahbar K, Ahmadzadehfar H, Kratochwil C, et al. German multicenter study investigating ^{177}Lu-PSMA-617 radioligand therapy in advanced prostate cancer patients. J Nucl Med. 2017;58:85–90.
12. Rahbar K, Schmidt M, Heinzel A, et al. Response and tolerability of a single dose of ^{177}Lu-PSMA-617 in patients with metastatic castration-resistant prostate cancer: a multicenter retrospective analysis. J Nucl Med. 2016;57:1334–8.
13. Yordanova A, Becker A, Eppard E, et al. The impact of repeated cycles of radioligand therapy using [^{177}Lu]Lu-PSMA-617 on renal function in patients with hormone refractory metastatic prostate cancer. Eur J Nucl Med Mol Imaging. 2017;44:1473–9.
14. Ahmadzadehfar H, Zimbelmann S, Yordanova A, et al. Radioligand therapy of metastatic prostate cancer using ^{177}Lu-PSMA-617 after radiation exposure to ^{223}Radichloride. Oncotarget. 2017;8:55567–74.
15. Rahbar K, Bode A, Weckesser M, et al. Radioligand therapy with ^{177}Lu-PSMA-617 as a novel therapeutic option in patients with metastatic castration resistant prostate cancer. Clin Nucl Med. 2016;41:522–8.
16. Ahmadzadehfar H, Wegen S, Yordanova A, et al. Overall survival and response pattern of castration-resistant metastatic prostate cancer to multiple cycles of radioligand therapy using [^{177}Lu]Lu-PSMA-617. Eur J Nucl Med Mol Imaging. 2017;44:1448–54.
17. Bräuer A, Grubert LS, Roll W, et al. 177Lu-PSMA-617 radioligand therapy and outcome in patients with metastasized castration-resistant prostate cancer. Eur J Nucl Med Mol Imaging. 2017;44:1663–70.

18. Delker A, Fendler WP, Kratochwil C, et al. Dosimetry for (^{177})Lu-DKFZ-PSMA-617: a new radiopharmaceutical for the treatment of metastatic prostate cancer. Eur J Nucl Med Mol Imaging. 2016;43:42.
19. Fendler WP, Rahbar K, Herrmann K, Kratochwil C, Eiber M. ^{177}Lu-PSMA radioligand therapy for prostate cancer. J Nucl Med. 2017;58:1196–200.
20. von Eyben FE, Kiljunen T, Joensuu T, Kairemo K, Uprimny C, Virgolini I. ^{177}Lu-PSMA-617 radioligand therapy for a patient with lymph node metastatic prostate cancer. Oncotarget. 2017;8:66112–6.
21. von Eyben FE, Roviello G, Kiljunen T, et al. Third-line treatment and ^{177}Lu-PSMA radioligand therapy of metastatic castration-resistant prostate cancer: a systematic review. Eur J Nucl Med Mol Imaging. 2018;45:496–508.
22. Hofman MS, Emmett L, Sandhu S, et al. (^{177}Lu)Lu-PSMA-617 versus cabazitaxel in patients with metastatic castration-resistant prostate cancer (TheraP): a randomised, open-label, phase 2 trial. Lancet (London, England). 2021;397(10276):797–804.
23. Sartor O, de Bono J, Chi KN, et al. Lutetium-177-PSMA-617 for metastatic castration-resistant prostate cancer. N Engl J Med. 2021;385:1091–103.
24. Sadaghiani MS, Sheikhbahaei S, Werner RA, et al. ^{177} Lu-PSMA radioligand therapy effectiveness in metastatic castration-resistant prostate cancer: an updated systematic review and meta-analysis. Prostate. 2022;82:826–35.
25. Ahmadzadehfar H, Eppard E, Kürpig S, et al. Therapeutic response and side effects of repeated radioligand therapy with ^{177}Lu-PSMA-DKFZ-617 of castrate-resistant metastatic prostate cancer. Oncotarget. 2016;7:12477–88.
26. Budäus L, Leyh-Bannurah SR, Salomon G, et al. Initial experience of (68)Ga-PSMA PET/CT imaging in high-risk prostate cancer patients prior to radical prostatectomy. Eur Urol. 2016;69:393–6.
27. Kulkarni HR, Singh A, Schuchardt C, et al. PSMA-based radioligand therapy for metastatic castration-resistant prostate cancer: the Bad Berka experience since 2013. J Nucl Med. 2016;57(Suppl 3):97S–104S.
28. Okamoto S, Thieme A, Allmann J, et al. Radiation dosimetry for ^{177}Lu-PSMA I&T in metastatic castration-resistant prostate cancer: absorbed dose in normal organs and tumor lesions. J Nucl Med. 2017;58:445–50.
29. Baum RP, Kulkarni HR, Schuchardt C, et al. ^{177}Lu-labeled prostate-specific membrane antigen radioligand therapy of metastatic castration-resistant prostate cancer: safety and efficacy. J Nucl Med. 2016;57:1006–13.
30. Kelk E, Ruuge P, Rohtla K, Poksi A, Kairemo K. Radiomics analysis for ^{177}Lu-DOTAGA-(l-y)fk(Sub-KuE) targeted radioligand therapy dosimetry in metastatic prostate cancer—a model based on clinical example. Life (Basel). 2021;11:170.
31. Kairemo K, Joensuu T. Lu-177-PSMA treatment for metastatic prostate cancer: case examples of major responses. Clin Translat Imaging. 2018;6:223–37.
32. Kairemo K, Kangasmäki A, Joensuu T, Seregard S. Eye symptoms in a patient with prostate cancer. Clin Nucl Med. 2020;45:370–1.

Part IV

Clinical Trials

Clinical Experience in ^{225}Ac-PSMA

15

^{225}Ac(Actinium-225)-PSMA (prostate-specific membrane antigen) is a radiopharmaceutical used in targeted alpha therapy (TAT). ^{225}Ac is promising due to its ability to cause irreparable double-strand DNA damage in cancer cells with minimal harm to surrounding healthy tissue. The alpha particles it emits are potent antitumor agents due to their high linear energy transfer (LET) and short tissue penetration.

In numerous clinical trials, ^{225}Ac-PSMA has shown high efficacy, particularly in patients who have failed conventional treatments. Studies demonstrate significant reductions in PSA (prostate-specific antigen) levels, with biochemical responses (PSA decline >50%) observed in a large percentage of patients. I have written a recent review with my German and South African colleagues [1].

The WARMTH Act study, a large-scale, real-world investigation, involving 488 patients, reported a PSA decline ≥50% in 57% of patients and a median overall survival (OS) of 15.5 months [2]. I had a privilege to write an editorial to this article [3].

In this chapter, the clinical use of ^{225}Ac-PSMA will be discussed.

Clinical Experience

Actinium-225 for PSMA-TAT ^{225}Ac has a half-life of 9.9 days and decays to produce four alpha particles with an energy of 5.8–8.4 MeV, with a tissue range of up to 85 μm [4]. This alpha emitter has been labeled to PSMA ligands as ^{225}Ac-PSMA for targeted alpha therapy (TAT). ^{225}Ac deposits high energy resulting in irreparable double-strand DNA destruction while sparing surrounding normal tissue making it an attractive antitumor agent. PSMA is a transmembrane protein highly expressed in prostate epithelial cells and is significantly

K. Kairemo, *Prostate Cancer from a Nuclear Oncology Perspective*,
https://doi.org/10.1007/978-3-031-90337-3_15

upregulated in prostate cancer, especially in metastatic disease. PSMA ligands, such as PSMA-617 or PSMA-I&T (Fig. 15.1), are used to deliver ^{225}Ac directly to the cancer cells, ensuring high precision and minimizing off-target effects. Clinical application of ^{225}Ac-PSMA TAT as last line of therapy in patients with mCRPC has demonstrated an excellent response, e.g., chemotherapy naive patients, although most clinical studies report it as third-line therapy or after a failure of ^{177}Lu-PRLT. Widespread application of ^{225}Ac-PSMA TAT is hampered by its salivary gland toxicity. The clinical studies are listed in Table 15.1, which are described in a more detailed manner in the following.

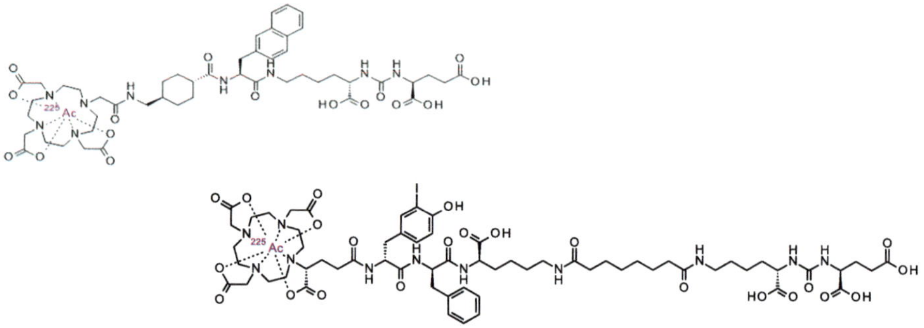

Fig. 15.1 Chemical structures of ^{225}Ac-PSMA-617 (left) and ^{225}Ac-PSMA-I&T (right)

Table 15.1 Clinical trials of Actinium-225-PSMA-targeted alpha therapy

	Number of patients	Activity per cycle/MBq	Biochemical response PSA_{50}	PFS/OS [mo]	Major toxicity	First author year [ref.#]
PSMA-617	2	100 kBq/kg	100% (2/2)		Xerostomia	Kratochwil 2016 [5]
PSMA-617	14	50–200 kBq/kg	44% (4/9)	na/8.5	Xerostomia	Kratochwil 2017 [6]
PSMA-617	40	100 kBq/kg	63% (24/38)	na/>12	Xerostomia	Kratochwil 2018 [7]
PSMA-617	17	4–8	88% (15/17)		Xerostomia	Sathekge 2019b [8]
PSMA-617	73	4–8	70% (51/73)	15.2/18.0		Sathekge 2020 [9]
PSMA-617	26	4–8	65% (17/26)	3.5/7.7	XerostomiaHb↓, WBC↓, plt↓	Feuerecker 2020 [10]
PSMA-617	28	100 kBq/kg	39% (11/28)	12/17	Xerostomia, fatigue	Yadav 2020 [11]
PSMA-617	13	6–8	69% (9/13)	na/8.5	Xerostomia	van der Doelen 2020 [12]
PSMA-617	11	100 kBq/kg	45% (5/11)		Xerostomia	Satapathy 2020 [13]

(continued)

Table 15.1 (continued)

	Number of patients	Activity per cycle/MBq	Biochemical response PSA_{50}	PFS/OS [mo]	Major toxicity	First author year [ref.#]
PSMA-617	20	5.3 (1.5–7.9)	65% (13/20)	4.7/11	Xerostomia	Khreish 2020 [14]
PSMA-617	15	2.7 ± 1.1	53% (8/15)	na/19.4	Xerostomia	Rosar 2021 [15]
PSMA-617	12	100 kBq/kg	50% (6/12)	4/10	Xerostomia	Sanli 2021 [16]
PSMA-617	38	100 kBq/kg	66% (25/38)	8/12	Xerostomia	Sen 2021 [17]
PSMA-617	53	8	91% (48/53)	20/>55	Xerostomia	Sathekge 2022 [18]
PSMA-617	106	8	80% (85/106)	14.0/15.0	Xerostomia	Lawal 2022 [19]
PSMA-617	21	8	86% (18/21)	>36/>36	Xerostomia	Sathekge 2023 [20]
PSMA-617	488	6–8	57% (278/488)	7.9/15.5	Xerostomia	Sathekge 2024 [2]
PSMA-I&T	1	8	100% (1/1)	na	Xerostomia	Ilhan 2020 [21]
PSMA-I&T	14	7.8	50% (7/14)	na	Xerostomia	Zacherl 2021 [22]
PSMA-I&T	25	100 kBq/kg	50% (10/20)	na	Xerostomia	Delpassand 2024 [23]

Updated from Kairemo et al. [1]

Clinical Efficacy

The first human studies with ^{225}Ac-PSMA were performed by Kratochwil et al. [5], who observed a complete biochemical response (PSA levels undetectable) in two patients who had previously failed multiple lines of therapy. Both patients demonstrated complete tumor responses on PET/CT imaging, and their PSA levels dropped below measurable thresholds after receiving 100 kBq/kg of ^{225}Ac-PSMA-617 every 8 weeks. Subsequent studies confirmed these findings in larger patient cohorts. For example, Feuerecker et al. [10] investigated 26 patients who had failed a median of 6 prior lines of therapy. The PSA decline exceeded 50% in 65% of patients, with 88% showing some PSA reduction.

The most extensive study to date, the WARMTH Act [2], included 488 patients across 4 countries (South Africa, India, Germany, and Australia). It showed a PSA decline of ≥50% in 57% of patients, with median overall survival (OS) of 15.5 months and progression-free survival (PFS) of 7.9 months. This study confirmed that ^{225}Ac-PSMA could effectively treat advanced prostate cancer even in late-stage disease when conventional therapies had failed.

In the literature, four meta-analyses have been published; the results have been listed in Table 15.2. All these meta-analyses had more than 200 pts and consisted of 6–10 original studies (Table 15.2). The populations overlapped in these studies although they had slightly different criteria—the combined data takes the overlap into account. The first meta-analysis included patients who had advanced, progressive mCRPC and who were ineligible for conventional radiotherapy [24]. Ma et al. [25] included patients who had failed conventional second- or third-line therapies. The patient inclusion criteria were not properly stated in [26], and in the study by Parida et al. [27], the patients had failed on multiple forms of conventional treatments which were not specified. These all studies were observational and retrospective—only single studies might have included prospective approach and mainly Ac-225-PSMA-617 was used. In the meta-analyses, only a single article with Ac-225-PSAM-I&T was included.

The results of these meta-analyses have been compared with those of the recent WARMTH Act study [2] consisting of 488 patients (Table 15.2). The results of meta-analyses give slightly better results, because they base on smaller and selected patient populations. The WARMTH Act study is a global real world evidence summary from four countries (South Africa, India, Germany, and Australia). This work was published in Lancet Oncology and commented in the editorial [3]. A comparison of these meta-analyses [24–27] shows response rates of 60–70%, with PFS ranging from 6 to 9.2 months and OS of 12–15 months. The therapeutic effects are more pronounced in smaller, more selective populations than in large-scale studies like the WARMTH trial [2], which includes more diverse patient groups.

Several clinical trials have documented the success of ^{225}Ac-PSMA in treating patients with advanced prostate cancer. For example, Kratochwil et al. reported complete responses in patients after multiple lines of failed therapies [7]. Moreover, Sathekge et al. noted an 82% PSA decline in chemotherapy-naïve patients [20].

Table 15.2 Combined meta-analyzes of Actinium-225-PSMA-targeted alpha therapy in comparison with the WARMTH Act trial

	Satapathy 2021 [24]	Ma 2022 [25]	Lee 2022 [26]	Parida 2023 [27]	Combined	Sathekge 2024 [2]
Patient number	256 (10)	201 (6)	263 (9)	226 (8)		488
Response >50%	63	66	61	60	62	57
Any response	67	87	84	81	82	73
Molecular response	74	54	n.a.	29	54	n.a.
PFS (months)	9.1	9.1	9.2	6	9.1	7.9
OS (months)	12.8	12.5	11.8	12.8	12.6	15.5
Xerostomia	73	77	63	74	73	68
Anemia	12.3	30.3 (7.5)	n.a. (14.4)	n.a. (10.8)	10.8	81 (13)
Leukocytopenia	8.3	n.a. (4.4)	n.a. (4.1)	5.9		44 (4)
Thrombocytopenia	6.3	n.a. (5.5)	n.a. (7.2)	4.7		54 (7)
Nephrotoxicity	3.8	n.a. (3.0)	n.a.	3.8	3.8	5

Modified from Vorster et al. [28]

The most common side effect is xerostomia (dry mouth), which is dose-limiting and often leads to discontinuation of therapy in up to 25% of patients. Other notable toxicities include anemia, leukocytopenia, and nephrotoxicity, though these are less frequent. Various strategies are being explored to mitigate xerostomia, such as reducing the activity of ^{225}Ac or using alternative therapies like ^{177}Lu-PSMA to reduce the radiation load on the salivary glands. Dosimetry studies show that salivary glands receive the highest radiation dose, which correlates with the high incidence of xerostomia. Efforts to optimize dosimetry are ongoing, though imaging-based dosimetry for alpha particles remains challenging. ^{225}Ac-PSMA is a highly effective therapy for patients with metastatic prostate cancer, especially those who have exhausted other treatment options. However, its widespread use is currently limited by side effects like xerostomia, necessitating ongoing research into dose optimization and combination therapies.

The results of 1174 therapy cycles in 488 patients were very convincing, because a substantial antitumor effect (prostate-specific antigen [PSA] decline of ≥50%) occurred in 278 (57%) patients, and a median overall survival of 15.5 months (95% CI 13.4–18.3) and progression-free survival of 7.9 months (6.8–8.9) were observed in this late stage of prostate cancer [2]. In these patients, multiple factors were found to be associated with overall survival and progression-free survival. These factors included, for example, PSA response, previous treatments (chemotherapy, prostate RLT, androgen blockade) received before ^{225}Ac-PSMA RLT, the type of metastases (e.g., liver, peritoneum), and the presence of anemia at baseline. In this study, it has been shown that ^{225}Ac-PSMA RLT works in distinguished institutions worldwide in clinical practice, including in patients with very advanced mCRPC disease and who have not responded to several previous therapies [2].

PMSA-617 has been the main theragnostic agent which has been under review in TAT in mCRPC; however, PSMA-I&T has been investigated in ^{177}Lu-PSMA radioligand therapy and did not show any inferiority in the literature when compared to ^{177}Lu-PSMA-617 [29]. The first clinical data using ^{225}Ac-PSMA-I&T showed highly comparable biochemical responses as after ^{225}Ac-PSMA-617 TAT [21, 22]. Zacherl et al. were the first to study a clinical cohort with PMSA-I&T in TAT [22]. Fourteen patients who were either not eligible for or had failed conventional therapy were included in the study with 79% of these patients having had received prior ^{177}Lu-PSMA radioligand therapy. ^{18}F-PSMA-1007 PET/CT was used to assess suitability for therapy [22]. This group demonstrated a PSA decline ≥50% of 45% and any PSA decline of 73% in the subgroup of patients who had received prior ^{177}Lu-PSMA radioligand therapy which is comparable with other groups which have investigated ^{225}Ac-PSMA therapy in patients who have failed ^{177}Lu-PSMA radioligand therapy [22]. Delpassand et al. [23] report at AACR conference that 35 patients had been injected with ^{225}Ac-PSMA-I&T in a trial by Fusion Pharmaceuticals, 25 patients had received all planned cycles, and 20 patients had been analyzed for response in this interim analysis. The PSA decline ≥50% was observed in 10 patients and PSA response in 14 patients [23].

Radioresistance Some patients exhibit radioresistance to PSMA-TAT due to mutations in DNA damage repair genes (e.g., BRCA1, BRCA2). Radioresistance as a result of mutations in the genes responsible for DNA repair has been thought to be the reason that some patients did not demonstrate a response to ^{225}Ac-PSMA TAT despite demonstrating tumor PSMA expression as evidenced by intense tumor uptake of tracer on PSMA PET/CT imaging [30]. Kratochwil et al. identified 10 patients out of 60 who presented with a poor response to ^{225}Ac-PSMA-617, despite sufficient tumor uptake in PSMA PET/CT [30]. They took CT-guided biopsies with histologic validation of the nonresponding lesions in seven of these nonresponding patients. Specimens were analyzed by next generation sequencing (NGS) interrogating 37 DNA damage-repair-associated genes. Seven tumor samples were analyzed, of which a total of 15 whole-gene deletions, deleterious or presumably deleterious mutations were found affecting TP53 (n = 3), CHEK2 (n = 2), ATM (n = 2), and BRCA1, BRCA2, PALB2, MSH2, MSH6, NBN, FANCB, and PMS1 (n = 1 each). The average number of deleterious or presumably deleterious mutations was 2.2 (range, 0–6) per patient. In addition, several variants of unknown significance in ATM, BRCA1, MSH2, SLX4, ERCC, and various FANC genes were detected. Patients with resistance to PSMA-TAT despite PSMA positivity frequently harbor mutations in DNA damage repair and checkpoint genes. These findings encourage future studies combining PSMA-TAT and DNA damage-repair–targeting agents such as PARP inhibitors. Radioresistance is a significant challenge in prostate cancer treatment. Because genetic analyses of tumor biopsies have revealed that mutations in DNA repair genes (e.g., TP53, BRCA1, BRCA2, ATM) are often associated with poor responses to ^{225}Ac-PSMA, these findings suggest that combining ^{225}Ac-PSMA with PARP inhibitors (which target DNA repair pathways) could help overcome radioresistance in these patients [30].

Toxicity and Treatment Optimization

Despite its efficacy, toxicity, particularly in the salivary glands and kidneys, limits the widespread use of ^{225}Ac-PSMA therapy.

^{225}Ac-PSMA TAT Toxicity Profile

Salivary Glands The most common and dose-limiting toxicity is xerostomia (dry mouth). In the clinical setting, several studies reported toxicity related to TAT with ^{225}Ac-PSMA-617/PSMA-I&T (Tables 15.1 and 15.2). Studies report that 10–25% of patients discontinue treatment due to severe xerostomia, caused by the high radiation dose absorbed by the salivary glands. Modifying doses, reducing the number of treatment cycles, and using protective interventions like **sialendoscopy** (a procedure to clear and irrigate salivary glands) have shown limited success in mitigating this side effect [31]. Xerostomia should, therefore, be prevented. Modification of the administered activity of ^{225}Ac-PSMA-617 and the number of cycles of TAT may decrease the side effects while still achieving response [9, 14]. Sialendoscopy with dilatation, saline irrigation, and steroid injection (prednisolone) have been investigated in patients with some but limited success [32]. Eleven men with metastatic castration-resistant prostate cancer underwent sialendoscopy and injection of both submandibular and both parotid glands before or after every cycle of ^{225}Ac-PSMA-617 TAT [32]. In all 11 patients, both parotid and both submandibular glands were affected by radiation sialadenitis [32]. Sialendoscopy had beneficial effects on salivary gland function and quality of life in patients undergoing ^{225}Ac-PSMA-617 RLT. However, even with sialadenoscopic support after multiple cycles of TAT, salivary gland function was reduced and xerostomia was present. Therefore, not only inflammation but also the direct effect of radiation is a putative cause of dry mouth [32]. Cooling techniques during therapy and botulinum toxin injections have also been explored to protect the salivary glands from radiation exposure. These strategies offer temporary relief but are not widely adopted [31]. Therefore, effective methods to reduce salivary toxicity are needed.

Kidneys Kidneys are at risk due to their physiological expression of PSMA and the excretion of radionuclides. While renal toxicity is less frequent than xerostomia, it is still a concern. Some patients have reported chronic kidney disease or worsened renal function following treatment [33].

If PSMA on the surface of cancer cells is not sufficiently internalized after binding of the ligand, TAT with ^{225}Ac with multiple unstable daughters might be suboptimal and toxic [7]. It has also been speculated that the radioactive daughters of ^{225}Ac, but not ^{225}Ac-PSMA-617, can accumulate in the tubular cells and irradiate the kidneys, leading to renal injury.

Hematologic Toxicity Anemia, leukopenia, and thrombocytopenia (low blood counts) are other side effects. However, the short range of alpha particles (47–85 μm) in tissue helps limit hematological toxicity, making it manageable in most patients. Still, individuals with bone marrow involvement or preexisting myelosuppression are more likely to develop these complications [19].

The summarized hematological toxicity data of ^{225}Ac-PSMA-PSMA-RLT from a meta-analysis is presented in Fig. 15.2.

General Safety Measures Though PSMA is highly expressed prostate cancer cells, physiological expression of PSMA is seen in the lacrimal glands, salivary glands, gastrointestinal tract, and renal tubular cells [1]. Binding to these nonmalignant tissue PSMA-expressing sites is responsible for the side effects that are seen with ^{225}Ac-PSMA therapy. Probably, therefore also xeropthalmia has been reported after ^{225}Ac-PSMA-TAT [34]. Safety measures that may be adopted to reduce the risk of developing nephrotoxicity include baseline screening, e.g., with ^{99m}Tc-MAG3

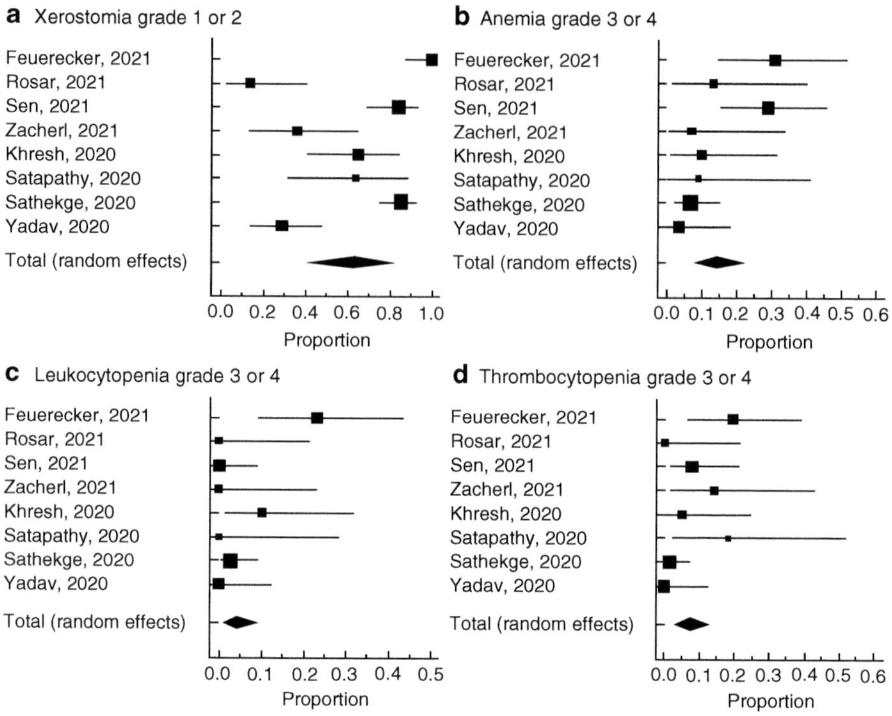

Fig. 15.2 Grade 1 and 2 xerostomia (**a**) and grade 3 and 4 hematologic adverse events after Ac-225-PSMA-RLT: anemia (**b**), leukopenia (**c**), thrombocytopenia (**d**). (Forest plot presentations from the meta-analysis by Lee and Kim [26]. Copyright from The Society of Nuclear Medicine)

renal scintigraphy: to exclude obstructive renal pathology (or correct it when feasible). Co-administration of normal saline with the radioligand is recommended. Patients with poor baseline renal function maybe at risk of developing severe nephrotoxicity [8]. Most patients have demonstrated favorable nephrotoxicity to ^{225}Ac-PSMA. However, it is known that with radionuclide therapy radiation, induced renal injury may develop at a delayed stage and thus be missed in the reported cohorts.

Salivary gland toxicity is the most common toxicity from TAT with ^{225}Ac-PSMA. Symptoms from xerostomia may range from mild symptoms to severe symptoms without requiring dietary changes to severe symptoms requiring nasogastric feeding or total parenteral nutrition. In a case series, salivary gland toxicity was the dose-limiting factor as patients refused any further treatment with ^{225}Ac-PSMA due to intolerable xerostomia [7]. Salivary gland toxicity is dose dependent—even irreversible severe xerostomia may develop when high cumulative activity is administered. To improve salivary gland toxicity, Sathekge et al. used a "dynamic de-escalation" where 8 MBq of ^{225}Ac-PSMA was the initial activity—a patient with three cycles (8, 6, and 6 MBq) is shown in Fig. 15.3. If the patient

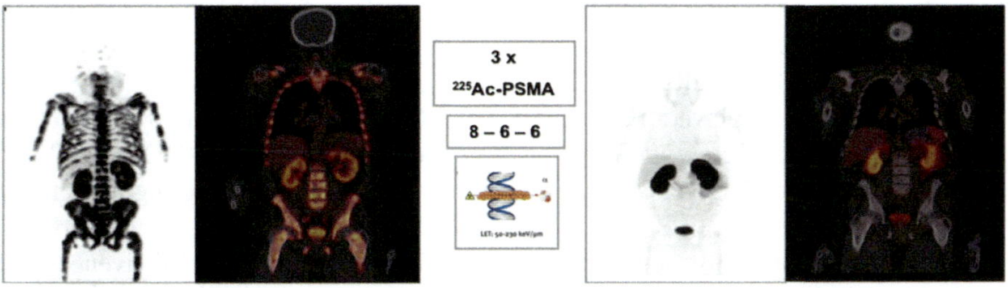

Fig. 15.3 A 67-year-old prostate cancer (GS 4 + 5) patient with a widespread skeletal disease. Complete visual response was observed after three cycles of ^{225}Ac-PSMA and no bone marrow toxicity. (Adopted from [35])

demonstrated a good response after the first cycle, then the subsequent activity was reduced by 2 MBq—this process is then repeated again prior to the third cycle down to 4 MBq. This approach resulted in patients reporting only grade 2 xerostomia and no need for withdrawal of treatment due to salivary gland toxicity [8]. Tandem administration of a reduced ^{225}Ac-PMSA and full dose ^{177}Lu-PMSA has also been used as an alternative approach to reduce the severity of salivary gland toxicity without compromising PSA response [14].

Dosimetric Aspects

Dosimetry studies have demonstrated that the salivary glands receive the highest absorbed dose of the nontarget organs [5]. The mechanism of PSMA uptake in the salivary glands has not been fully understood—to date, several interventions have been reviewed to improve patient quality of life; however, these attempts at preventing salivary gland toxicity have been unsuccessful. These strategies have been discussed earlier, and in order to predict the grade of salivary gland toxicity, the absorbed radiation dose should be measured.

Relative Biological Effectiveness (RBE) The basis for clinical dosimetry calculations has been the relative biological effectiveness (RBE = 5) found in an experimental study in a mouse model using immunohistochemical γH2AX-foci formation as an indicator for the amount of DNA double-strand breaks [36]. The response to internal radiotherapy between α- and β-emission (^{225}Ac/^{177}Lu) as a biological consequence of different ionization densities along a particle track was measured in somatostatin expressing AR42J cells which were incubated with octreotate analogs ^{225}Ac-DOTATOC and ^{177}Lu-DOTATOC up to 48 h. The cell viability was analyzed using the common MTT assay. DNA double-strand breaks were quantified by immunofluorescence staining of γH2AX foci, and cell cycle was analyzed by flow cytometry. In vivo uptake of both radiolabeled somatostatin analogues into subcutaneously growing AR42J tumors and the number of cells displaying γH2AX-foci was measured [36].

^{225}Ac-DOTATOC resulted in ED_{50} values of 14 kBq/ml after 48 h, whereas ^{177}Lu-DOTATOC displayed ED_{50} values of 10 MBq/ml. The number of DNA double-strand breaks grew with increasing concentration of ^{225}Ac-DOTATOC and similarly with ^{177}Lu-DOTATOC when applying a factor of 700-fold higher activity compared to ^{225}Ac [36].

Ruigrok et al. [36] evaluated the relative biological effectiveness of [^{225}Ac]Ac-PSMA-I&T and [^{177}Lu]Lu-PSMA-I&T by assessing in vitro binding characteristics, dosimetry, and therapeutic efficacy. In the PSMA-expressing PCa cell line, PC3-PIP binding and displacement assays were performed, which revealed similar binding characteristics between [^{225}Ac]Ac-PSMA-I&T and [^{177}Lu]Lu-PSMA-I&T. The cells treated with [^{225}Ac]Ac-PSMA-I&T had slower DSB repair kinetics compared to cells treated with [^{177}Lu]Lu-PSMA-I&T, when the number of 53BP1 foci, a marker for the number of DNA double-strand breaks (DSBs), was assessed. Additionally, clonogenic survival assays showed that specific targeting with [^{225}Ac]Ac-PSMA-I&T and [^{177}Lu]Lu-PSMA-I&T caused a dose-dependent decrease in survival. Lastly, after dosimetric assessment, the relative biological effectiveness (RBE) of [^{225}Ac]Ac-PSMA-I&T was found to be **4.2** times higher compared to [^{177}Lu]Lu-PSMA-I&T [37].

Dose Finding The clinical dosimetry basis and dose finding study was performed by using the isotopes ^{225}Ac and ^{177}Lu by Kratochwil et al. [5]. A dosimetry estimate was calculated on the basis of time-activity curves derived from serially obtained ^{177}Lu-PSMA-617 scans extrapolated to the physical half-life of ^{225}Ac, assuming instant decay of unstable daughter nuclides. Salvage therapies empirically conducted with 50 (n = 4), 100 (n = 4), 150 (n = 2), and 200 kBq/kg (n = 4) of 225Ac-PSMA-617 were evaluated retrospectively regarding toxicity and treatment response. Eight of 14 patients received further cycles in either 2- or 4-month intervals with identical or de-escalated activities.

From this study, the following dosimetry estimates were observed for 1 MBq of ^{225}Ac-PSMA-617 assuming a relative biologic effectiveness of 5: 2.3 Sv for salivary glands, 0.7 Sv for kidneys, and 0.05 Sv for red marrow that are composed of 99.4% α-, 0.5% β-, and 0.1% photon radiation, respectively [5]. In Table 15.3, the absorbed radiation dose estimates for ^{225}Ac-PSMA-617 are shown together with ^{131}I-"PSMA" and ^{177}Lu-PSMA-617 doses [5]. We see that mean dose for salivary glands is approximately 70% higher with ^{225}Ac-PSMA-617 than with ^{177}Lu-PSMA-617, and red marrow dose 85% higher, respectively. Note that Table 15.3 uses RBE 4.2, because this number is based on prostate cancer models in animals and in vitro experiments.

In clinical application, severe xerostomia became the dose-limiting toxicity if treatment activity exceeded 100 kBq/kg per cycle. At 100 kBq/kg, the duration of prostate-specific antigen decline was less than 4 months, but if therapy was repeated

Table 15.3 Dosimetry in critical organs with Ac-225-PSMA-617 and other PSMA-radionuclide therapies

	Kratochwil [5]	Zechmann [38]	Kratochwil [39]
Dose-limiting organ	^{225}Ac-PSMA-617 ($Sv_{RBE=4.2}$/7.4 MBq)[a]	^{131}I-MIP-1095 (Gy/3.7GBq)[a]	^{177}Lu-PSMA-617 (Gy /7.4 GBq)[a]
Salivary glands	14.5	17.1	10.2
Kidneys	4.60	5.37	5.55
Red marrow	0.31	1.15	0.22

Basic data from [5], recalculated using RBE = 4.2
[a]The activities represent typical therapy doses

every 2 months, patients experienced additive antitumor effects. Treatment activities of 50 kBq/kg were without toxicity but induced insufficient antitumor response in these high-tumor-burden patients. Remarkable antitumor activity by means of objective radiologic response or tumor marker decline was observed in 9 of 11 evaluable patients [5]. For advanced-stage patients, a treatment activity of 100 kBq/kg of ^{225}Ac-PSMA-617 per cycle repeated every 8 weeks presents a reasonable trade-off between toxicity and biochemical response.

Gamma Imaging The clinical dosimetry for ^{225}Ac is cumbersome. Even though dosimetry in clinical radionuclide therapy practice is mandatory according to EU guidelines, there are no tools available for clinical practice. One attempt has been shown in the literature. Because the ^{225}Ac decay chain shows a noticeable gamma emission (440 keV, 25.9%; 218 keV, 11.4%) (Fig. 15.4), it may be used for SPECT imaging. However, recommended low therapeutic activities (4–8 MBq) limit the clinical applicability of SPECT, although initial attempts for ^{225}Ac imaging exist. Gosewisch et al. [40] reported a mCRPC patient (65 years), whose imaging of the abdomen was performed at 24 h p.i. after therapeutic activity of 8.1 MBq ^{225}Ac-PSMA-I&T on a SPECT/CT camera (γ-energy 440 keV; window 20%). Final absorbed dose assessment was performed by combining the single ^{225}Ac image with the effective half-life information determined from a previous ^{177}Lu-PSMA-I&T imaging sequence. This resulted in an absorbed dose of 0.18 and 0.17 $Sv_{(RBE=5)}$/MBq for the left and right kidney, respectively, compared with 0.27 and 0.24 Gy/GBq for the preceding ^{177}Lu cycle (6.2 GBq). A comparison with the pre-therapy ^{18}F-PSMA-I&T PET/CT demonstrates that ^{225}Ac SPECT imaging for this patient was able to locate a small lesion in the right hip. The ^{225}Ac-absorbed dose was determined as 0.26 $Sv_{(RBE=5)}$/MBq, compared with 0.35 Gy/GBq for ^{177}Lu-PSMA-I&T.

In summary, the precise dosimetry for clinical practice is extremely complex and time consuming. Additionally, it is based on several assumptions, because only two of the actual alpha decays can be imaged quantitatively in patients. On the other hand, the clinical data speaks for itself, and major essential threats or hazards have been observed in the clinical practice globally [3].

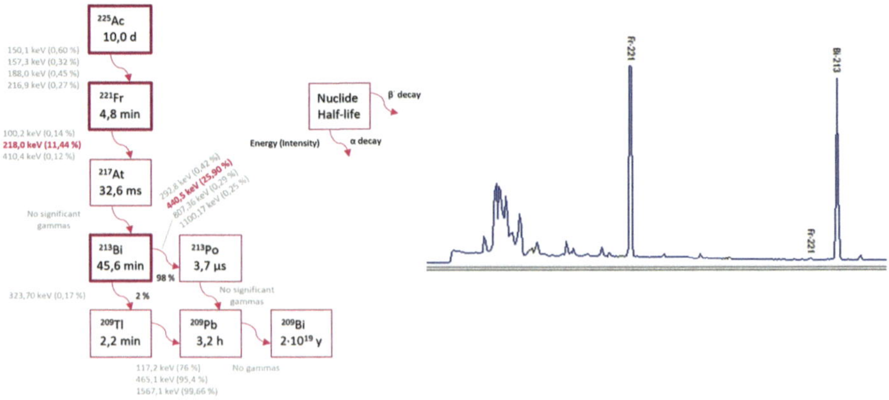

Fig. 15.4 Ac-225 decay scheme with essential gamma energies (left) and gamma spectrum

Conclusive Remarks

^{225}Ac-PSMA represents a highly promising therapy for mCRPC, especially in patients who have exhausted conventional options. Its efficacy is notable, particularly in reducing PSA level and controlling tumor progression, even in heavily pretreated patients. However, its clinical adoption is limited by significant side effects, particularly xerostomia, and the need for more precise dosimetry. Research into combination therapies and protective measures for nontarget organs will be critical in optimizing its clinical use.

References

1. Kairemo K, Kgatle M, Bruchertseifer F, Morgernstern A, Sathekge MM. Design of ^{225}Ac-PSMA for targeted alpha therapy in prostate cancer. Ann Transl Med. 2024; https://doi.org/10.21037/atm-23-1842.
2. Sathekge MM, Lawal IO, Bal C, et al. Actinium-225-PSMA radioligand therapy of metastatic castration-resistant prostate cancer (WARMTH Act): a multicentre, retrospective study. Lancet Oncol. 2024;25:175–83.
3. Kairemo K. Targeted alpha therapy: a new tool for advanced prostate cancer. Lancet Oncol. 2024;25(2):148–9.
4. Morgenstern A, Apostolidis C, Kratochwil C, Sathekge M, Krolicki L, Bruchertseifer F. An overview of targeted alpha therapy with (^{225})actinium and (^{213})bismuth. Curr Radiopharm. 2018;11(3):200–8.
5. Kratochwil C, Bruchertseifer F, Giesel FL, et al. ^{225}Ac-PSMA-617 for PSMA-targeted alpha-radiation therapy of metastatic castration-resistant prostate cancer. J Nucl Med. 2016;57:1941–4.
6. Kratochwil C, Bruchertseifer F, Rathke H, et al. Targeted alpha-therapy of metastatic castration-resistant prostate cancer with (^{225}) Ac-PSMA-617: dosimetry estimate and empiric dose finding. J Nucl Med. 2017;58:1624–31.

7. Kratochwil C, Bruchertseifer F, Rathke H, et al. Targeted alpha-therapy of metastatic castration-resistant prostate cancer with (^{225}) Ac-PSMA-617: swimmer-plot analysis suggests efficacy regarding duration of tumor control. J Nucl Med. 2018;59:795–802.
8. Sathekge M, Bruchertseifer F, Knoesen O, et al. (^{225})Ac-PSMA-617 in chemotherapy-naive patients with advanced prostate cancer: a pilot study. Eur J Nucl Med Mol Imaging. 2019;46:129–38.
9. Sathekge M, Bruchertseifer F, Vorster M, et al. Predictors of overall and disease-free survival in metastatic castration-resistant prostate cancer patients receiving (^{225}) Ac-PSMA-617 radioligand therapy. J Nucl Med. 2020;61:62–9.
10. Feuerecker B, Tauber R, Knorr K, et al. Activity and adverse events of actinium-225-PSMA-617 in advanced metastatic castration-resistant prostate cancer after failure of lutetium-177-PSMA. Eur Urol. 2021;79(3):343–50.
11. Yadav MP, Ballal S, Sahoo RK, Tripathi M, Seth A, Bal C. Efficacy and safety of (^{225}) Ac-PSMA-617 targeted alpha therapy in metastatic castration-resistant prostate cancer patients. Theranostics. 2020;10:9364–77.
12. van der Doelen MJ, Mehra N, van Oort IM, et al. Clinical outcomes and molecular profiling of advanced metastatic castration-resistant prostate cancer patients treated with ^{225}Ac-PSMA-617 targeted alpha-radiation therapy. Urol Oncol. 2020;39(10):1–10.
13. Satapathy S, Mittal BR, Sood A, et al. Health-related quality-of-life outcomes with actinium-225-prostate-specific membrane antigen-617 therapy in patients with heavily pre-treated metastatic castration-resistant prostate cancer. Indian J Nucl Med. 2020;35:299–304.
14. Khreish F, Ebert N, Ries M, et al. (^{225}) Ac-PSMA-617/ (^{177}) Lu-PSMA-617 tandem therapy of metastatic castration-resistant prostate cancer: pilot experience. Eur J Nucl Med Mol Imaging. 2020;47:721–8.
15. Rosar F, Krause J, Bartholomä M, et al. Efficacy and safety of [^{225}Ac]Ac-PSMA-617 augmented [^{177}Lu]Lu-PSMA-617 radioligand therapy in patients with highly advanced mCRPC with poor prognosis. Pharmaceutics. 2021;13:722.
16. Sanli Y, Kuyumcu S, Simsek DH, et al. ^{225}Ac-prostate-specific membrane antigen therapy for castration-resistant prostate cancer: a single-center experience. Clin Nucl Med. 2021;46:943–51.
17. Sen I, Thakral P, Tiwari P, et al. Therapeutic efficacy of ^{225}Ac-PSMA-617 targeted alpha therapy in patients of metastatic castrate resistant prostate cancer after taxane-based chemotherapy. Ann Nucl Med. 2021;35:794–810.
18. Sathekge MM, Bruchertseifer F, Lawal IO, et al. Treatment of brain metastases of castration-resistant prostate cancer with (^{225})Ac-PSMA-617. Eur J Nucl Med Mol Imaging. 2019;46:1756–7.
19. Lawal IO, Morgenstern A, Vorster M, et al. Hematologic toxicity profile and efficacy of [^{225}Ac]Ac-PSMA-617 α-radioligand therapy of patients with extensive skeletal metastases of castration-resistant prostate cancer. Eur J Nucl Med Mol Imaging. 2022;49(10):3581–92. https://doi.org/10.1007/s00259-022-05778-w2022.
20. Sathekge M, Bruchertseifer F, Vorster M, et al. ^{225}Ac-PSMA-617 radioligand therapy of de novo metastatic hormone-sensitive prostate carcinoma (mHSPC): preliminary clinical findings. Eur J Nucl Med Mol Imaging. 2023;50(7):2210–8. https://doi.org/10.1007/s00259-023-06165-9. Epub ahead of print. PMID: 36864360
21. Ilhan H, Gosewisch A, Böning G, et al. Response to (^{225}) Ac-PSMA-I&T after failure of long-term (^{177}) Lu-PSMA RLT in mCRPC. Eur J Nucl Med Mol Imaging. 2021;48:1262–3.
22. Zacherl MJ, Gildehaus FJ, Mittlmeier L, et al. First clinical results for PSMA targeted alpha therapy using (^{225}) Ac-PSMA-I&T in advanced mCRPC patients. J Nucl Med. 2021;62:669–74.
23. Delpassand ES, Hashmi MJ, Kazakin J, et al. Preliminary efficacy and safety results from the TATCIST trial: a PSMA-directed targeted alpha therapy with FPI-2265 (225Ac-PSMA-I&T) for the treatment of metastatic castration-resistant prostate cancer. Abstracts the American Association for Cancer Research (AACR) annual meeting; April 5–10, 2024; San Diego, CA.

24. Satapathy S, Sood A, Das CK, Mittal BR. Evolving role of ^{225}Ac-PSMA radioligand therapy in metastatic castration-resistant prostate cancer—a systematic review and meta-analysis. Prostate Cancer Prostatic Dis. 2021;24(3):880–90.
25. Ma J, Li L, Liao T, Gong W, Zhang C. Efficacy and safety of ^{225}Ac-PSMA-617-targeted alpha therapy in metastatic castration-resistant prostate cancer: a systematic review and meta-analysis. Front Oncol. 2022;3(12):796657. https://doi.org/10.3389/fonc.2022.796657.
26. Lee DY, Kim YI. Effects of ^{225}Ac-labeled prostate-specific membrane antigen radioligand therapy in metastatic castration-resistant prostate cancer: a meta-analysis. J Nucl Med. 2022;63(6):840–6.
27. Parida GK, Panda RA, Bishnoi K, Agrawal K. Efficacy and safety of actinium-225 prostate-specific membrane antigen radioligand therapy in metastatic prostate cancer: a systematic review and metanalysis. Med Princ Pract. 2023;32(3):178–91.
28. Vorster M, Sathekge M. Advances in PSMA alpha theragnostics. Semin Nucl Med. 2024;S0001-2998(24):00029–1.
29. Fendler WP, Rahbar K, Herrmann K, Kratochwil C, Eiber M. ^{177}Lu-PSMA radioligand therapy for prostate cancer. J Nucl Med. 2017;58(8):1196–200.
30. Kratochwil C, Giesel FL, Heussel CP, et al. Patients resistant against PSMA-targeting a-radiation therapy often harbor mutations in DNA damage-repair–associated genes. J Nucl Med. 2020;61:683–8.
31. Langbein T, Chausse G, Baum RP. Salivary gland toxicity of PSMA radioligand therapy: relevance and preventive strategies. J Nucl Med. 2018;59:1172–3.
32. Rathke H, Kratochwil C, Hohenberger R, et al. Initial clinical experience performing sialendoscopy for salivary gland protection in patients undergoing (^{225}) Ac-PSMA-617 RLT. Eur J Nucl Med Mol Imaging. 2019;46:139–47.
33. Gallyamov M, Meyrick D, Barley J, Lenzo N. Renal outcomes of radioligand therapy: experience of ^{177}lutetium—prostate specific membrane antigen ligand therapy in metastatic castrate-resistant prostate cancer. Clin Kidney J. 2019;13:1049–55.
34. de Medeiros RB, Grigolon MV, Araújo TP, Srougi M. Metastatic castration-resistant prostate cancer (mCRPC) treated with ^{225}Ac-PSMA-617. Case report. Braz J Oncol. 2019;15:1–9.
35. Sathekge MM, Bruchertseifer F, Vorster M, Morgenstern A, Lawal IO. Global experience with PSMA-based alpha therapy in prostate cancer. Eur J Nucl Med Mol Imaging. 2021;49:30–46.
36. Graf F, Fahrer J, Maus S, , et al. DNA double strand breaks as predictor of efficacy of the alpha-particle emitter Ac-225 and the electron emitter Lu-177 for somatostatin receptor targeted radiotherapy. PLoS One 2014, 9(2), e88239.
37. Ruigrok EAM, Tamborino G, de Blois E, et al. In vitro dose effect relationships of actinium-225- and lutetium-177-labeled PSMA-I&T. Eur J Nucl Med Mol Imaging. 2022;49:3627–38.
38. Zechmann CM, Afshar-Oromieh A, Armor T, et al. Radiation dosimetry and first therapy results with a (124)I/(131)I-labeled small molecule (MIP-1095) targeting PSMA for prostate cancer therapy. Eur J Nucl Med Mol Imaging. 2014;41:1280–92.
39. Kratochwil C, Giesel FL, Stefanova M, et al. PSMA-targeted radionuclide therapy of metastatic castration-resistant prostate cancer with ^{177}Lu-labeled PSMA-617. J Nucl Med. 2016;57:1170–6.
40. Gosewisch A, Schleske M, Gildehaus FJ, et al. Image-based dosimetry for ^{225}Ac-PSMA-I&T therapy using quantitative SPECT. Eur J Nucl Med Mol Imaging. 2021;48:1260–1.

16 Multicenter Trials of Prostate Radioligand Therapy (PRLT) in Castration-Resistant Cancer

My own nonprofit organization, i.e., the World Association of Radiopharmaceutical and Molecular Therapy (WARMTH), has conducted in mCRPC patients altogether three major global trials which were published in high-ranked journals. The first two were retrospective trials using ^{177}Lu-PSMA-617 (the same compound as Pluvicto®), both published in the *European Journal of Nuclear Medicine and Molecular Imaging* [1, 2]. In these studies, there were more than 400 patients treated, and factors predicting outcome and excellent results could be confirmed before official registration trials, using real-world evidence data. The third WARMTH trial describing targeted alpha therapy using ^{225}Ac-PSMA-617 was published in The Lancet Oncology in February 202 [3]. In this retrospective study with 488 patients from 4 continents, Sathekge et al. reported an excellent outcome—more than half of the advanced stage patients responded, and limited adverse effects were observed, and multiple factors affecting response could be identified. Additionally, I was requested to provide a commentary for The Lancet Oncology [4]. Besides these trials, a global trial with mCRPC patients with predominantly lymph node metastases is presented.

The first study reported by Ahmadzadehfar et al. (2021) assesses prior therapies' prognostic impact on overall survival (OS) in patients with metastatic castration-resistant prostate cancer (mCRPC) treated with the radioligand ^{177}Lu-PSMA-617 [1]. The multicenter, retrospective "617 trial" analyzed data from 631 mCRPC patients across 11 clinics, and all participants had been treated with either abiraterone or enzalutamide before starting ^{177}Lu-PSMA-617, but chemotherapy history varied. Patients were grouped based on prior chemotherapy exposure—those who did not have it or those with contraindications. The median OS across 416 analyzed patients was 11.1 months. Patients with prior chemotherapy had a shorter median OS (10.9 months for one-line chemotherapy and 8.9 months for two lines) than those without any chemotherapy history (14.6 months). Patients who avoided chemotherapy but had no contraindications had the longest OS at 15.8 months, while those with contraindications had an OS of 14.0 months.

K. Kairemo, *Prostate Cancer from a Nuclear Oncology Perspective*,
https://doi.org/10.1007/978-3-031-90337-3_16

Significant negative predictors of OS included prior chemotherapy, presence of bone and liver metastases, and poorer ECOG performance status. In particular, patients with bone metastases had a median OS of 10.8 months, while those without bone involvement showed significantly higher survival times. Liver metastases further shortened OS to 6.0 months compared to 13.0 months in patients without liver involvement. 71.8% of patients experienced a decline in prostate-specific antigen (PSA) levels after the first treatment cycle, and 41.5% saw a decline of 50% or more.

A decline in PSA levels was associated with longer OS: patients with ≥50% PSA decline had a median OS of 14.3 months compared to 7.2 months for those with rising PSA. Prior treatment with abiraterone or enzalutamide did not significantly impact OS. Patients undergoing concurrent enzalutamide treatment during radioligand therapy had a slightly shorter OS (10.8 months) than those with a history of enzalutamide alone (12.3 months). Patients with prior radium-223 treatment showed a marginally shorter OS (10.8 months) compared to those without radium-223 exposure.

Our study highlighted that avoiding chemotherapy and having minimal metastasis (e.g., no liver involvement) correlate with longer survival in mCRPC patients receiving ^{177}Lu-PSMA-617. A PSA decline following the first treatment cycle also serves as a positive prognostic indicator for survival.

This study emphasized the role of chemotherapy history and metastasis location in determining patient outcomes with radioligand therapy, suggesting that earlier application of ^{177}Lu-PSMA-617 in selected patients could potentially optimize survival.

Figure 16.1 demonstrates how the location of metastases affects survival. From the figure, it can be seen that the presence of skeletal and liver metastases is negative prognosticator, whereas the presence of lymph node or lung metastases does not affect survival. Our patients had a median age of 71.9 years, and median baseline PSA value of 177 ng/ml. 92.8% had bone metastases, while 20.9% had liver metastases. The detailed data and findings are based on retrospective analyses and need further validation through prospective trials like the phase III VISION and TheraP trials [5, 6].

We made an additional WARMTH multicenter study to assess how the extent of bone metastases impacts overall survival (OS), treatment response, and hematotoxicity in metastatic castration-resistant prostate cancer (mCRPC) patients treated with the radioligand ^{177}Lu-PSMA-617 [2].

This was a retrospective, multicenter analysis of subgroup of the WARMTH 617 trial including 319 mCRPC patients with documented bone lesion counts and a minimum 6-month follow-up post-therapy onset. We classified by bone lesion count: <6 lesions, 6–20 lesions, >20 lesions, or diffuse involvement. The median age of the patients was 72 years and the median baseline PSA level is 191 μg/L. 93.7% of the patients had bone metastases, with 21% having <6 lesions, 16% having 6–20 lesions, 30.7% having >20 lesions, and 26% with diffuse bone involvement. 56.1% of patients had received both abiraterone and enzalutamide before ^{177}Lu-PSMA-617,

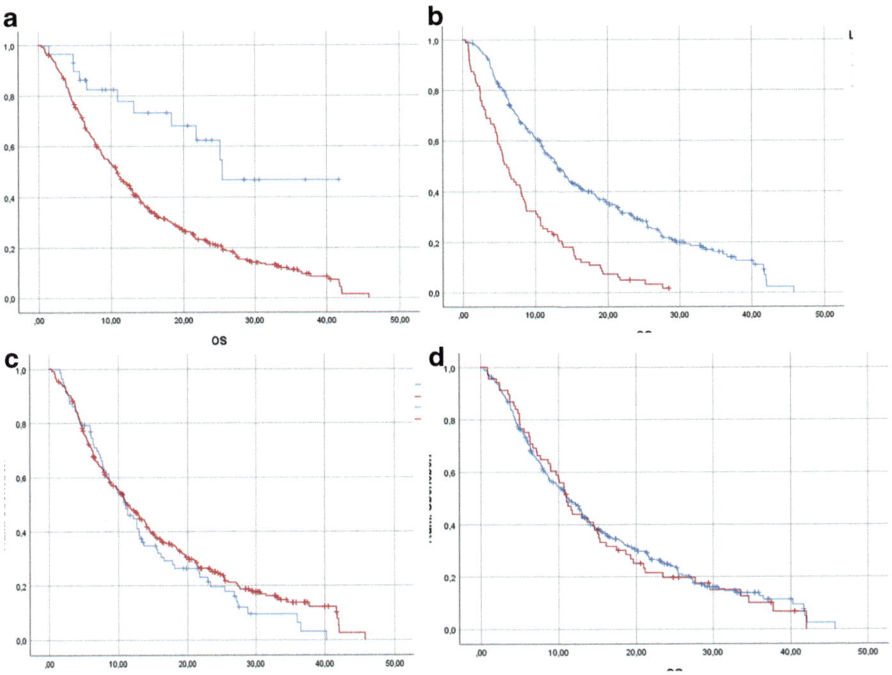

Fig. 16.1 Kaplan-Meier plots for bone metastases (**a**), liver metastases (**b**), lumph node metastases (**c**), and lung metastases (**d**). (Curves **a** and **b** from [1]; **c** and **d** have not been published, but data from [1]). Red graph = present, blue graph = absent

76.2% had undergone first-line chemotherapy with docetaxel, and 24.1% had prior Ra-223 therapy (median six cycles) [2].

Alltogether 72.8% of the patient population showed a PSA decline, and 43.6% out of them achieved a ≥ 50% reduction. No significant correlation between the extent of bone metastases and PSA response was found. Median OS varied by bone lesion count: it was 18.3 months when <6 lesions; with 6–20 lesions, 13.0 months; and with >20 lesions, 10.8 months. When diffuse involvement was present, then OS was 8.2 months [2].

Patients without bone metastases had the longest OS at 25.5 months ($p < 0.0001$). Prior Ra-223 therapy correlated with improved OS across all bone involvement subgroups. Most pronounced benefits: when the patients had 6–20 lesions, the OS extended from 12.1 to 16.4 months ($p = 0.038$) [2].

Diffuse involvement: OS extended from 7.1 to 11.0 months ($p = 0.034$). Presence of liver metastases was a significant negative prognostic factor for OS in all bone involvement subgroups. Increased incidence of anemia and thrombocytopenia correlated with higher bone lesion counts. Grade 3 or 4 anemia and thrombocytopenia occurred in 10% and 3.4% of patients, respectively. No patients developed severe leukopenia (grade 3 or 4), even in the diffuse bone involvement group.

The extent of bone involvement in mCRPC patients undergoing 177Lu-PSMA-617 treatment correlates negatively with OS but does not significantly impact PSA response. Prior Ra-223 therapy shows a potential OS benefit, especially in patients with moderate to high bone involvement. Increased hematotoxicity was observed in patients with high bone burden, though severe cases remained uncommon.

As seen (Fig. 16.1), the presence of lymph node disease is not a negative prognosticator for ^{177}Lu-PSMA radioligand therapy—we made a retrospective cohort study evaluating LuPRLT for mCRPC patients with predominantly lymph node metastases. Our article entitled "^{177}Lu-PSMA Radioligand Therapy of Predominant Lymph Node Metastatic Prostate Cancer" by von Eyben et al. (2019) [7] focused on Lu-177 PSMA radioligand therapy (LuPRLT) for metastatic castration-resistant prostate cancer (mCRPC) with lymph node metastases (LNM). This study was conducted across six institutions in Europe and Australia—the study included 45 patients with LNM, some of whom also had limited bone metastases. The study focused on PSA response, progression-free survival (PFS), overall survival (OS), and adverse effects of LuPRLT in patients previously treated with conventional therapies.

The median age of the patients was 61 years (IQR, 57–66 years) with a median baseline PSA level of 18 μg/L (IQR, 3.3–39 μg/L). Thirty-five patients had only LNM, while ten had LNM with up to two bone metastases. Patients received either LuPSMA I&T or LuPSMA-617—median administered Lu-177 activity was 14.5 GBq (IQR: 12.2–20.4 GBq); patients received a median of three cycles (IQR: 2–3) at approximately 8-week intervals.

The median maximum PSA decline was 92% (IQR: 70–99%), with 80% of patients showing a >50% decline; PSA median PSA progression-free survival (PFS) was 16 months; median PFS for PSMA PET/CT imaging was 18 months.

Overall survival (OS) was generally better in patients with LNM alone than those with additional bone metastasis ($p = 0.046$). Patients receiving cumulative Lu-177 activity of ≥14.8 GBq showed a longer PFS than those with lower doses ($p = 0.03$). Docetaxel-naïve patients had longer PFS compared to those who were docetaxel-resistant ($p = 0.049$). Patients who relapsed after LuPRLT and received a "rechallenge" with LuPRLT or Actinium-based RLT showed improved OS compared to those receiving alternative therapies ($p = 0.045$).

Adverse effects were mild and transient, with no severe hematologic or non-hematologic side effects reported. Australian patients frequently reported fatigue, and some reported nausea and vomiting.

Patients from both regions had similar outcomes in terms of PSA decline, PFS, and OS. Eurasian patients had more prior treatments compared to Australian patients, possibly due to differing healthcare practices. The study's retrospective design limits control over variables and the ability to infer causality. With only 45 patients, findings may require validation in larger, randomized trials.

WARMTH conducted a multicenter retrospective study examining the efficacy and safety of Actinium-225-PSMA radioligand therapy (^{225}Ac-PSMA RLT) for metastatic castration-resistant prostate cancer (mCRPC).

This study, conducted across multiple centers globally, investigated ^{225}Ac-PSMA as a novel therapy for mCRPC, focusing on patient outcomes and treatment-induced toxicities. It involved 488 patients treated from January 1, 2016, to May 31, 2023, with the primary outcomes being overall survival (OS) and progression-free survival (PFS).

The median age in this patient population was 68.1 years (±8.8 years), and the median baseline prostate-specific antigen (PSA) was 169.5 ng/mL with an interquartile range (IQR) of 34.6–519.8 ng/mL.

The patients received a median of two cycles of ^{225}Ac-PSMA (IQR: 2–4).

Their median overall survival (OS) was 15.5 months (95% CI: 13.4–18.3 months), and their median progression-free survival (PFS) was 7.9 months (95% CI: 6.8–8.9 months).

PSA Response: ≥50% PSA decline was observed in 57.0% of patients (278 out of 488). Any PSA decline was achieved in 73.4% of patients after at least one cycle of treatment.

Side Effects

Xerostomia (Dry Mouth): Sixty-eight percent of patients reported xerostomia after the first cycle, with this side effect seen in all patients who received more than seven cycles.

Bone Marrow Toxicity: Grade ≥ 3 anemia occurred in 13.1% of patients; grade ≥ 3 leukopenia was observed in 3.9% of patients; grade ≥ 3 thrombocytopenia was found in 6.6% of patients.

Renal Toxicity: Grade ≥ 3 renal impairment affected 4.5% of patients.

Patients with liver or peritoneal metastases had a significantly shorter OS and PFS. Prior taxane chemotherapy, androgen-receptor-axis inhibitors, or Lutetium-177 PSMA therapy were associated with lower survival and progression-free rates.

The study concludes that 225Ac-PSMA is an effective option for heavily pretreated mCRPC patients, with notable PSA response and survival times, although xerostomia remains a prevalent side effect. Severe hematologic and renal toxicities were comparatively rare, suggesting the therapy is relatively safe for advanced mCRPC cases.

In conclusion, PSMA-TAT showed promising efficacy and an acceptable safety profile in treating metastatic prostate cancer. A significant PSA response was reported in a substantial proportion of patients, from heavily pretreated cohorts to earlier disease settings. Adverse events are generally mild and manageable. This treatment can exert impressive therapeutic effects in this challenging scenario. These findings together with optimised treatment protocols in randomised controlled trials, will lead toward the prompt implementation of PSMA-TAT in clinical practice.

Conclusive Remarks

The retrospective multicenter analyses regarding Lutetium-177 (^{177}Lu)-PSMA RLT in mCRPC by the World Association of Radiopharmaceutical and Molecular Therapy (WARMTH) community found multiple factors associated with overall survival and progression-free survival and were also able to predict overall survival and progression-free survival before actual randomized controlled registration trial TheraP and VISION reported data. In the third WARMTH study, the beta-emitting radionuclide ^{177}Lu was replaced with the alpha-emitter ^{225}Ac. This study on ^{225}Ac-PSMA RLT is a continuation of the WARMTH multicenter trials: on the basis of a retrospective analysis with a wide clinical experience, multiple factors associated with overall survival and progression-free survival for ^{225}Ac-PSMA RLT can be predicted before official registration trial report data.

The additional multicenter study presented in this chapter suggests that ^{177}LuPRLT is a promising therapy for mCRPC patients with lymph node-predominant metastasis, providing significant PSA response and prolonged survival with manageable side effects. The findings encourage further prospective, randomized trials to validate ^{177}LuPRLT's efficacy and safety in this patient group, too.

It is obvious that both ^{177}Lu-PSMA RLT and ^{225}Ac-PSMA RLT are considerable and even preferred treatment modalities in metastatic castration-resistant prostate cancer. It remains to be seen in what extent they are going to be used earlier.

References

1. Ahmadzadehfar H, Rahbar K, Baum RP, et al. Prior therapies as prognostic factors of overall survival in metastatic castration-resistant prostate cancer patients treated with [^{177}Lu]Lu-PSMA-617. A WARMTH multicenter study (the 617 trial). Eur J Nucl Med Mol Imaging. 2021;48:113–22.
2. Ahmadzadehfar H, Matern R, Baum RP, et al. The impact of the extent of the bone involvement on overall survival and toxicity in mCRPC patients receiving ^{177}Lu-PSMA-617: a WARMTH multicentre study. Eur J Nucl Med Mol Imaging. 2021;48:4067–76.
3. Sathekge MM, Lawal IO, Bal C, et al. Actinium-225-PSMA radioligand therapy of metastatic castration-resistant prostate cancer (WARMTH Act): a multicentre, retrospective study. Lancet Oncol. 2024;25:175–83.
4. Kairemo K. Targeted alpha therapy: a new tool for advanced prostate cancer. Lancet Oncol. 2024;25:148–9.
5. Sartor O, de Bono J, Chi KN, et al. Lutetium-177-PSMA-617 for metastatic castration-resistant prostate cancer. N Engl J Med. 2021;385:1091–103.
6. Hofman MS, Emmett L, Violet J, et al. TheraP: a randomized phase 2 trial of ^{177} Lu-PSMA-617 theranostic treatment vs cabazitaxel in progressive metastatic castration-resistant prostate cancer (Clinical Trial Protocol ANZUP 1603). BJU Int. 2019;124(Suppl 1):5–13.
7. von Eyben FE, Singh A, Zhang J, et al. ^{177}Lu-PSMA radioligand therapy of predominant lymph node metastatic prostate cancer. Oncotarget. 2019;10:2451–61.

Meta-Analyses and Systematic Reviews (Own Experience) in Prostate Cancer

17

Meta-analysis is a synthesis of quantitative data from multiple independent studies addressing a research question. An important part of this method involves computing a combined effect size across all of the studies. As such, this statistical approach involves extracting effect sizes and variance measures from various studies. By combining these effect sizes, the statistical power is improved and can resolve uncertainties or discrepancies found in individual studies. Meta-analyses may be used for shaping treatment guidelines and influencing health practice. Meta-analyses are often, but not always, important components of a systematic review.

Network meta-analysis is a technique for comparing multiple treatments simultaneously in a single analysis by combining direct and indirect evidence within a network of randomized controlled trials. In this chapter, a few own systematic reviews are presented, in different stages of prostate cancer development demanding a treatment strategy as a part of own personal journey with prostate cancer (as a patient and as a doctor).

Local Therapy

Own examples of early phase of prostate are related to radiation therapy and active surveillance.

EBRT

External beam radiotherapy (EBRT) for prostate cancer can be performed with a high dose of 86 Gy; however, one-tenth or more of the patients will develop recurrence. Prostate cancer is mainly multifocal, but a dominant intraprostatic lesion (DIL) is often the site of local recurrence after EBRT. We undertook a systematic review and meta-analysis to clarify whether functional imaging might identify the DIL and whether a RT boost to the DIL might be increased to an ultrahigh dose level

K. Kairemo, *Prostate Cancer from a Nuclear Oncology Perspective*,
https://doi.org/10.1007/978-3-031-90337-3_17

of 90 Gy without increased toxicity. Of 62 selected studies, 13 reported the size of the DIL. The mean of the median DIL volumes was 2.4 cm^3 (95% confidence interval, 0.9–4.4 cm^3). Eighteen diagnostic studies with 1205 patients evaluated the diagnostic accuracy using multiparametric MRI for intraprostatic cancer lesions. Evaluating 14,654 prostate segments, the diagnostic accuracy was 77% [1].

Eleven therapeutic studies with 988 patients reported a RT boost for the DIL. The summary boost dose for the DIL was a mean of 89 Gy in five studies using intensity modulated RT (calculated as the equivalent dose in 2-Gy fractions) and a mean of 141 Gy in four studies using a combination of EBRT and brachytherapy ($P < 0.018$, t-test). In one therapeutic study, 239 patients had a 98% 10-year disease-free survival rate. Many of our therapeutic studies used a boost dose to the DIL of >90 Gy. The reported boost for DIL is effective and safe [1].

Many studies treated the DIL with an ultrahigh boost dose of >90 Gy. The reported boost to the DIL was effective and safe. Nevertheless, many studies that had detected the DIL using mp-MRI performed radical prostatectomy of the whole prostate [1].

This means, for the clinical practice, that RT can be used to give a boost to the whole prostate; however, most patients can tolerate only a radiation dose <86 Gy. Mp-MRI is becoming widely used to detect significant intraprostatic lesions and the DIL. The role of PET has been discussed in Chap. 11.

In general, the DIL constitutes only a small part of the prostate; thus, a boost to the DIL and a combination of EBRT and brachytherapy are options for increasing the radiation dose to the DIL to ultrahigh levels of 90 Gy, with respect for the constraints by the organs at risk. The therapeutic studies performed a boost to the DIL with a radiation dose of 196 Gy. One study reported a 98% 10-year disease-free survival rate after the boost to the DIL. Three percent of the reported patients had long-term rectal toxicity grade 2, and 12% had long-term genitourinary toxicity grade 2 [1].

Dose escalation is not indicated for patients with low-risk Pca; however, the results from the meta-analysis could have an effect on use of focal therapy and definitive RT for patients with primary Pca.

Active Surveillance After Radical Prostatectomy

The systematic review by von Eyben et al. (2024) investigates the prognostic value of ultrasensitive PSA (uPSA) assays in monitoring early prostate cancer recurrence post-radical prostatectomy (RP) [2]. The review includes 115 studies with 67,479 prostate cancer (Pca) patients, out of which 14,965 experienced PSA recurrence (PSAR) and 2663 patients died [2].

Patients with the lowest post-surgery PSA nadir (undetectable or very low levels) have better survival outcomes and a significantly reduced risk of PSAR. The cumulative significance for separating PSAR-prone from non-PSAR-prone patients based on PSA nadir reached (cumulative p value <3.7 × 10^{-12}) indicating a robust correlation between low nadir and reduced mortality risk. Among RP patients with PSA nadirs below 10 ng/L, the lowest rates of recurrence and improved 5-year survival rates were observed, indicating that uPSA measurements are critical in predicting longer-term outcomes [2].

Starting SRT at PSA levels below 0.5 μg/L (500 ng/L) substantially improves metastasis-free survival (MFS) and overall survival (OS). Data indicate that patients who received SRT at PSA levels between 30 and 50 ng/L benefited most, showing up to a 20% improvement in 5-year MFS rates compared to patients who started SRT at higher PSA levels [2]. An additional benefit was observed in patients who started SRT at PSA nadir levels as low as 1–10 ng/L, where the likelihood of progression to metastasis was lowest. This suggests that SRT initiation at very low PSA levels may be optimal for long-term control. Ultrasensitive PSA assays demonstrated high diagnostic accuracy, especially for negative predictive value (NPV). Studies show that uPSA tests at thresholds of 0.001–0.1 μg/L have up to a 95% NPV in detecting early biochemical recurrence before clinical progression, supporting the use of uPSA for close monitoring after RP [2]. Out of the 76 studies on clinical outcomes, uPSA assays consistently identified PSAR in patients up to 2 years before conventional PSA tests, showing the importance of uPSA in early detection and timely SRT intervention.

In patients considered PSAR-prone, PSA increased to above 50 ng/L before SRT, compared to non-PSAR-prone patients who had PSA levels fluctuating around 30 ng/L post-RP. These findings emphasize the significance of PSA kinetics (rates of change) in identifying high-risk patients for recurrence. During the first year post-RP, PSAR-prone patients exhibited steadily rising PSA levels, in contrast to stable or declining PSA in non-PSAR patients; thus, PSA kinetics can be a reliable early indicator for recurrence and need for SRT [2]. Short PSADT was correlated with increased risk of metastasis and poor OS. Patients with PSADT under 6 months were found to have a 1.5-fold higher risk of recurrence and death compared to patients with slower PSA doubling. As a result, PSADT, alongside PSA nadir, serves as a useful stratification tool for guiding early SRT and assessing patient prognosis [2].

This comprehensive review supports the adoption of uPSA assays for more accurate detection of biochemical recurrence in Pca patients post-RP. uPSA monitoring allows for timely initiation of SRT at optimal PSA levels, improving survival outcomes. The evidence suggests a potential shift in PSA-based recurrence guidelines, emphasizing early SRT initiation and continuous monitoring using ultrasensitive PSA measurements [2]. In summary, ultrasensitive PSA assays significantly enhance early detection of recurrence, and timely salvage radiotherapy at low PSA levels (<50 ng/L) improves survival outcomes for prostate cancer patients after radical prostatectomy.

Third-Line Therapies for mCRPC

PRLT (Prostate Radioligand Therapy)

There is a controversy as to the relative efficacy of ^{177}Lu prostate-specific membrane antigen (PSMA) radioligand therapy (RLT) and third-line treatment for patients with metastatic castration-resistant prostate cancer (mCRPC). The aim of our systematic review was to elucidate whether ^{177}Lu-PSMA RLT and third-line treatment have similar effects and adverse effects (PROSPERO trial) [3]. The review followed Preferred Reporting Items for Systematic Reviews and Meta-Analysis (PRISMA) guidelines, and the meta-analysis used the random-effects model.

Twelve studies including 669 patients reported ^{177}Lu-PSMA RLT. Overall, 43% of the patients had a maximum decline of PSA of ≥50% following treatment with ^{177}Lu-PSMA RLT. The treatment with ^{177}Lu-PSMA-617 and ^{177}Lu-PSMA for imaging and therapy (I&T) had mainly transient adverse effects. Sixteen studies including 1338 patients reported third-line treatment [3]. Overall, 22% of the patients had a best decline of PSA of ≥50% following third-line treatment. After third-line treatment with enzalutamide and cabazitaxel, adverse effects caused discontinuation of treatment for 10–23% of the patients. ^{177}Lu-PSMA RLT gave a best PSA decline ≥50% more often than third-line treatment (mean 44% versus 22%, p = 0.0002, t-test) [3]. Figure 17.1 demonstrates these results by the forest plots for the frequency of a best PSA decline of >50% in 12 articles for Lu-177-based treatments (on the left) and in 16 articles for third-line treatments—enzalutamide, abiraterone,

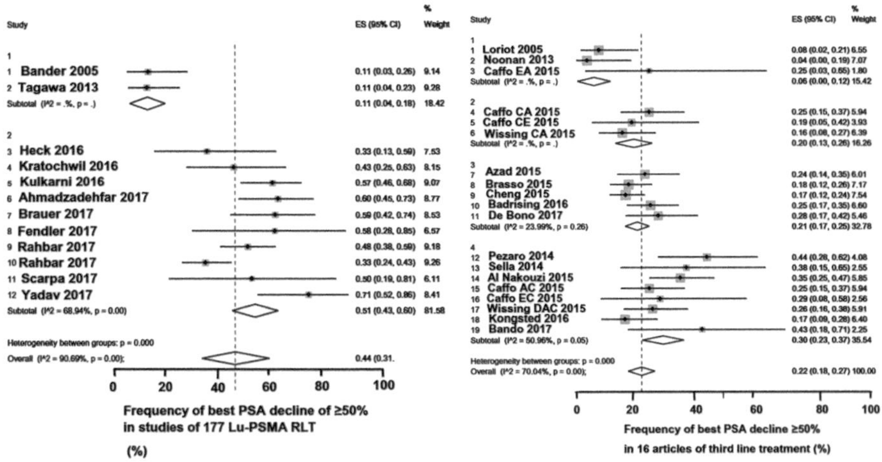

Fig. 17.1 Forest plot showing the frequency of a best PSA decline of >50% in 12 articles; articles with ^{177}Lu-PSMA-J591 antibody and 10 articles with ^{177}Lu-RLT (PSMA-617 or PSMA-I&T) on the left. Forest plot showing the frequency of a best PSA decline of >50% in 16 articles with third-line treatment (enzalutamide, abiraterone, cabazitaxel) on the right. Forest plots show best PSA decline >50% with the 95% confidence interval. ^{177}Lu-PSMA RLT gave a best PSA decline of >50% in 44% patients, whereas third-line treatment PSA decline > 50% only in 22% patients. (Modified from [3])

cabazitaxel (on the right) [3]. ^{177}Lu-PSMA RLT gave objective remission more often than third-line treatment (overall 31 of 109 patients versus 43 of 275 patients, $p = 0.004$, $\chi 2$-test). Median survival was longer after ^{177}Lu-PSMA RLT than after third-line treatment, but the difference was not statistically significant (mean 14 months versus 12 months, $p = 0.32$, t-test) [3]. Adverse effects caused discontinuation of treatment more often for third-line treatment than for ^{177}Lu-PSMA RLT (22 of 66 patients versus 0 of 469 patients, $p < 0.001$, $\chi 2$-test) [3].

In summary, as for patients with mCRPC, treatment with ^{177}Lu-PSMA-617 RTL and ^{177}Lu-PSMA I&T gave better effects and caused fewer adverse effects than third-line treatment [3]. Our systematic review and meta-analysis had limitations. The articles mainly used ^{177}Lu-PSMA RLT for patients with end-stage Pca. So, the review did not evaluate the efficacy for patients in an earlier phase of PC. Background factors may be important for overall survival after third-line treatment, but the articles rarely reported these characteristics. The articles summarized overall survival from start of ^{177}Lu-PSMA RLT or start of third-line treatment and not from a common point in the progression of the disease such as the diagnosis of mCRPC. As the articles had a short follow-up, our review did not assess long-term effects and adverse effects of ^{177}Lu-PSMA RLT.

Network meta-analysis is a technique for comparing multiple treatments simultaneously in a single analysis by combining direct and indirect evidence within a network of randomized controlled trials.

A network meta-analysis (NMA) is an advanced statistical method that synthesizes evidence from multiple studies comparing different interventions. Unlike traditional meta-analyses, which only compare two treatments at a time (pairwise comparisons), NMAs can evaluate multiple treatments simultaneously by creating a network of comparisons. This method allows for a more comprehensive assessment of available evidence, especially in cases where direct comparisons between treatments may be limited or unavailable. In summary, a network meta-analysis provides a robust framework for comparing multiple treatments by synthesizing direct and indirect evidence. Its capacity to rank treatments and inform evidence-based decision-making makes it a valuable tool in clinical research, despite its reliance on specific statistical assumptions.

We applied a network meta-analysis (NMA) for evaluating the effectiveness and safety of third-line treatments for metastatic castration-resistant prostate cancer (mCRPC), focusing particularly on ^{177}Lu-PSMA-based radioligand therapy (PRLT) in comparison with other treatments.

The NMA included 3958 patients across 7 randomized controlled trials (RCTs), evaluating 8 third-line treatments including PRLT, cabazitaxel, and abiraterone [4]. The setup is shown in Fig. 17.2.

PSA Response PRLT data in this NMA was based on VISION and TheraP trials [5, 6], and it demonstrated a significantly higher probability of achieving a prostate-specific antigen (PSA) decline of $\geq 50\%$, showing a 1.3-fold increase in response rate compared to treatments like cabazitaxel and abiraterone. PRLT was estimated to be the most effective treatment in achieving PSA response with a 97.6% likelihood of being the best option. The PSA response data is shown in Fig. 17.3 [4].

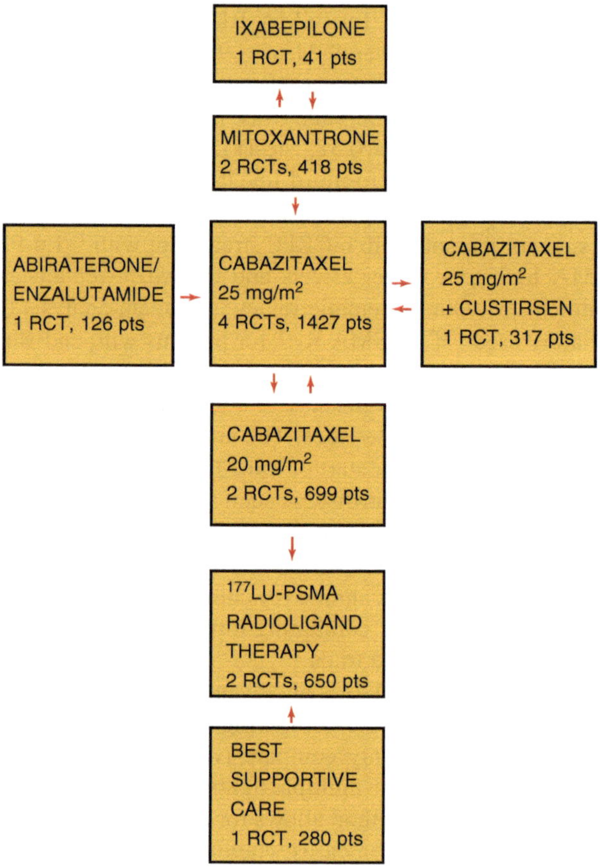

Fig. 17.2 The network meta-analysis (NMA) for evaluating the effectiveness and safety of third-line treatments for mCRPC, eight different treatments to mCRPC; ^{177}Lu-RLT (PRLT), ixabepilone, mitoxantrone, cabazitaxel (20 mg/m^2 and 25 mg/m^2), alternative abiraterone or enzalutamide, and best supportive care. The third-line treatments connect the randomized controlled clinical trials in a network with a ladder and a star configuration without any loops. A single arrow between two treatments points to the most effective treatment, and double arrows indicate non-inferiority between the treatments [4]

Progression-Free Survival (PFS) PRLT improved radiographic progression-free survival (rPFS), with a 1.1-fold increase in 6-month progression-free survival compared to cabazitaxel. In terms of ranking, PRLT was rated as the top third-line treatment for prolonging rPFS among the available options.

Overall Survival (OS) PRLT in the VISION trial resulted in a median overall survival of 15.3 months, slightly outperforming other third-line treatments (e.g., cabazitaxel with median OS of 13–14 months). For patients who had failed abiraterone or enzalutamide treatments, cabazitaxel showed better survival outcomes, though PRLT achieved a slight overall survival advantage when measured at the 12-month mark.

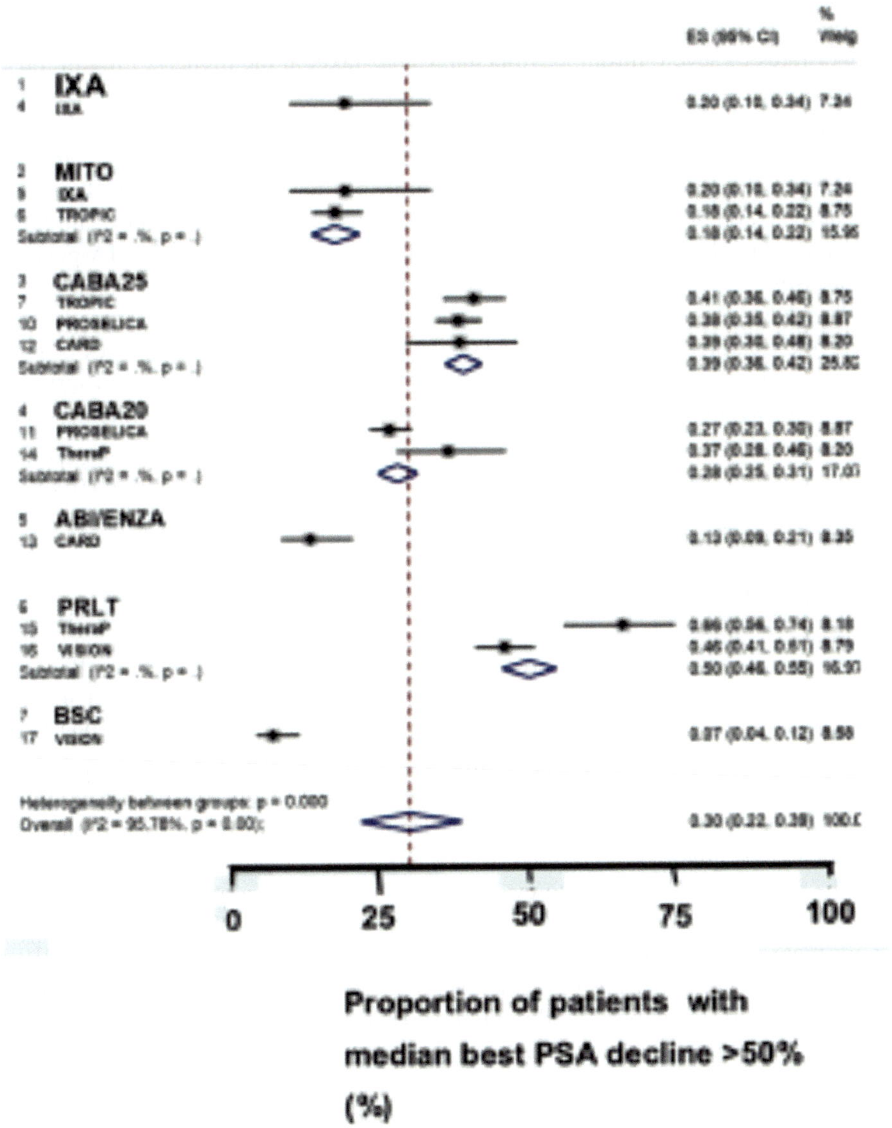

Fig. 17.3 Forest plot showing the frequency of a best PSA declinc of >50% from eight different treatments to mCRPC; ^{177}Lu-RLT (PRLT) resulted in the best decline of >50%. IXA denotes ixabepilone, MITO to mitoxantrone, CABA to cabazitaxel, and ABI/ENZA to alternative abiraterone or enzalutamide. Forest plots show best PSA decline >50% with 95% confidence interval. (Modified from [4])

Adverse Effects PRLT presented a more favorable safety profile with fewer instances of severe leukopenia compared to cabazitaxel, although it did lead to higher rates of severe thrombocytopenia. Cabazitaxel at the higher 25 mg/m^2 dose had a higher discontinuation rate due to adverse effects, while PRLT and ixabepilone also showed relatively high discontinuation rates (Fig. 17.3).

PRLT was the highest ranked for PSA response and progression-free survival, indicating strong potential as an effective third-line treatment for mCRPC. For overall survival, combination therapy of cabazitaxel with custirsen ranked best, although PRLT remained a favorable option particularly for patients with PSMA-positive metastases.

This NMA highlights that PRLT is a highly effective and comparatively safe third-line treatment option for mCRPC, demonstrating superior outcomes in PSA response and progression-free survival and slight improvements in overall survival. Its efficacy supports its use as a preferred option among third-line treatments, especially for patients who are PSMA-positive.

Third-Line Therapies

Radiation Sensitizers

Metastatic castration-resistant prostate cancer (mCRPC) is particularly challenging to treat, as it becomes resistant to traditional androgen receptor-targeted therapies. In recent years, poly (ADP-ribose) polymerase (PARP) inhibitors (PARPis) have emerged as a promising treatment option, especially for patients with homologous recombination repair (HRR) gene mutations. PARPis work by inhibiting DNA repair mechanisms, leading to cancer cell death by preventing the repair of double-stranded DNA breaks.

The aim of our NMA was to evaluate the efficacy and safety of four PARPis—olaparib, niraparib, rucaparib, and talazoparib—in the treatment of mCRPC. A network meta-analysis (NMA) was conducted based on six high-quality phase II/III randomized controlled trials (RCTs), involving a total of 3205 patients. The following outcomes were analyzed: radiographic progression-free survival (rPFS), overall survival (OS), adverse events (AEs), and severe adverse events (grade ≥ 3 AEs) [7].

The analysis used Bayesian statistical methods with a random-effects model to allow indirect comparisons between treatments. The studies reported on rPFS, OS, and adverse events. The quality of the studies was assessed using the Cochrane Risk-of-Bias 2 tool. Two separate network meta-analyses were performed due to differences in trial designs. These compared four PARPis for mCRPC patients [7].

Progression-Free Survival (rPFS) Olaparib significantly improved rPFS compared to niraparib and talazoparib, with a hazard ratio (HR) of 0.67 (95% confidence interval: 0.46–0.96). Talazoparib had the highest probability of being the preferred treatment for rPFS (58.6%), followed by olaparib (35.5%). Rucaparib and olaparib were nearly equivalent in improving rPFS, with olaparib having a slight advantage [7].

Overall Survival (OS) No statistically significant differences in OS were observed among olaparib, niraparib, and talazoparib [7]. However, the OS data were immature, and ongoing trials may provide more clarity in the future.

Adverse Events (AEs) All PARPis, including olaparib, niraparib, and talazoparib, were associated with increased rates of severe (grade $\geq$ 3) AEs. Talazoparib had the highest risk of severe AEs (HR 3.7), but there were no statistically significant differences between olaparib and placebo [7].

Olaparib had the best safety profile, with the highest probability (3.5%) of being the safest treatment option for severe AEs [7].

Ranking Probabilities and SUCRA Analysis For radiographic progression-free survival (rPFS), talazoparib had the highest SUCRA (the surface under the cumulative ranking) value (0.82), followed by olaparib (0.74). In terms of adverse events, olaparib ranked highest for safety with a SUCRA value of 0.57. Based on the comprehensive results, olaparib performed best in both efficacy and safety [7].

This analysis suggests that olaparib may offer the best combination of improved rPFS and a favorable safety profile for mCRPC patients compared to other PARPis. Olaparib can be considered a first-line treatment option, particularly for patients with BRCA or HRR mutations, though treatment decisions should still be individualized based on patient characteristics and potential adverse effects [7].

The use of PARPis significantly alters the treatment landscape for mCRPC, particularly for patients with homologous recombination repair mutations. The importance of genetic profiling in treatment decisions is emphasized, but further research is needed to develop optimal treatment strategies for these patients.

Conclusive Remarks

Focal boost to the dominant intraprostatic lesion (DIL) which is often the site of local recurrence after EBRT is a relevant treatment option.

Ultrasensitive PSA assays significantly enhance early detection of recurrence, and timely salvage radiotherapy at low PSA levels (<50 ng/L) improves survival outcomes for prostate cancer patients after radical prostatectomy.

In metastatic disease, our meta-analyses show that already retrospective studies with ^{177}Lu-PSMA RLT had better effects and caused less adverse effects than newest third-line treatments.

Randomized controlled clinical trials with ^{177}Lu-PSMA RLT within an NMA highlighted that PRLT is a highly effective and comparatively safe third-line treatment option for mCRPC, demonstrating superior outcomes in PSA response and progression-free survival and slight improvements in overall survival. Therefore, the PRLT option should be preferred option among third-line treatments, especially in PSMA-positive mCRPC patients. Out of PARP inhibitors, olaparib may offer a best advantageous combination of improved PFS and a favorable safety profile for mCRPC patients.

References

1. von Eyben FE, Kiljunen T, Kangasmaki A, Kairemo K, von Eyben R, Joensuu T. Radiotherapy boost for the dominant intraprostatic cancer lesion—a systematic review and meta-analysis. Clin Genitourin Cancer. 2016;14:189–97.
2. von Eyben FE, Kairemo K, Kapp DS. Prostate-specific antigen as an ultrasensitive biomarker for patients with early recurrent prostate cancer: how low shall we go? A systematic review. Biomedicines. 2024;12(4):822.
3. von Eyben FE, Roviello G, Kiljunen T, et al. Third-line treatment and ^{177}Lu-PSMA radioligand therapy of metastatic castration-resistant prostate cancer: a systematic review. Eur J Nucl Med Mol Imaging. 2018;45:496–508.
4. on Eyben FE, Kairemo K, Paller C, et al. ^{177}Lu-PSMA radioligand therapy is favorable as third-line treatment of patients with metastatic castration-resistant prostate cancer. A systematic review and network meta-analysis of randomized controlled trials. Biomedicines. 2021;9(8):1042.
5. Sartor O, de Bono J, Chi KN, et al. Lutetium-177-PSMA-617 for metastatic castration-resistant prostate cancer. N Engl J Med. 2021;385:1091–103.
6. Hofman MS, Emmett L, Violet J, et al. TheraP: a randomized phase 2 trial of ^{177} Lu-PSMA-617 theranostic treatment vs cabazitaxel in progressive metastatic castration-resistant prostate cancer (Clinical Trial Protocol ANZUP 1603). BJU Int. 2019;124(Suppl 1):5–13.
7. Huang Y, He H, Liang L, et al. Efficacy and safety of PARP inhibitors in the treatment of prostatic cancer: a systematic review and network meta-analysis. Chin Clin Oncol. 2024;13:64.

Part V

Own Cancer Career

18 Own History of Cancer Suspicions

History of Cancer Suspicions

For the first time cancer was suspected in 2010. In January, 2010, I was from Finland at a congress (Clinical Applications of Nanotechnologies in the Field of Cancer) in Montpellier, France. I went there to speak about targeting intelligent nanoparticles in cancer treatment. Just before my presentation, entitled "Multimodality Imaging in Oncology Utilizing Targeted Drug Delivery systems," I received a call to Lappeenranta's occupational health service regarding my laboratory results. At the time of the call, I was already on stage. This was a routine control checkup for hospital personnel. I had to call the nurse back immediately after my presentation, and I learned that my tumor marker CA 19-9 was clearly elevated, actually 65 (reference range < 27 IU/l); I knew which tests had been taken from me and I asked her to tell me the numerical values. This marker is associated, e.g., with pancreatic and colon cancer. The next presentation in the congress was about the treatment of pancreatic cancer with a poor prognosis, and I took exceptionally accurate notes and I still remember how I was sweating. Then, during the next break, I called the occupational health doctor in Finland and asked him to make referrals to Helsinki University Central Hospital for both internal medicine and surgery for suspected pancreatic cancer. Then back home, I went through numerous laboratory and imaging tests and endoscopy examinations, some even twice. I underwent MRI, CT, PET (Fig. 18.1), and ultrasound examinations, which did not show any findings suggestive of cancer. During the 6 months when all the tests were done, the marker also normalized and the investigations were terminated. I learned to understand what it felt like to live in uncertainty for half a year.

In June 2014, I had a tonsillectomy due to a small tumor that was barely visible on the MRI images. The study was conducted due to a marginal finding in the occupational health inspection. No significant findings and malignancy were found in histopathology. This was my first surgery ever.

Then the prostate cancer story started in mid-March 2022. I got an invitation to participate in prostate cancer screening study. The study included initially serum

K. Kairemo, *Prostate Cancer from a Nuclear Oncology Perspective*,
https://doi.org/10.1007/978-3-031-90337-3_18

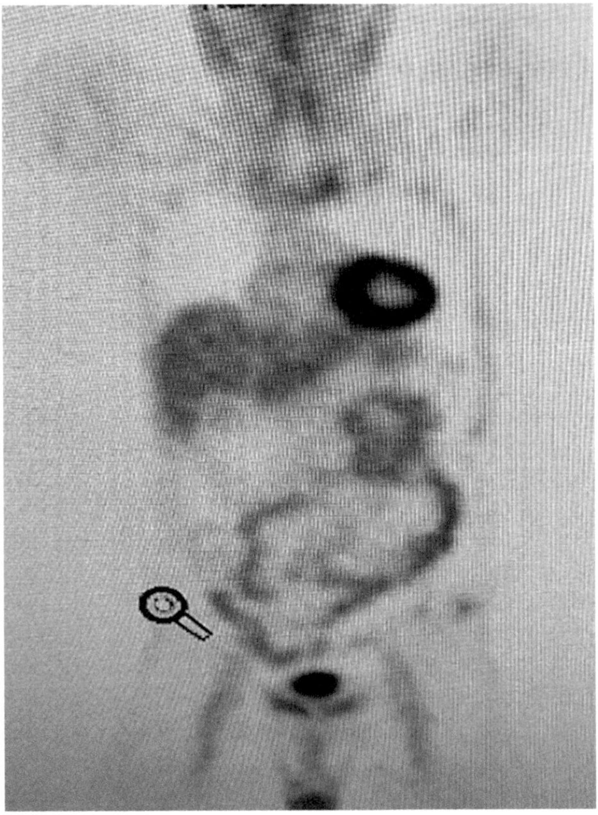

Fig. 18.1 FDG-PET study II-2010, where no malignancy was observed

and urine samples and possible prostate biopsies and imaging studies if a prostate cancer was suspected. My 4K test (consisting of four biomarkers: total PSA, free PSA, intact PSA, and human kallikrein2 (hK2)) was suspicious 12% (reference range: <10%) like the S-PSA value of 7.9. I got next an invitation to the pelvic MRI. This was supposed to take place in 6–12 weeks. At that time, there was a lot of care debt due to the SARS-CoV-2 pandemic and additionally nurses went on strike. I was not worried because I still thought that my laboratory values were due to hyperplasia. Finally, I had this 3T-MRI in September. The report stated enlargement in the prostate but no signs of malignancy. My prostate size was 51 cm^3. My S-PSA value was 7.6 at the same time, and free PSA was 1.58 and PSA ratio was 21% (reference value >15%). Based on these findings, a whole body CT and prostate biopsies were programmed within a month. Thirteen sectorial transrectal biopsies were taken and eight samples were positive for prostate cancer. The CT did not reveal any prostate cancer related spread.

The treatment consultation was scheduled for the beginning of December. I myself was puzzled by the findings, which is why I wanted to order an additional PSMA-PET examination at a private hospital. I had to pay for this study, even though I myself had established the study in Finland. Fortunately, the tracers were being changed, so I was able to have two different PET scans on consecutive days. I myself had emphasized in my previous presentations that these markers work differently in primary tumors.

In my case, my disease classification came out as T2b, but if I had believed the official PET scan, it would have been T2a, and if I had believed the official MRI statement, it would have been T0 or Tx. I analyzed my MRIs myself at the end of November and noted that a centimeter-diameter tumor can be seen on the left.

Well, 2 h before the treatment consultation, it was canceled by a text message. At this point, I sent a friendly letter to the chief physicians of the clinic and the two urologists who wrote the referrals. In the letter I stated that I have a GS7 prostate cancer, which should be treated with ADT in combination of VMAT and brachytherapy. My own diagnosis T2bN0M0 was based on MRI, CT, and 2 PSMA-PET imaging studies and the histology from 13 biopsies. I did not mention that the radiology report was consistent with the T0N0M0 diagnosis.

I got an appointment within 2 weeks for a treatment consultation in Vantaa (another city next to Helsinki). However, the time was changed to Helsinki a day earlier. I wandered at the urology clinic for 2 h until I realized that there was no appointment. A text message was sent to me, confirming that appointment time was an error. Finally, I got an extra appointment for the next day, where I came with my wife. One of the four doctors who received my letter, the only doctor who had responded positively to my message and agreed with my diagnosis, promised to see me. During the reception, I found out that hormone therapy could be started on the same day, and it would take 6–8 months to start radiation therapy. I understood that I have prostate cancer which has to be treated. The sooner the treatments start, the better the prognosis. In my case, it took 9 months from the start of hormone therapy alone to the suspicion of cancer. According to the urologist, even surgical treatment cannot cure (remove) my disease, which I agreed with.

Of course, the hormone treatment did not start on the same day, but on the same week (Degarelix® injection). I was really worried about the delay in starting the radiation treatment, which is why I contacted the Docrates Cancer Hospital. I got an appointment there to start external radiation therapy within a week. This was preceded by the installation of gold anchors in the prostate for radiotherapy. I also wanted the PSA value not to be taken the next day because I have just had an intraprostatic procedure. After all, that S-PSA was clearly artificially elevated due to damage in prostate cells, up to 13.2.

It was 1 week before the Christmas when my radiation therapy started, and by Christmas, I got 5 out of 20 planned radiation therapy cycles. On Christmas Eve, I was very tired and had a lot of side effects related to the therapy: dysuria, pollacisuria, hematuria, diarrhea, steatorrhea, melaena, and pain in the pelvic region. In the morning of Christmas Eve, I decided to go to the pharmacy and started medication (tamsulosin, a selective $\alpha_{1A/1D}$-adrenoceptor antagonist reduces tension of the smooth muscles in the prostate and the urethra; tadalafil, a selective phosphodiesterase-5, leading to increased levels of cGMP in the corpus cavernosum leading to smooth muscle relaxation and vasodilation; pain medication). My children and grandchildren were happy when I could be present at the Christmas Eve. I had

Table 18.1 The patient history

	Clinical tests		
Time [months]	S-PSA	Procedure	Finding
0	7.9	4K test	Suspicious 12% (<10%)
6	7.6	3T MRI	Prostate size 51 cm^3
7	1.22	Free PSA	$T_{2b}N_0M_0$
7	0.54	Transrectal biopsies (13)	Free 1.58
8	0.06	Whole body CT	PSA ratio 21% (>15%)
8	0.11	^{18}F-PSMA-1007-PET	GS 3 + 4 (25%);
8	0.41	^{18}F-DCFPyL-PET	Eight samples/139 mm
9		Gold anchor, 3 T MRI	$T_0N_0M_0$
10		VMAT, ADT	SUV_{max} 14.8, $T_{2b}N_0M_0$
10.5		VMAT ready	SUV_{max} 11.9, $T_{2a}N_0M_0$
11		PSA test	Pr 62 Gy, SV 49.4 Gy,
12		Brachytherapy	LN 44 Gy
17		TRUS	18/20 cycles
19		PSA test	15 Gy, 17 needles
		PSA test	Prostate size 28 cm^3
		PSA test	ADT continues

This 67-year-old male with GS7 PCa was treated with ADT and with a combination of VMAT and brachytherapy. The dose lineation was based on ^{18}F-PSMA-1007-PET

Abbreviations: *4K*: total PSA, free PSA, intact PSA, and human kallikrein2, *ADT* androgen deprivation therapy, *CT* computed tomography, *GS* Gleason score, *LN* lymph nodes, *PCa* prostate cancer, *PET* positron emission tomography, *Pr* prostate, *SUV* standard uptake value, *SV* seminal vesicles, *TNM* TNM classification, *TRUS* transrectal ultrasonography, *VMAT* volumetric modulated arc radiotherapy

severe urinary retention, but medication relieved my symptoms. After Christmas 2022, my VMAT therapies continued, and a single brachytherapy session was planned for the beginning of February 2023.

The time course of my history is presented in Table 18.1. The major findings are listed as well in Table 18.1. The diagnostic procedures and treatments are discussed separately later.

Prostate Cancer Diagnosis

The case history is described earlier. The imaging findings are summarized in Fig. 18.1. The results of diagnostic studies are listed in Table 18.1. In summary, this 67-year-old male was diagnosed with GS7 prostate cancer, and he was treated with ADT in combination of VMAT and brachytherapy. The diagnosis T2bN0M0 was based on MRI, CT, and two PSMA-PET imaging studies, and the histology was obtained from 13 biopsies.

The MRI study report did not explain any other pathology in the prostate besides the large size. However, there is an apical cancer extending to the capsule (Fig. 18.1) which can be seen both in T1- and T2-weighed images. Its classification is PIRADS 4/5. In this case, I would consider to be a victim of medical malpractice. I also found that whole body CT to exclude or confirm prostate cancer metastases is not anymore appropriate. There are multiple PET studies available as discussed in this book elsewhere which perform better than CT in evaluation of metastatic sites of prostate cancer.

The prostate biopsies taken revealed a prostate. A total of 12 sectorial biopsies were taken, and they contained 8 mm cancer in a total of 139 mm sample biopsies. Additionally, a biopsy was taken for the screening study.

There was 4 mm cancer in the left apex, 2.5 mm in the left middle sections, and 1 mm in the left basis. On the right, there is 0.5 mm cancer in the apex. The Gleason score was 3 + 4 in 25% of samples.

Fortunately, I was puzzled with these findings in contrast to the imaging results. Therefore, I wanted to have PET confirmation for my own disease.

The first PET study with ^{18}F-PSMA-1007-PET revealed two intraprostatic foci with SUVmax up to 14.8. The ^{18}F-DCFPyL-PET on the following day showed one intraprostatic focus with SUVmax 11.9 (in the left apex). Biopsies showed PCa on both sides as discussed earlier. The tumors were larger in PET as compared to the MRI 3 months earlier.

The dose lineation for VMAT and brachytherapy was based on ^{18}F-PSMA-1007-PET. The studies and PSA values are listed in Table 18.2. The PET imaging is shown in Fig. 18.2. The radiation therapy plans are shown in Fig. 18.3. The PSA

Table 18.2 S-PSA during the treatments (hormone therapy + EBRT + brachy)

Date Study	S-PSA	Comment
March 2022	7.9	4K test 12% (>10%)
September 2022 MRI		51 cm^3 T2bN0 Report T0M0(!)
October 2022	7.6	Free 1.58 PSA-ratio 21% (>15%)
October 2022 Biopsy		GS 3 + 4 (25%); 8/139 mm R_{ap} 0.5(1), L_{ap} 4(2), L_{mi}2.5(2), L_{ba}1(1)
November Whole body CT		N0M0
Nov 22022 ^{18}F-PSMA-1007		$L_{ap/mi}$, R_{ap} SUVmax 14.8 T2bN0
Nov 2022 ^{18}F-DCFPyL		Lap SUVmax 11.9 T2aN0 (!)
Dec the 15th 2022 Start of 20 cycles of EBRT and HT	13.2	Cold anchor deposited Dec the 14th (iatrogenic elevation of S-PSA)
Jan the 16th 2023 Second HT	1.22	2 VMAT cycles left
Jan the 25th 2023	0.54	
Feb the 3rd 2023 Brachytherapy		
Feb the 24th 2023	0.06	PSA-nadir after radiation therapies
July 2023	0.11	
September 2023	0.41	PSA-stabilized after hormone and radiation therapies

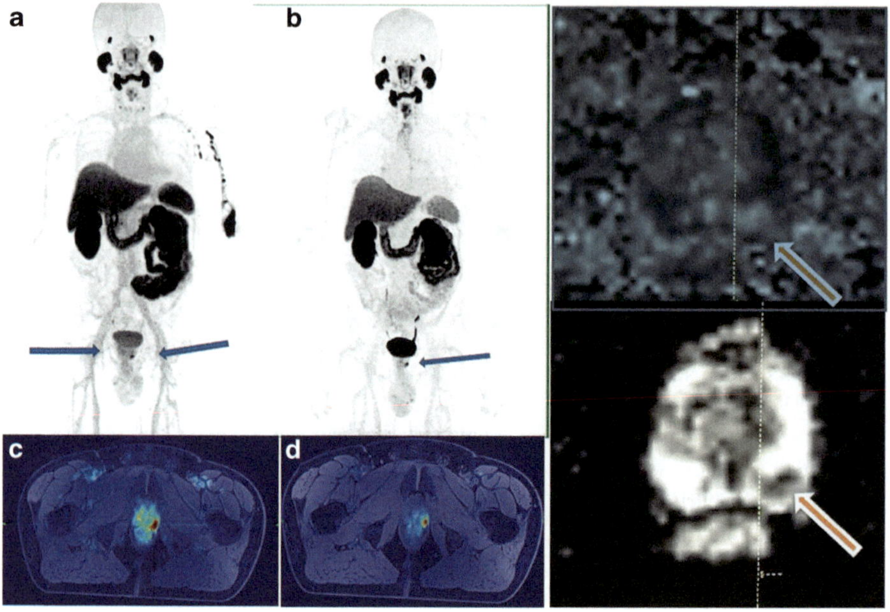

Fig. 18.2 An example of a patient case, where radiation dose planning is based on two PET studies in a primary disease. Diagnostic imaging. On the left, ^{18}F-PSMA-1007-PET demonstrates prostatic disease (two lesions), in panel **a** (MIP image) and panel **c** (fusion image). In the ^{18}F-DCFPyL-PET studies, only one lesion is shown, in panel **b** (MIP image) and panel **d** (fusion image). The lesions are shown with blue arrows in the MIP images (**a** and **b**). SUV_{max} values were 14.7 and 11.8. On the right, the 3T-MRI studies are shown in T1- and T2-weighed images—a PIRADS 4/5 tumor, approximately 1 cm in diameter, is seen in the left apical region with capsular contact (white/orange arrows)

response in this patient was more 90%, it decreased from 7.6 to 0.06 μg/L. The prostate size decreased from 51 cm^3 (MRI) to 28 cm^3 (US).

Treatments and Active Surveillance

As written previously, I was diagnosed with GS7 prostate cancer, stage T2bN0M0, and the idea was to treat it with ADT in combination of VMAT and brachytherapy. The staging was based on MRI, CT, and two PSMA-PET imaging studies, and histology was obtained from prostate biopsies.

The first PET study with ^{18}F-PSMA-1007-PET revealed two intraprostatic foci with SUVmax up to 14.8. The ^{18}F-DCFPyL-PET on the following day showed one intraprostatic focus with SUVmax 11.9 (in the left apex). Biopsies showed PCa on both sides.

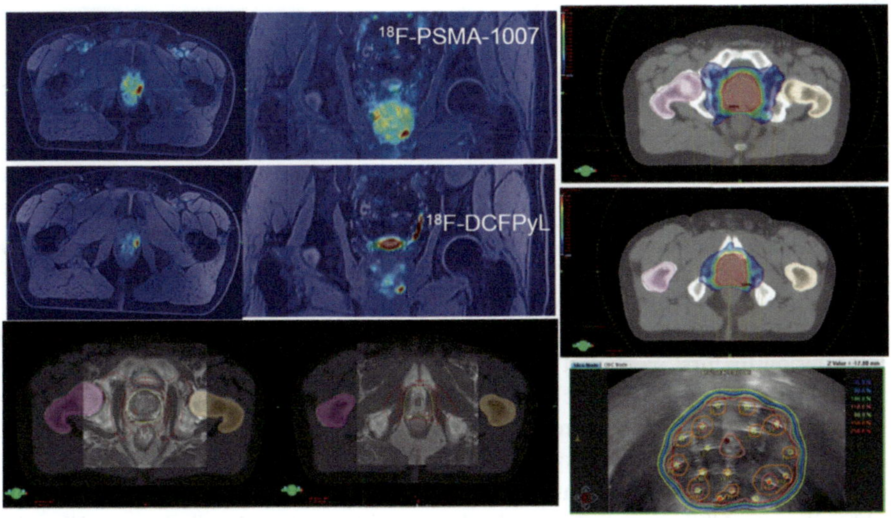

Fig. 18.3 An example of a patient case, where radiation dose planning is based on two PET studies in a primary disease. Dose planning studies and dose distributions in VMAT and brachytherapy. On the left in the upper panel ^{18}F-PSMA-1007-PET findings and in the middle panel ^{18}F-DCFPyL-PET findings in the transaxial and coronal PET/CT fusion images are shown. On the left, in the lower panel, transaxial dose distributions are shown on MRI. On the right, in the upper and middle panel, dose distribution is shown at two levels and in the lower panel the local doses in the HDR brachytherapy. The dose planning was based on ^{18}F-PSMA-1007-PET, and doses to the prostate, seminal vesicles, and pelvic lymph nodes were 62 Gy, 49.4 Gy, and 44 Gy, respectively. The HDR brachytherapy dose was 15 Gy using 17 needles. In this patient, there was >90% biochemical response in 3 months

The dose lineation for external beam radiotherapy (VMAT as known as RapidArc) and intraprostatic brachytherapy was based on ^{18}F-PSMA-1007-PET. The dose planning PET studies and dose distribution images for the radiation therapy plans are shown Fig. 18.1. The ADT started in mid-December 2022 with degarelix (Firmagon®) and continued with Triptorelin® in mid-January 2023. The VMAT was given in 20 cycles, starting in mid-December 2022 and ending in mid-January 2023. The planned total cumulative doses to the prostate, seminal vesicles, and pelvic lymph nodes were 62 Gy, 49.4 Gy, and 44 Gy, respectively. The HDR brachytherapy was performed in the beginning of February 2023, and the total dose to the prostate was 15 Gy using 17 needles. The high dose brachytherapy utilizes Ir-192 irradiation locally. Figure 18.1 demonstrates the positioning of needles in the transrectal US image. The prostate volume in this study was 28 cm^3, whereas it was 51 cm^3 5 months earlier in the MRI. The best PSA-response in this patient was more than 90%, it decreased from 7.6 to 0.06 µg/L.

It is noteworthy that I gave an invited plenary lecture in the Austrian Nuclear Medicine Conference between my VMAT and brachytherapy.

Symptoms

I had frequent urination even before radiotherapy, approximately twice a night due to enlarged prostate. Within 1 week during the external beam radiotherapy, the symptoms worsened, up to two to seven times at night. Tamsulosin and tadalafil were started, which brought some minor relief. The water intake was 1.5–2 liters per day. During the last week, I woke up 4 times a night to urinate, and I urinate in average 13 times during the day. I could not empty the bladder properly. For example, as measured, there was 215 ml of urine in the bladder when checked by ultrasound—after urinating, there was still 131 ml of residual urine.

The bowel movements were regular. During radiation therapy, the stool loosened a little during the first week, but there was no need for antidiarrheal medicine. A few times, there was a little bit of clear blood with the intestinal mucus—with no hemorrhoids. Blood came from the rectum during the first 3 weeks, but no more blood at during the last fourth week. Also, mucus has not come out significantly from the rectum.

One month after the subsequent brachytherapy, the urologist wrote: "A fit 67-year-old colleague. GS7 prostate cancer. Ended up with combined radiotherapy. First, he received external radiation therapy in a private cancer hospital, and then we had 15 Gy HDR brachytherapy for the entire prostate area. The treatment was combined with a total of 4 months of neoadjuvant treatment (chemical castration). After brachytherapy, there was macroscopic hematuria for 3 weeks, which has now subsided. No other local symptoms. Now PSA 0.06 (nadir). Hormone therapy does not continue."

Half a year later, after the 4 months of adjuvant hormone therapy, the symptoms had been corrected. Dysuria, pollacisuria, and hematuria were related to radiotherapy. There was even a need for catheterization for a while due to urinary retention. Then there were no significant urinary problems—I could sleep.

Active Surveillance

Then it became the time of active surveillance. Personally, I was following the PSA doubling time; it changed from 0.06 to 0.11 in 2 months and then from 0.11 to 0.41 in 5 months. I was a little bit worried, but realistic. I also checked S-testosterone levels—it remained stable in two measurements within 6 weeks. The PSA values also started to stabilize—now the latest value a year later is 0.47. It is normal for the PSA to rise after the end of the hormonal effect, but level is of course individual. The PSA curve is shown in Fig. 18.4.

A year after the brachytherapy, the urinary symptoms worsened. I had to urinate 5–11 times per night, up to 15–20 times a day. For this pollacisuria, a new medication, mirabegron, was started. It is a selective agonist of beta-3 adrenergic receptors, which relaxes detrusor smooth muscle during the storage phase of the urinary bladder fill-void cycle, which increases the bladder's storage capacity, thereby alleviating feelings of urgency and frequency. This medication has helped after 6 months of use. I have to wake up three to five times per night. A ^{68}Ga-PSMA-11 PET MIP image (Fig. 18.5) demonstrates a substantial urinary retention in ureters and in the

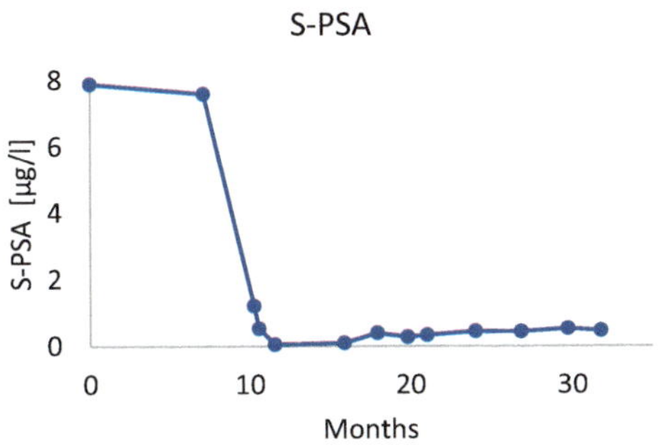

Fig. 18.4 The behavior of the serum PSA values in this patient. The follow-up from the suspicion of PCa (month 0) and hormone and radiation therapies started 9 months later: VMAT (month 9) and brachytherapy (month 11). The PSA nadir 0.06 µg/L was achieved in 12 months. The PSA reached the value 0.41 µg/L in 18 months—after that, it has been fluctuating from 0.29 to 0.53 µg/L up to 30 months' follow-up from the beginning

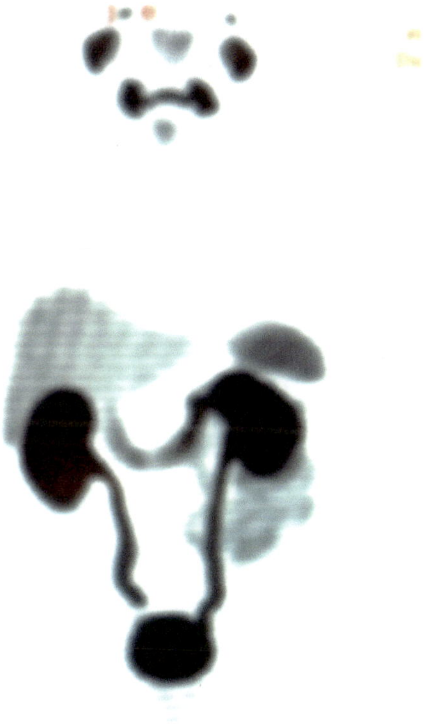

Fig. 18.5 The ^{68}Ga-PSMA-11 PET (MIP image) of the same patient as in Fig. 18.2 16 months after brachytherapy and external beam radiation therapy. The major side effects were associated with dysuria and pollacisuria. In the PET/CT study, there were no signs of recurrence, but remarkable urinary retention in spite of voiding before the imaging session

urinary bladder in spite of immediate voiding before the study. In this PET/CT study, there were no signs of recurrence.

I have not had substantial urinary incontinence. There are three mechanisms for controlling urination. These include the sphincter around the bladder neck, muscle fibers in the prostate gland, and the detrusor muscle that is used to consciously stop or start the urine stream. An enlarged prostate might cause an urge to void frequently. This is usually due to an irritated bladder muscle and inadequate emptying of the bladder. I have heard from prostatectomized patients that it may take months before these urge symptoms disappear after removing the prostate. Incontinence is rather frequent in older men. Anyway, my symptoms are related to an irradiated bladder and partially destroyed prostate gland. The sphincter functionality, however, could be saved, at least partially, in spite of the fact that the bilateral tumor was located mainly apically.

So here we are. I am mostly suffering pollacisuria. Hopefully new medication will help or then I have to stop drinking (water). This was the situation in November 2024. Now, this condition, postradiation cystitis, has significantly relieved with medication: with alpha-blockers or phosphodiesterase-5 inhibitors, which facilitate bladder emptying; 5-alpha reductase inhibitors, which reduce the size of the prostate gland; beta-3 agonists or anticholinergics, which reduce the symptoms of overactive bladder. Additionally intravesical instillations of hyaluronic acid have been given.

Public Appearance Because of Nuclear Oncology (Pictorial Essay)

19

In 1974, I started my university career in the Department of Chemical Engineering at Helsinki University of Technology, resulting in MSc (Eng) degree in 1980. I started my medical studies in 1979 (picture as medical student in 1985; Fig. 19.1). I completed my MD degree in 1986 and EU orientation internship phase in 1987 and got MD, PhD (D.Med. Sci) degree in 1993. I took Medical Specialist training in Clinical Chemistry (examination in 1994), Nuclear Medicine (1996), Health Care Administration (2002) and Pharmaceutical Medicine (2006), all at University of Helsinki HU (Central Hospital).

I got a lot of publicity in the biggest newspaper (*Helsingin Sanomat*) in Finland in 1993 (Fig. 19.2), because of my dissertation about Mab imaging in cancer. After that I started to avoid publicity, because I could not arrange new imaging or therapy opportunities for cancer patients.

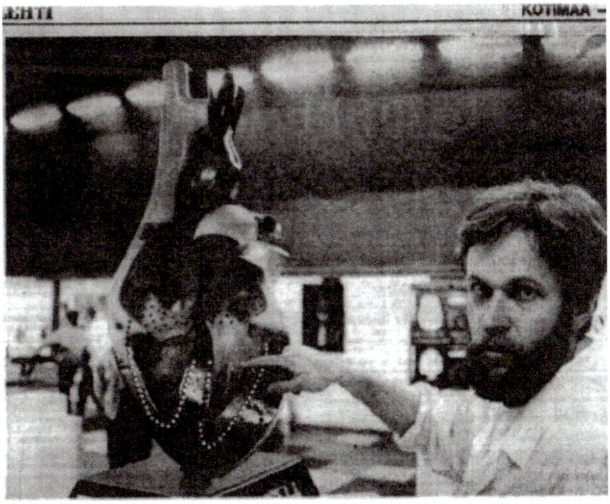

Fig. 19.1 Guide in the Medical Exhibition for Science Center Heureka, Aamulehti Newspaper, in 1985

K. Kairemo, *Prostate Cancer from a Nuclear Oncology Perspective*,
https://doi.org/10.1007/978-3-031-90337-3_19

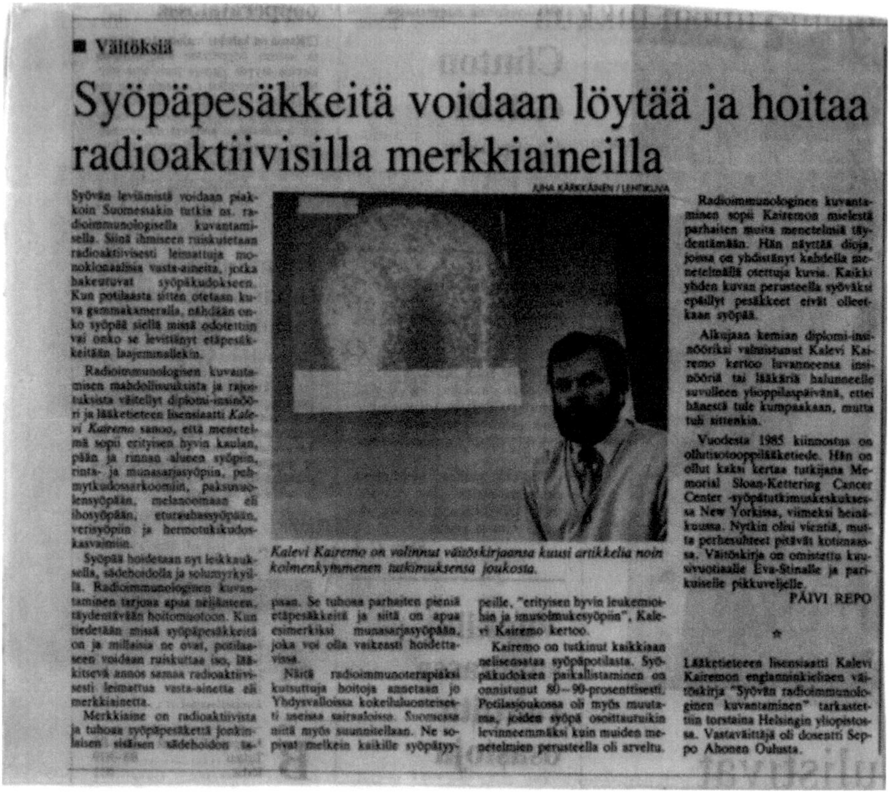

■ Väitöksiä

Syöpäpesäkkeitä voidaan löytää ja hoitaa radioaktiivisilla merkkiaineilla

Syövän leviämistä voidaan pian Suomessakin tutkia ns. radioimmunologisella kuvantamisella. Siinä ihmiseen ruiskutetaan radioaktiivisesti leimattuja monoklonaalisia vasta-aineita, jotka hakeutuvat syöpäkudokseen. Kun potilaasta sitten otetaan kuva gammakameralla, nähdään onko syöpä siellä missä odotettiin vai onko se levittänyt etäpesäkkeitään laajemmallekin.

Radioimmunologisen kuvantamisen mahdollisuuksista ja rajoituksista väitellyt diplomi-insinööri ja lääketieteen lisensiaatti *Kalevi Kairemo* sanoo, että menetelmä sopii erityisen hyvin kaulan, pään ja rinnan alueen syöpiin, rinta- ja munasarjasyöpiin, pehmytkudossarkoomiin, paksusuolensyöpään, melanoomaan eli ihosyöpään, eturauhassyöpään, verisyöpiin ja hermotukikudoskasvaimiin.

Syöpää hoidetaan nyt leikkauksella, sädehoidolla ja solumyrkyillä. Radioimmunologinen kuvantaminen tarjoaa apua neljänteen, täydentävään hoitomuotoon. Kun tiedetään missä syöpäpesäkkeitä on ja millaisia ne ovat, potilaaseen voidaan ruiskuttaa iso, lääkitsevä annos samaa radioaktiivisesti leimattua vasta-ainetta eli merkkiainetta.

Merkkiaine on radioaktiivista ja tuhoaa syöpäpesäkkeitä jonkinlaisen sisäisen sädehoidon tapaan. Se tuhoaa parhaiten pieniä etäpesäkkeitä ja siitä on apua esimerkiksi munasarjasyöpään, joka voi olla vaikeasti hoidettavissa.

Näitä radioimmunoterapiaksi kutsuttuja hoitoja annetaan jo Yhdysvalloissa kokeiluluonteisesti useissa sairaaloissa. Suomessa niitä myös suunnitellaan. Ne sopivat melkein kaikille syöpätyypeille, "erityisen hyvin leukemioihin ja imusolmukesyöpiin", Kalevi Kairemo kertoo.

Kairemo on tutkinut kaikkiaan neljisensataa syöpäpotilasta. Syöpäkudoksen paikallistaminen on onnistunut 80–90-prosenttisesti. Potilasjoukossa oli myös muutamia, joiden syöpä osoittautuikin levinneemmäksi kuin muiden menetelmien perusteella oli arveltu.

Kalevi Kairemo on valinnut väitöskirjaansa kuusi artikkelia noin kolmenkymmenen tutkimuksensa joukosta.

Radioimmunologinen kuvantaminen sopii Kairemon mielestä parhaiten muita menetelmiä täydentämään. Hän näyttää dioja, joissa on yhdistänyt kahdella menetelmällä otettuja kuvia. Kaikki yhden kuvan perusteella syöväksi epäillyt pesäkkeet eivät olleetkaan syöpää.

Alkujaan kemian diplomi-insinööriksi valmistunut Kalevi Kairemo kertoo isovanhempiensa insinööriä tai lääkäriä halunneelle suvulleen ylioppilaspäivänä, ettei hänestä tule kumpaakaan, mutta tuli sittenkin.

Vuodesta 1985 kiinnostus on ollut isotooppilääketiede. Hän on ollut kaksi kertaa tutkijana Memorial Sloan-Kettering Cancer Center -syöpätutkimuskeskuksessa New Yorkissa, viimeksi heinäkuussa. Nytkin olisi vientiä, mutta perhesuhteet pitävät kotimaassa. Väitöskirja on omistettu kuusivuotiaalle Eva-Stinalle ja parikuiselle pikkuveljelle.

PÄIVI REPO

*

Lääketieteen lisensiaatti Kalevi Kairemon englanninkielinen väitöskirja "Syövän radioimmunologinen kuvantaminen" tarkastettiin torstaina Helsingin yliopistossa. Vastaväittäjä oli dosentti Seppo Ahonen Oulusta.

Fig. 19.2 "Cancer can be detected and found with radioactive drugs," my dissertation, Newspaper Helsingin Sanomat in 1993

I had had a postdoctoral research fellowship at Memorial Sloan-Kettering Cancer Center (MSKCC) from 1989 to 1991 and again in 1993 in New York. I had an interview in the Finnish newspaper in New York as well (Fig. 19.3).

In 1994, I was appointed to a position of Associate Professor in Experimental Nuclear Medicine at HU. In 1999, this was upgraded to a clinical position, Associate Professor in Nuclear Medicine and Clinical Chemistry. Then I got a Professorship in Clinical Chemistry at the Norwegian University of Science and Technology (1998–1999), Professor in Nuclear Medicine at Uppsala University Hospital in Sweden (2001–2005), and Head of the Nuclear Medicine Division, Department of Oncology at Helsinki University Central Hospital (2004–2009).

In 2010–2018, I was the Chief of Nuclear Medicine and Molecular Radiotherapy (Theragnostics) at the Docrates Cancer Center, in Helsinki. Since 2015, I have been a Visiting Professor in the Nuclear Medicine Department of the University of Texas MD Anderson Cancer Center.

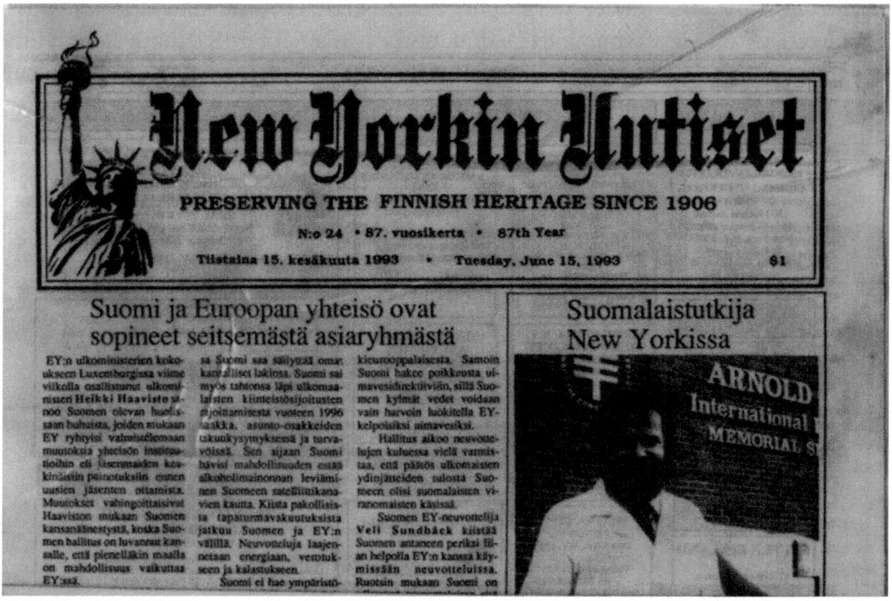

New Yorkin Uutiset

PRESERVING THE FINNISH HERITAGE SINCE 1906

N:o 24 • 87. vuosikerta • 87th Year

Tiistaina 15. kesäkuuta 1993 • Tuesday, June 15, 1993 $1

Suomi ja Euroopan yhteisö ovat sopineet seitsemästä asiaryhmästä

Suomalaistutkija New Yorkissa

Fig. 19.3 A Finnish researcher at Memorial Sloan-Kettering Cancer Center, the front page of New York Times (in Finnish) in 1993

Pharmaceutical Industry I have also held posts in industry, as Medical Director of CTT Cancer Targeting Technologies (2001–2006), Medical Director of Imanext Ltd. (2006–2008), and Clinical Director at Advanced Accelerator Applications SA (AAA), a joint French-Italian company. CTT was a Finnish biotech company focusing in targeted drug delivery with intelligent nanoparticles and phage display technology. Imanext was a contract research organization focusing in tailored imaging services for pharmaceutical industry, having research sites in 38 countries. AAA is now a Novartis Company, but in 2009 I was involved with initiating clinical services and designing phase I trials, such as LutaThera® which in 8 years became a blockbuster product. Occasionally, I have also acted as Consultant in MAP Medical Technologies Oy in Helsinki (now part of Curium Pharma).

Authority Service I also acted as Chief Physician in the National Radiation and Nuclear Safety Authority (STUK) in 2000 by introducing national guidelines regarding the use radioactive compounds according to the EU Directive for Medical Radiation Safety. In my research, I have developed and investigated multiple tumor-seeking compounds, including monoclonal antibodies, specific phage display peptides, and cytotoxic drugs. I also have coordinated multiple EU research program proposals in 1995–2004, and the most important of these activities was the European Union COST Action Project (BM 0607, Targeted Radionuclide Therapy) where I was the National Coordinator and Management Committee Member for 2007–2011.

For industry, I have been developing intelligent targeting nanoparticles which contained cytotoxic compounds and/or tracers (also for MRI, optical or ultrasound imaging). The key targets were MMP's and leukocyte integrins. I have been involved with, e.g., radiation sensitizing, hypoxia, angiogenesis, and apoptosis related targeting approaches. I also worked with gene therapy radionuclide applications (nanotargeting). In the clinic, I was developing PET tracers for oncology, actually by introducing more than ten new tracers into clinical practice (compassionate use) in Finland. One of the foci was early response evaluation in clinical cancer therapy.

For scientific periodicals, I have edited several special issues. Some examples are as follows:

1. For *Current Radiopharmaceuticals*, two special issues, i.e., the very first issue vol. 1 (1) in 2008 with a special emphasis on "The Role of Radiopharmaceuticals in Drug Discovery" and for the second time vol. 8 (1) in 2015 with special topics in "PET/CT in External Beam Radiation Therapy Dose Planning."
2. For *Diagnostics (Basel)*, multiple special issues in 2015–2020: two of them dealt with early response evaluation.
3. For *Current Pharmaceutical Design*, two special issues: the last dealt with "Targeted Drug Delivery and Theragnostics" (picture of the journal flyer in Fig. 19.4).
4. Two for *International Journal of Molecular Sciences* entitled "Targeted Therapies in Cancer: Radionuclides, Multi-Omics and Nanomedicine" and "Selected Papers from the 12th Targeted Alpha Therapy Congress."
5. One for *Life*.
6. One for *Acta Oncology*.

Besides a few patents, I have published more than 250 original articles in peer-reviewed journals (PubMed 190+, RG 280+). I also received the Lifetime Achievement Award from the World Association of Radiopharmaceutical and Molecular Therapy (WARMTH) in 2012.

Own Congresses I have arranged multiple international medical congresses in Finland, Sweden, and Denmark. In Uppsala, I arranged two International Congresses in Nuclear Medicine (2002) and Radiobiology (2003). I acted as President of an International Conference for Pharmaceutical Development in Copenhagen in 2007. At Docrates Cancer, I hosted four international conferences about nuclear oncology, nuclear endocrinology, and emergency oncology and theragnostics (2012–2016). Most importantly, I was the President of the seventh International Conference on Radiopharmaceutical Therapy held in November 2012 in Levi in the Finnish Lapland. In 2014, I also hosted ISORBE Symposium and Workshop "Cell Labelling and Cell Therapies" in Helsinki. My latest own arrangement was the International Symposium on Radiopharmaceutical Therapy (WARMTH) in November 2018 in Helsinki (the congress flyer is shown in Fig. 19.5). The Levi Congress group photo is shown in Fig. 19.6.

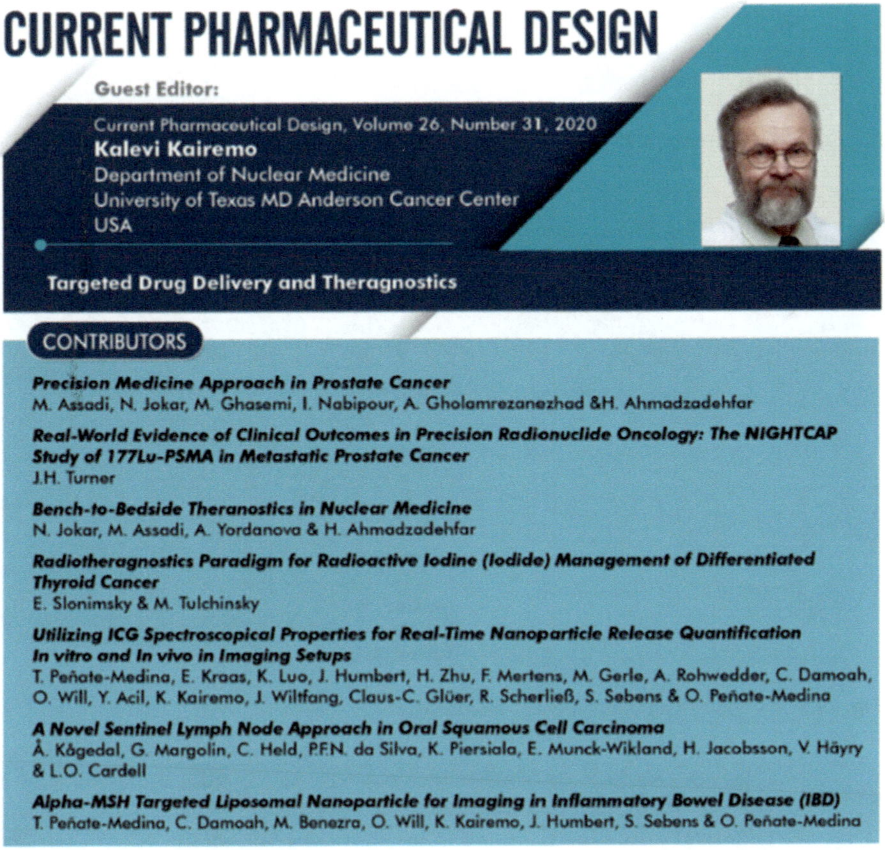

Fig. 19.4 Example of a Special Issue flyer

Clinical Work My work has been mostly semi-clinical, meaning that I have not met all the patients to whom I have given a diagnostic report. Patients whom I treated I have met at the time of administration, but I have not always been able to follow them. My early clinical career was fully patient-oriented. I worked in primary healthcare centers in Helsinki regions. Most of the compulsory EU training I spent in surgery and internal medicine which I did in Ekenäs is Swedish. Most of my training in nuclear medicine and clinical chemistry took place in Helsinki University Central Hospital (Central Laboratory, Radiology and Oncology departments) and in Helsinki City Hospitals in 1985–1998. Then I went to Trondheim University Hospital in Norway (1998–1999) and to Uppsala University Hospital in Sweden (2001–2005). I also acted as Chief Physician in Kymenlaakso Central Hospital (Kotka) and South Karelia Central Hospital (Lappeenranta) in 2006–2010. Clinical highlights were multiple, but I never could imagine to end up on a front page of tabloid papers both in Sweden (*Aftonbladet*) and Finland (*Iltasanomat*) and only because of success in new patient treatments for prostate cancer. I started targeted

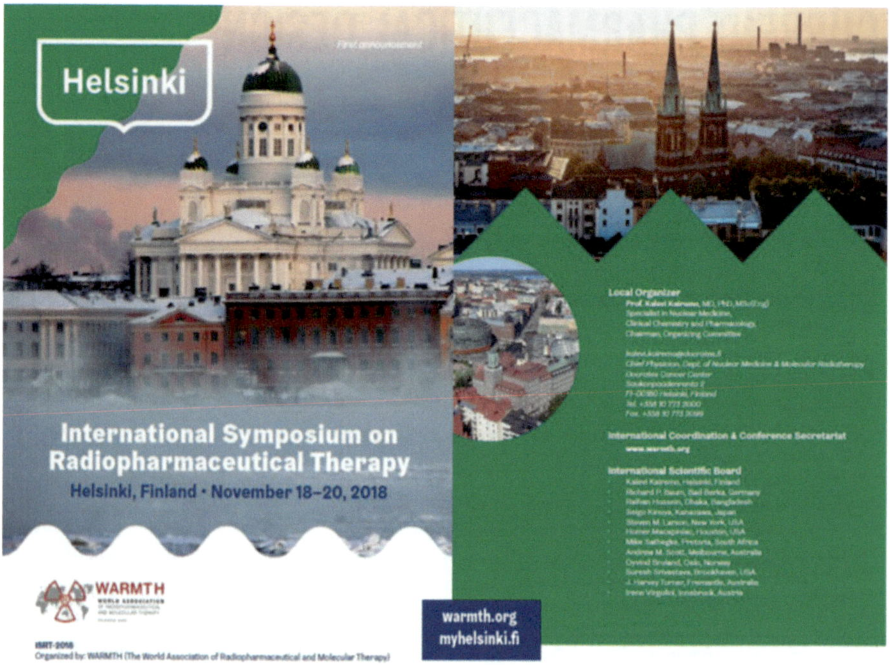

Fig. 19.5 Example of an International Congress flyer

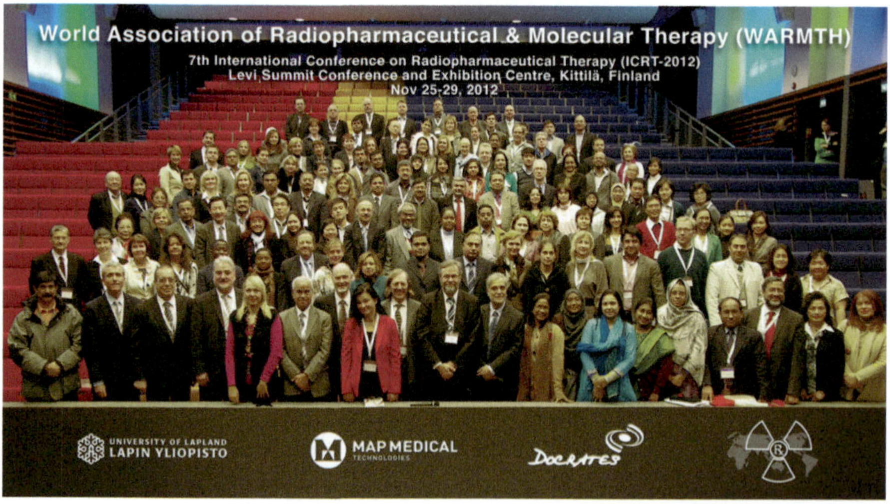

Fig. 19.6 The picture was taken on the last day of the International Congress of Radiopharmaceutical Therapy by WARMTH in Lapland. This was held in Levi in the Finnish Lapland (beyond Arctic Circle in November in 2012) There were 312 registered participants from 72 nationalities. There was 1½ m snow outside, and temperature varied from +1 to −24 °C, no sunlight at that time of the year

radionuclide therapies very early, in the early 1990s radioimmunotherapy in Helsinki, In-111- and Y-90-octreotate therapies both in Helsinki and Uppsala. Lu-177-octreotate was started in the late 2000s. I continued in 2010 at Docrates in Helsinki and introduced more than ten radiopharmaceuticals into clinical practice in Finland. We started very early with Ra-223, Lu-177-octreotate, and Lu-177-PSMA. This meant that I got many foreign patients for treatments. I also introduced multiple PET tracers for oncology routine practice. For prostate cancer, we used choline, fluciclovine, NaF, and multiple PSMA tracers. This allowed us to perform accurate diagnostics, especially in prostate cancer patients. Figures 19.7 and 19.8 show patients who wanted to be interviewed by tabloid newspapers. Figure 19.7 presents a Swedish patient who got a miracle response, reported by a Finnish newspaper, and Fig. 19.8 is another Swedish patient who got Lu-177 as first-line treatment with an excellent response in a Swedish tabloid paper (*Aftonbladet*). Then I was invited to start to set up new methods in other hospital abroad. This activity gave me a lot of international experience.

Science I had the privilege to introduce approximately 20 monoclonal antibodies into clinical practice in the late 1980s and 1990s in multiple indications. SPECT imaging with Tc-99 m, In-111, I-123, or I-131-labeled antibody fragments was used. Furthermore, I introduced radioimmunotherapy in the early 1990s in Finland with Y-90- and I-131-labeled antibodies.

I worked with the theragnostic concept in vitro, in vivo, ex vivo (e.g., radioimmunochemistry), in vivo (Dx), in vivo (Tx), and in vivo (Rx) ever since the late 1980s. One of my initiatives was Auger-chemotherapy in the clinics. I also tested

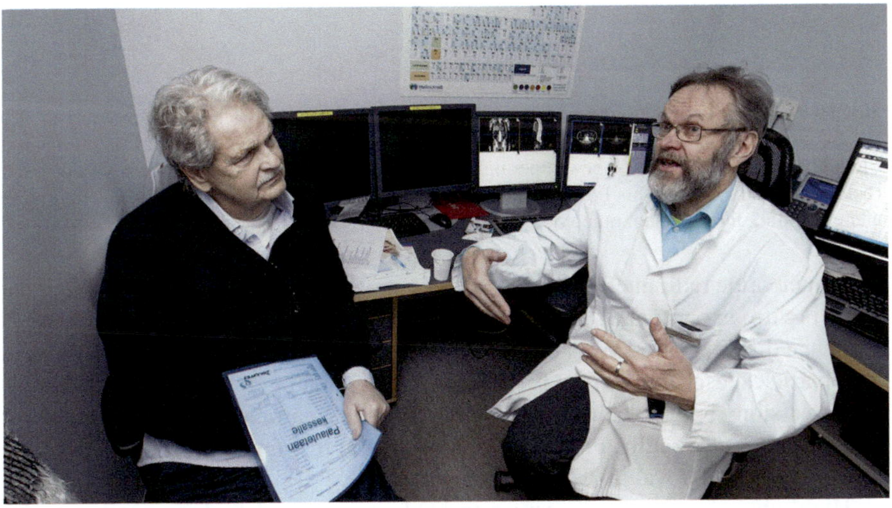

Fig. 19.7 A Swedish PCa patient with me. Picture from the website of a Finnish tabloid newspaper (*Iltasanomat*) stating that he was cured of hopeless cancer in Finland with a medicine that requires a substance from a nuclear reactor (2018)

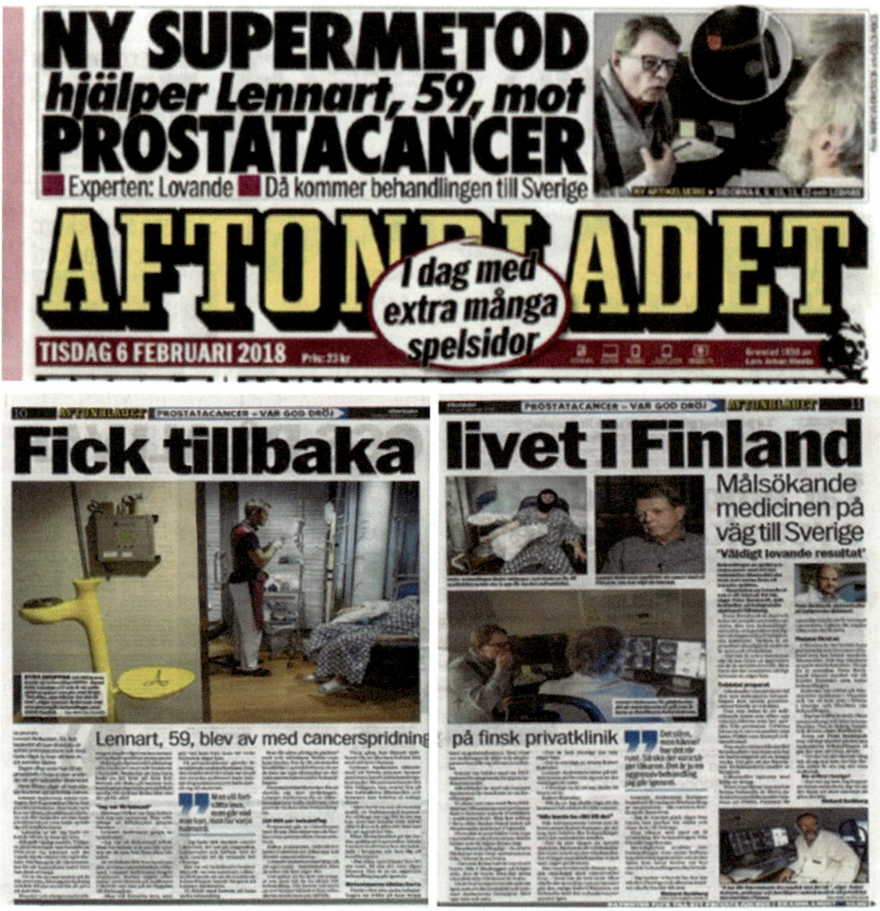
NY SUPERMETOD
hjälper Lennart, 59, mot
PROSTATACANCER
Experten: Lovande Då kommer behandlingen till Sverige
AFTONBLADET
I dag med extra många spelsidor
TISDAG 6 FEBRUARI 2018
PROSTATACANCER – VAR GOD DRÖJ
Fick tillbaka livet i Finland
Målsökande medicinen på väg till Sverige
"Väldigt lovande resultat"
Lennart, 59, blev av med cancerspridning på finsk privatklinik

Fig. 19.8 Example of a tabloid paper reporting radionuclide therapies and therapy tourism. The front cover of *Aftonbadet* in Sweden. I am sitting with the patient who brought the journalist to Finland. (Above): The title "A new super method is helping against prostate cancer" Middle pages (below): the title "He got his life back in Finland." I am sitting with the patient, showing images and explaining the excellent outcome

oligonucleotide radionuclide therapy (radionanotargeting) in theoretical setting and some in vitro experiments.

Phage display peptide was in use in preclinical setting. They were used to target nanoparticles, especially in the CTT Biotech Co. Then I got involved with commercial precision radiomolecular oncology using beta particles to target peptides at AAA in St Genis Pouilly, France; their first clinical theragnostic product LutaThera got marketing approval in 2017.

Highlights of my scientific career probably came very late. I was interviewed in the top journal of my discipline *Journal of Nuclear Medicine* by the Editor-in-Chief Johannes Czernin (Fig. 19.9), where we discuss multiomics, theranostics, and

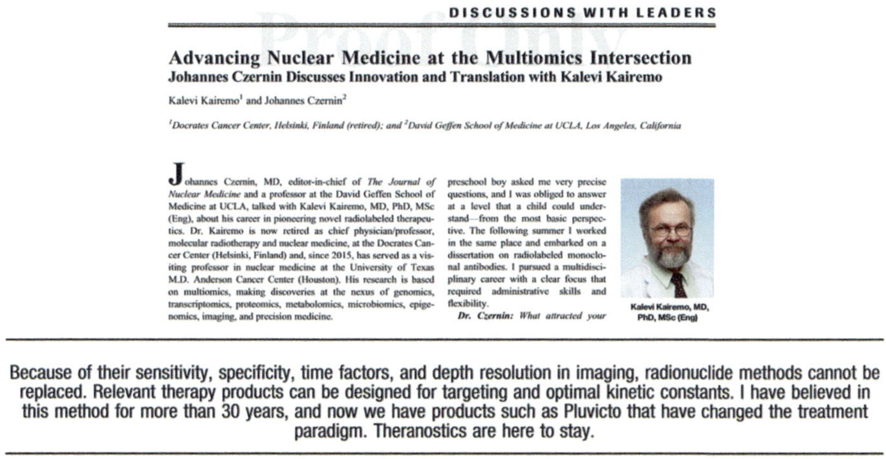
DISCUSSIONS WITH LEADERS

Advancing Nuclear Medicine at the Multiomics Intersection

Johannes Czernin Discusses Innovation and Translation with Kalevi Kairemo

Kalevi Kairemo[1] and Johannes Czernin[2]

[1]Docrates Cancer Center, Helsinki, Finland (retired); and [2]David Geffen School of Medicine at UCLA, Los Angeles, California

Johannes Czernin, MD, editor-in-chief of *The Journal of Nuclear Medicine* and a professor at the David Geffen School of Medicine at UCLA, talked with Kalevi Kairemo, MD, PhD, MSc (Eng), about his career in pioneering novel radiolabeled therapeutics. Dr. Kairemo is now retired as chief physician/professor, molecular radiotherapy and nuclear medicine, at the Docrates Cancer Center (Helsinki, Finland) and, since 2015, has served as a visiting professor in nuclear medicine at the University of Texas M.D. Anderson Cancer Center (Houston). His research is based on multiomics, making discoveries at the nexus of genomics, transcriptomics, proteomics, metabolomics, microbiomics, epigenomics, imaging, and precision medicine.

preschool boy asked me very precise questions, and I was obliged to answer at a level that a child could understand—from the most basic perspective. The following summer I worked in the same place and embarked on a dissertation on radiolabeled monoclonal antibodies. I pursued a multidisciplinary career with a clear focus that required administrative skills and flexibility.

***Dr. Czernin:** What attracted your*

Kalevi Kairemo, MD, PhD, MSc (Eng)

Because of their sensitivity, specificity, time factors, and depth resolution in imaging, radionuclide methods cannot be replaced. Relevant therapy products can be designed for targeting and optimal kinetic constants. I have believed in this method for more than 30 years, and now we have products such as Pluvicto that have changed the treatment paradigm. Theranostics are here to stay.

Fig. 19.9 Front page of my interview by Johannes Czernin in the *Journal of Nuclear Medicine*. It discusses some aspects of my career, including multiomics, theranostics, and international collaboration. The raised text (below) is from the interview and related to Lu-177-PSMA treatment in prostate cancer. (J. Nucl. Med. 2023; 64(11): 1671–1673 [1])

international collaboration, because I was elected as President of the World Association of Radiopharmaceutical and Molecular Therapy WARMTH for 2024–2025 [1]. The raised text mentioned Lu-177-PSMA and my multidisciplinary 30-year career in the field.

Very soon after my interview in the *JNM*, I got an invited editorial in The Lancet Oncology [2]. I have been working with alpha particles for more than 30 years. When WARMTH published the results of the global WARMTH Act study, I was very pleased to give an invited commentary (Fig. 19.10).

Alpha therapy has been close to my heart in clinical settings as well. At MD Anderson Cancer Center (MDACC) in Houston, I developed response criteria for metastasized osteosarcoma with $Na^{18}F$. These criteria were for alpha-emitter bone therapy (^{223}Ra), also used in the treatment of skeletal metastases in prostate cancer. I even edited a book about sodium fluoride ($Na^{18}F$) imaging with Homer A. Macapinlac from MDACC. The cover is shown in Fig. 19.11. I also had several guest lectures while I was staying in Texas. An example of advertising is shown below (Fig. 19.12). We are not used to advertise scientific lectures like that.

But this was when all these techniques were quite new in the United States, and we Europeans were frontrunners in this field.

I have done extensive traveling. I am also a member of Maailmanmatkaajat (Globetrotters Finland) where the minimum requirement is 70 countries. I have visited more than 120 UN member states, but I am not interested of travel itself or country count. There has to be several reasons for me to visit a new place. Very much of traveling has been due to participating in conferences, international collaboration, and hospital visits. I have started or I have been helping colleagues (hands on) to set up new therapies in multiple places. Typical to me, I was in tabloid

Comment

Targeted alpha therapy: a new tool for advanced prostate cancer

The study by Mike M Sathekge and colleagues in *The Lancet Oncology*[1] is the largest investigation to demonstrate the antitumour effect and toxicity of alpha-emitting Actinium-225 (^{225}Ac) prostate-specific membrane antigen (PSMA) radioligand therapy (RLT) in metastatic castration-resistant prostate cancer (mCRPC). Before this study, the largest published single institution experience had included 106 patients.[2] Sathekge and colleagues[1] now report 488 patients from countries in four continents: South Africa (n=248), Australia (n=57), India (n=111), and Germany (n=72). The results of 1174 therapy cycles (a median of two cycles [IQR 2–4] per patient) are very convincing, because a substantial antitumour effect (prostate-regarding Lutetium-177 (^{177}Lu)-PSMA RLT in mCRPC by the WARMTH community[3,4] found multiple factors associated with overall survival and progression-free survival and were also able to predict overall survival and progression-free survival before actual registration trials (TheraP[5] and VISION[6]) reported data. In the present study,[1] the beta-emitting radionuclide ^{177}Lu was replaced with the alpha-emitter ^{225}Ac. This study on ^{225}Ac-PSMA RLT[1] is a continuation of the WARMTH multicentre trials: on the basis of a retrospective analysis with a wide clinical experience, multiple factors associated with overall survival and progression-free survival for ^{225}Ac-PSMA RLT can be predicted before official registration trials report data.

Lancet Oncol 2024
Published Online
January 10, 2024
https://doi.org/10.1016/S1470-2045(23)00672-1
See Online/Articles
https://doi.org/10.1016/S1470-2045(23)00638-1

Fig. 19.10 K.Kairemo. Targeted alpha therapy: a new tool for advanced prostate cancer. (Lancet Oncology 2024; 25: 148–9 [2])

paper in Estonia when we administered the very first Lu-177-PSMA treatment in Baltic states (Fig. 19.13).

Retrospectively, I feel that I have had a visionary, systematic, and productive trailblazer career in spite of limited local resources and remote Arctic location. I have always believed in education and resilient learning of new things. I am honored that I found my focus early, and in order to accomplish something, even the details matter. I am very thankful to my wife, children, and grandchildren—without their support, nothing would have happened. To the international community who helped me to create this book, I cannot verbally express my real gratitude. On the next page, I show a few patient examples (from Canadian patient journals: ePatient (Nuclear Medicine [4]), Canadian PSMA guidelines [5], and Le Patient (General Medicine) [6]) who have been treated successfully with radionuclide therapies. Figures 19.14a and 19.14b show my interview and major PET and PSA responses in biochemical recurrences. Figure 19.15 is Canadian guideline team (for patients), and Figs. 19.16a and 19.16b are another interview for wider audience and superresponse by imaging. Without my own delayed cancer diagnosis (knowledge about it), this book would never have been made.

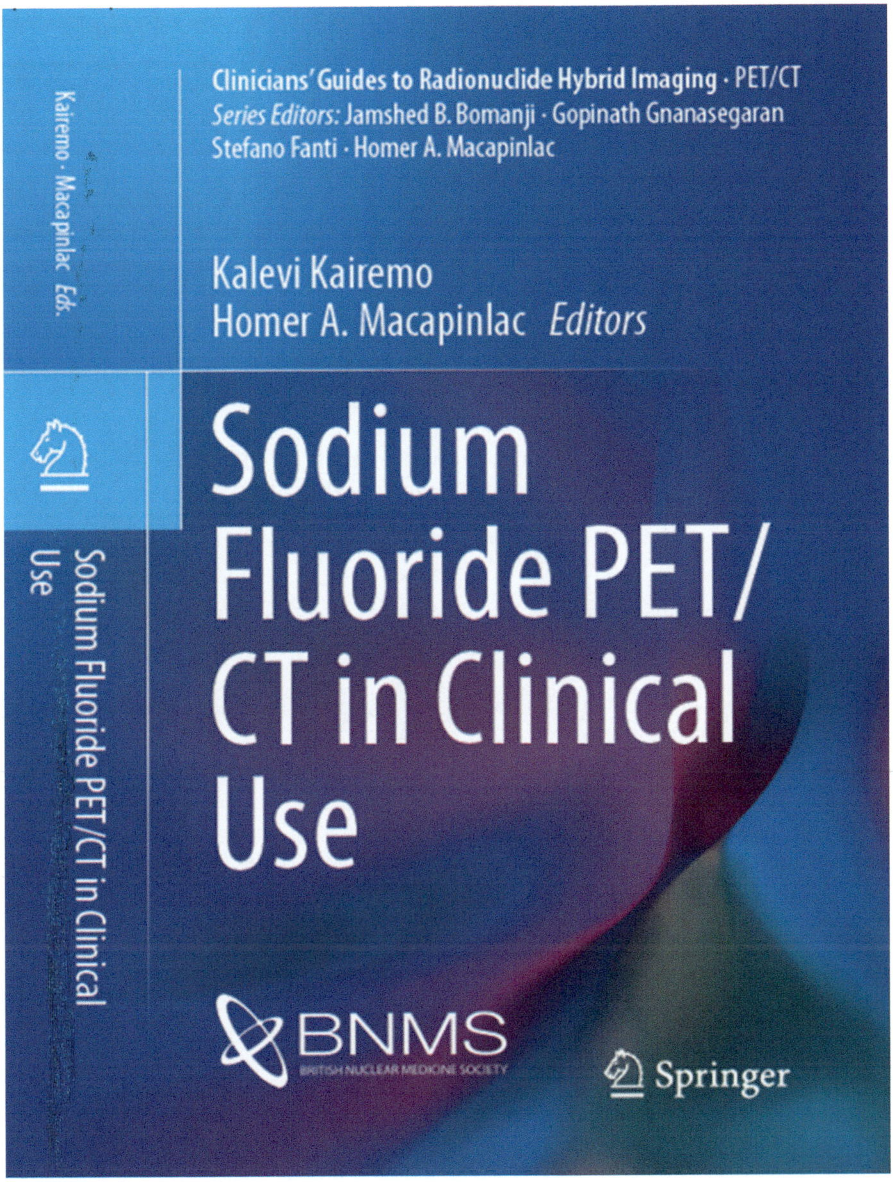

Fig. 19.11 The cover of my Springer ^{18}F-NaF-PET book [3]

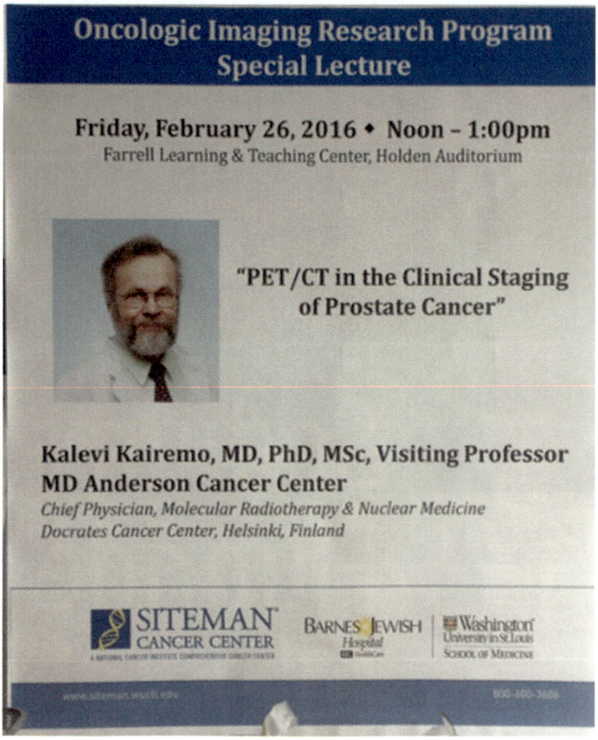

Fig. 19.12 Example of a big wall poster of a guest lecture, St Louis, MO 2016

Ida-Tallinna Keskhaigla alustas uut tüüpi ravi kaugelearenenud eesnäärmevähiga patsientidele (3)

Toimetas Sirje Maasikamäe, 20. detsember 2018, 15:31

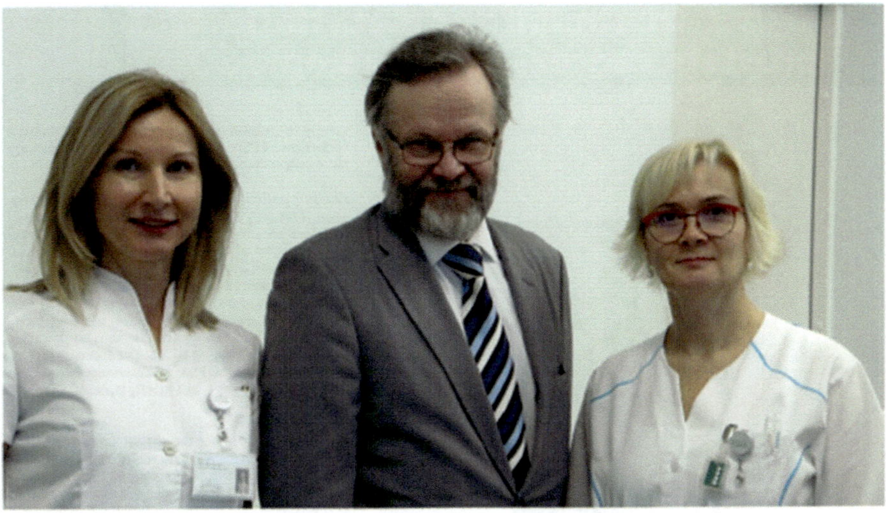

ITK radioloog-vanemarst Eve Kelk, Helsingi Ülikooli nukleaarmeditsiini professor Kalevi Kairemo ja ITK nukelaarmeditsiinikeskuse juhataja Anne Poksi. ITK

Ida-Tallinna Keskhaigla alustas täna Eestis esimesena uut tüüpi ravi kaugelearenenud eesnäärmevähiga patsientidele.

Sama meetodit kasutatakse Põhjamaades veel vaid Soomes. Esimest isotoopravi protseduuri 177Lu-PSMA-ga oli Ida-Tallinna Keskhaiglas nõustamas ja toetamas nukleaarmeditisiini professor Kalevi Kairemo Helsingist.

Uut tüüpi ravist on eriti suur abi patsientidele, kellel esineb haiguse progressioon vaatamata pidevale hormoon- ja keemiaravile või kes keemiaravi enam ei talu selle kõrvaltoimete tõttu.

Fig. 19.13 Together with Estonian doctors after the first ^{177}Lu-PSMA-treatment in Tallinn in 2018 (Õhtuleht). (T book [3])

a

Kalevi Kairemo

Department of Nuclear Medicine and Molecular Radiotherapy, Docrates Cancer Center, Helsinki, Finland

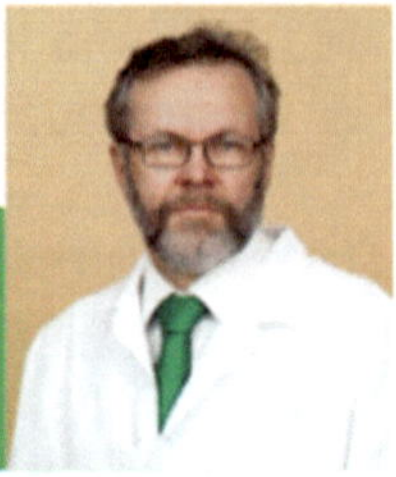

THERAGNOSTICS: Lu-177-PSMA treatment for metastatic prostate cancer – case examples

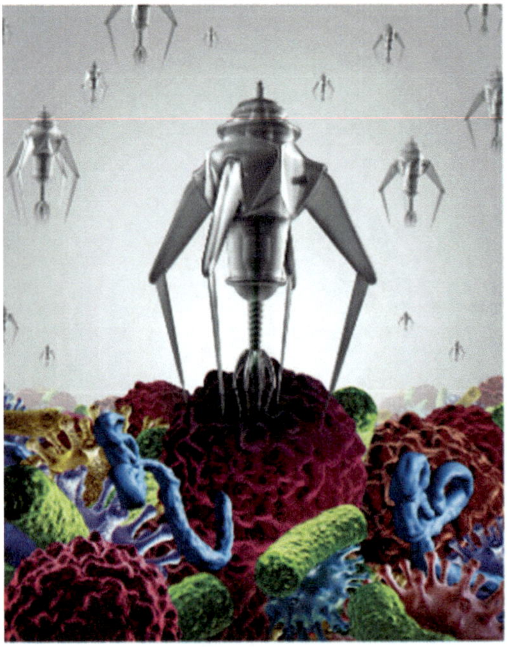

Prostate specific membrane antigen (PSMA) is a membrane glycoprotein with enzymatic activity (as explained in vol.1 no.2 by Jean-Luc Urbain). It is highly expressed in high-risk prostate cancer and therefore PSMA could be a basis for theragnostics. ^{177}Lu-PSMA radioligand therapy is mainly used for patients with end-stage prostate cancer, but it can be used earlier. I describe here three patients: one patient with a multiple recurrences and one with extensive metastastic disease during the first visit, and one patient where it was used as first-line treatmen. All these patients demonstrated a major response with ^{177}Lu-PSMA radioligand therapy, i.e. complete response by imaging and substantial reduction of PSA. ^{177}Lu-PSMA radioligand therapy gave only mild adverse effects.

Our first patient had hypertension and diabetes for years. Primarily PSA increased from 4.6 to 17 ng/ml within 6 months. Diagnosis was done based on second round of biopsies 16 years ago when GS 6 (3+3) prostate adenocarcinoma was found in both lobes. Hormonal therapy was started with leuprorelin and bicalutamide. Prostatectomy was performed 6 months later. Tumor was very large and it was infiltrating also to seminal vesicles, consistent with staging pT3b. The full case history including serum PSA behavior is shown schematically in Fig. 1, but briefly the case history is as follows.

One year later he got external beam radiation therapy to prostate fossa up to 70 Gy, bicalutamide and casodex were used for 3 years, until goserelin was started for 2 years. Bicalutamide was re-started one year later due to PSA increase (up to 4.1 ng/ml). Degarelix was introduced 2 years later for one year. Simultaneously, choline-PET-positive para-iliac and paracaval lymph nodes were irradiated up to 70/2 Gy. However, in PSA continued to increase up to 24 ng/ml and 7 cycles of docetaxel were given with partial response. Four months later, skeletal metastases were found in MRI, and palliative radiotherapy to lumbosarcal region was given. Histrelin acetate device was implanted for castration. Abiraterone and denosumab were started, but they were stopped due to the pain in muscles and joints in four months. The castration implant removed and abiraterone started again for 4 months. Denosumab was also started and continued for more than a year.

Degarelix was restarted, but it was changed to leuprorelin due to local and systemic reaction. He also got radiation therapy to choline positive upper retroperitoneal and mediastinal lymph nodes. Enzalutamide was also started but it had to be stopped in one month due to epileptic seizure. Six month later, dexamethasone combined with cyclophosphamide started to improve immunogenic response, but it had to be stopped due to the diarrhea, swelling and infection. Abiraterone started again, but four months later PSA was 33 ng/ml. On the same day in Ga-68-PSMA-PET-CT at

44

Fig. 19.14a Interview with case presentations (ePatient) [4]

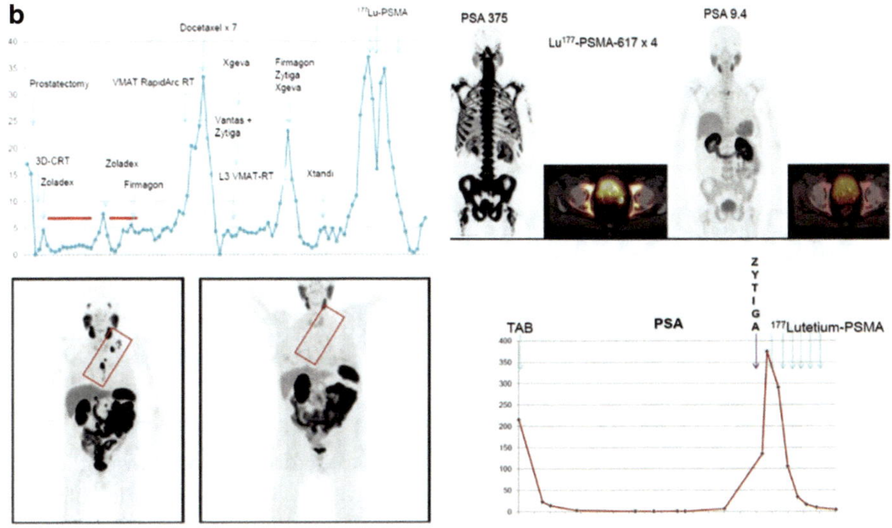

Fig. 19.14b Two cases with excellent responses (ePatient): On the left after the fifth relapse; on the right, after the first [4]. PSA curves and PSMA-PET, before/after [4]

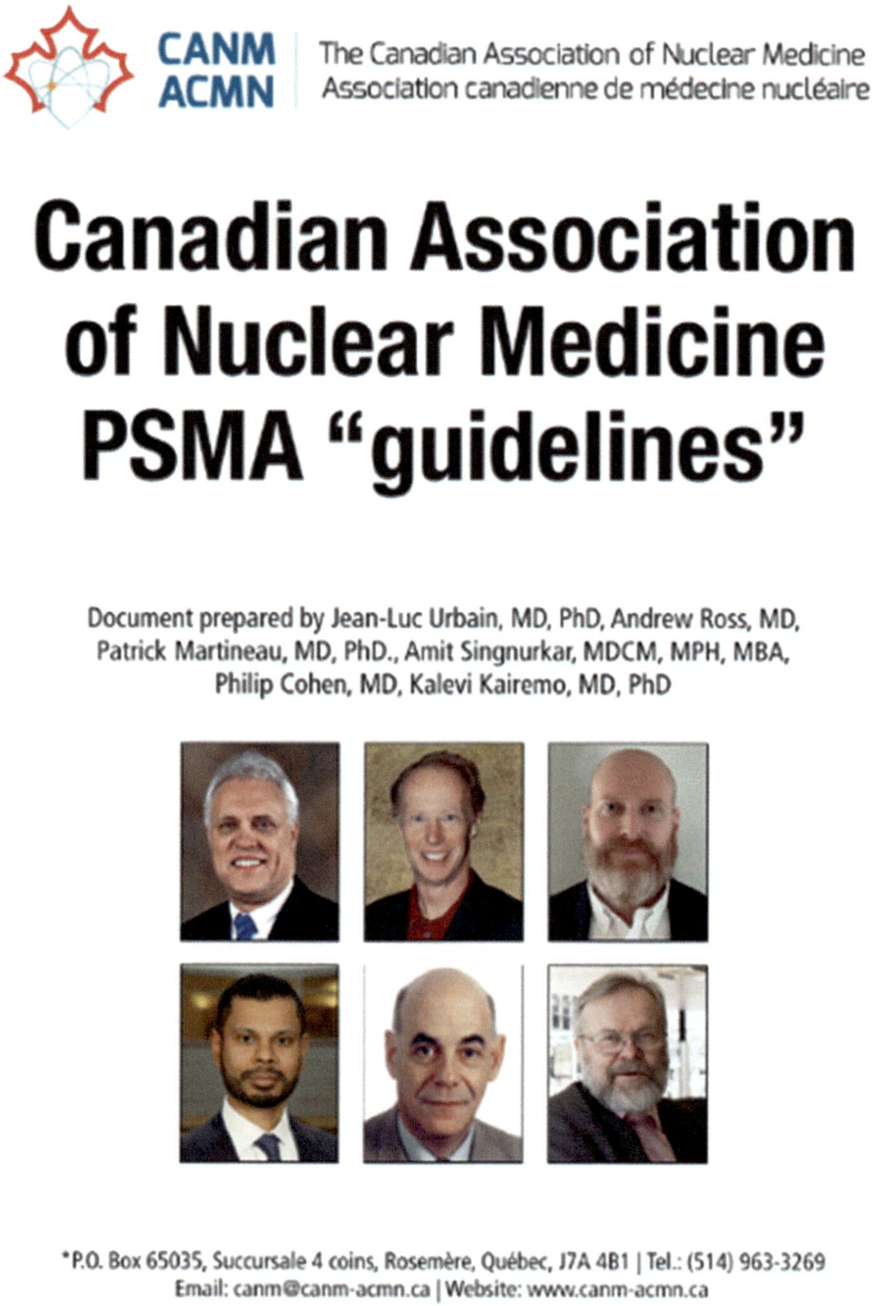

Fig. 19.15 Canadian PSMA guideline team [5]

a

THERA(G)NOSTICS IN PROSTATE CANCER -"PROSTAGNOSTICS"

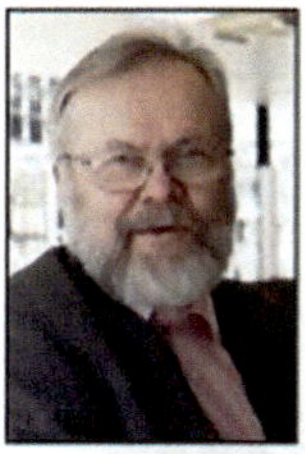

Kalevi Kairemo,
MD, PhD, MSc(Eng),
Professor
Consultant in Nuclear
Medicine, Clinical
Chemistry, Pharmaceutical
Medicine & Health Care
Administration
President 2024-5, World
Association of
Radiopharmaceutical and
Molecular Therapy
WARMTH

"Theranostics has rapidly developed into a viable option for the simultaneous implementation of cancer diagnostics and customized treatment (precision oncology). Theranostics is based on labeling the same molecule with both a diagnostic (most often positron-emitting) and a therapeutic (beta-emitting) isotope."

Theranostics is a giant leap forward in nuclear medicine. What is theranostics? Theranostics simply means combining therapy and diagnosis.

Theranostics has rapidly developed into a viable option for the simultaneous implementation of cancer diagnostics and customized treatment (precision oncology). Theranostics is based on labeling the same molecule with both a diagnostic (most often positron-emitting) and a therapeutic (beta-emitting) isotope. In this case, the treatment dose can be tailored exactly according to the patient, and the actual treatment dose can also be imaged.

Of course, this concept is not new to nuclear medicine. Rather, it has been used for decades to treat thyroid diseases; the first radioiodine therapy was given in 1940's. In recent years, however, theranostics have been successfully used for a whole range of other tumor diseases. These primarily include neuroendocrine tumors and prostate cancer. The effectiveness of the therapy of neuroendocrine tumors with radioactively labeled analogues of the peptide hormone somatostatin was definitely demonstrated in the randomized study, which got the FDA approval in 2017.

The effectiveness of the therapy of neuroendocrine tumors with radioactively labeled analogues of the peptide hormone somatostatin was definitely demonstrated in the NETTER-1 registration trial. This study led to the approval of the ligand ^{177}Lu-DOTA-TATE in Europe and the USA (LutaThera®).

Theranostics (or theragnostics) refers to a close connection between diagnostics and the resulting therapy. In principle, any combination of diagnostics and therapy can be used, e.g. a laboratory value and the resulting consequences for drug therapy. However, the term theranostics is increasingly being used specifically for nuclear medicine imaging and therapy using the same or two very similar radiopharmaceuticals. In parallel, positron-labelled somatostatin analogues ^{68}Ga-DOTA-TATE and 68Ga-DOTA-TOC were approved for neuroendocrine tumor imaging and patient selection for radionuclide therapy.

The VISION and TheraP trials with the aim of approving a radioactively labeled PSMA ligand for the treatment of metastatic prostate cancer were completed in 2021. After these phase III studies on the diagnosis and treatment of prostate cancer using PET/CT and radioactively labeled PSMA ligands, the therapeutic compound ^{177}Lu-PSMA-617 got its approval by 2022 both in Europe and the USA.

The prostate-specific membrane antigen (PSMA) has recently been established as a predictive biomarker for the staging of prostate cancer, as the expression of PSMA correlates with the severity of the disease. At the same time, its extracellular domain (i.e. surface structures) offers an excellent target for the radiopharmaceutical development of PSMA-targeting inhibitors, which can be used for both diagnostic imaging and therapeutic purposes. The abbreviation PSMA stands for prostate-specific membrane antigen. Like PSA, it is a protein (an enzyme) that the body can produce itself and therefore a known substance to the human organism. The PSMA uptake also occurs on the surface of healthy prostate cells, but only in small quantities. Significantly more PSMA - around 1000 times more - can be detected on prostate cancer cells and metastases. The more aggressive a man's prostate cancer is (the higher the Gleason score), the greater the amounts of PSMA are on the cancer cells. In the rest of the body, however, the protein is almost non-existent.

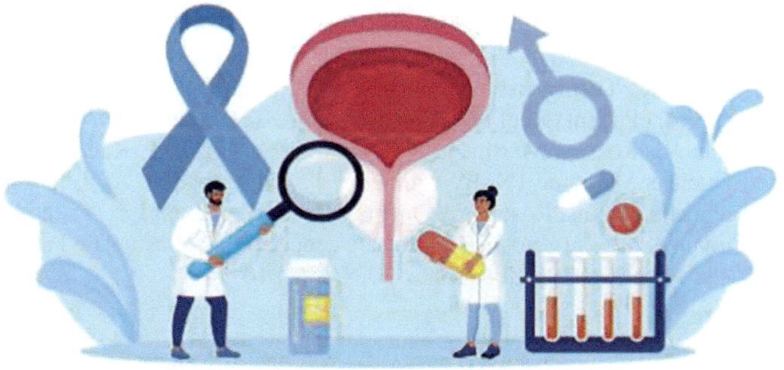

Fig. 19.16a Interview with case presentations (Le Patient) [6]

b

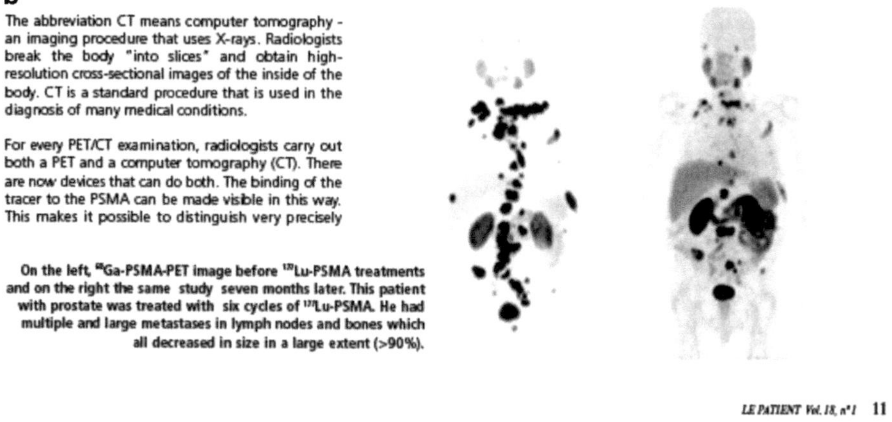

The abbreviation CT means computer tomography - an imaging procedure that uses X-rays. Radiologists break the body "into slices" and obtain high-resolution cross-sectional images of the inside of the body. CT is a standard procedure that is used in the diagnosis of many medical conditions.

For every PET/CT examination, radiologists carry out both a PET and a computer tomography (CT). There are now devices that can do both. The binding of the tracer to the PSMA can be made visible in this way. This makes it possible to distinguish very precisely

On the left, ^{68}Ga-PSMA-PET image before ^{177}Lu-PSMA treatments and on the right the same study seven months later. This patient with prostate was treated with six cycles of ^{177}Lu-PSMA. He had multiple and large metastases in lymph nodes and bones which all decreased in size in a large extent (>90%).

LE PATIENT Vol. 18, n°1 **11**

Fig. 19.16b A case with excellent response (Le Patient) [6]

References

1. Kairemo K, Czernin J. Advancing nuclear medicine at the multiomics intersection: Johannes Czernin discusses innovation and translation with Kalevi Kairemo. J Nucl Med. 2023;64:1671–3.
2. Kairemo K. Targeted alpha therapy: a new tool for advanced prostate cancer. Lancet Oncol. 2024;25:148–9.
3. Kairemo K, Macapinlac H, editors. Sodium fluoride PET/CT in clinical use. Clinicians' guides to radionuclide hybrid imaging. Cham: Springer; 2020. https://doi.org/10.1007/978-3-030-23577-2_7. (Print ISBN 978-3-030-23576-5), 2020 Springer Nature Switzerland AG
4. Kairemo K. Theragnostics: Lu-177-PSMA treatment for metastatic prostate cancer—case examples, ePatient. Nucl Med Mol Imaging. 2023;7(1):44–6.
5. Urbain JL, Ross A, Martineau P, Singnurkar A, Cohen P, Kairemo K. Canadian Association of Nuclear Medicine PSMA "guidelines", The Canadian Association of Nuclear Medicine, Succursale 4 coins, Rosemère, Québec, J7A 4B1, Canada.
6. Kairemo K. Thera(g)nostics in prostate cancer-prostagnostics Le Patient -Le seul magazine de tous le sprofessionells de la sante. 2024;18(1):10–1.

Appendix (Table A.1, Fig. A.1, Table A.2)

Table A.1 Histopathological grading of prostatic carcinoma

ISUP grade	Gleason scores	Definition
Grade 1	2–6	Only individual discrete well-formed glands
Grade 2	3 + 4 = 7	Predominantly well-formed glands with lesser component of poorly formed/fused/cribriform glands
Grade 3	4 + 3 = 7	Predominantly poorly formed/fused/cribriform glands with lesser component of well-formed glands
Grade 4	4 + 4 = 8	Only poorly formed/fused/cribriform glands
	3 + 5 = 8	Predominantly well-formed glands and lesser component lacking glands (or with necrosis)
	5 + 3 = 8	Predominantly lacking glands (or with necrosis) and lesser component of well-formed glands
Grade 5	9–10	Lacking gland formation (or with necrosis) with or without poorly formed/fused/cribriform glands

Modified from [1]

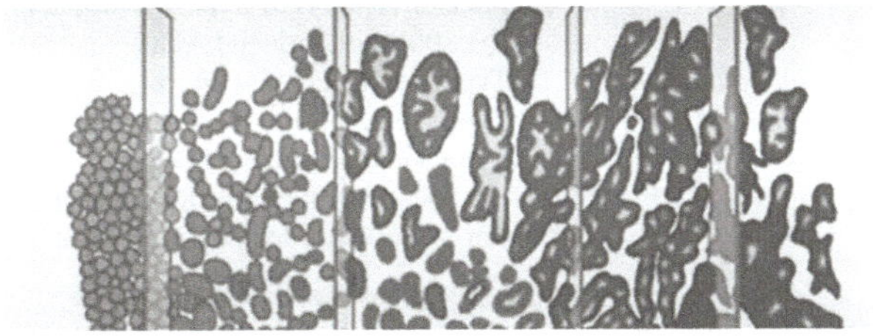

Fig. A.1 Schematic presentation of ISUP score from 1 (most left) to 5 (most right)

K. Kairemo, *Prostate Cancer from a Nuclear Oncology Perspective*,
https://doi.org/10.1007/978-3-031-90337-3

For morphological imaging and for the classification, the MRI evaluation Prostate Imaging Reporting and Data System (PI-RADS) has been developed [2–4] (Fig. A.2 and Table A.3).

Table A.2 PI-RADS scoring system

	Criteria	Score
T2WI (T2 weighed imaging) for the peripheral zone (PZ)	Uniform high signal intensity (SI)	1
	Linear, wedge shaped, or geographic areas of lower SI, usually not well demarcated	2
	Intermediate appearances not in categories 1/2 or 4/5	3
	Discrete, homogeneous low signal focus/mass confined to the prostate	4
	Discrete, homogeneous low signal intensity focus with extracapsular extension/invasive behavior or mass effect on the capsule (bulging), or broad (>1.5 cm) contact with the surface	5
T2WI (T2 weighed imaging) for the transition zone (TZ)	Heterogeneous TZ adenoma with well-defined margins: "organized chaos"	1
	Areas of more homogeneous low SI, however well marginated, originating from the TZ/BPH	2
	Intermediate appearances not in categories 1/2 or 4/5	3
	Areas of more homogeneous low SI, ill defined: "erased charcoal sign"	4
	Same as 4, but involving the anterior fibromuscular stroma or the anterior horn of the PZ, usually lenticular or water drop shaped	5
Diffusion weighted imaging (DWI)	No reduction in ADC compared with normal glandular tissue. No increase in SI on any high b-value image (≥b800)	1
	Diffuse, hyper SI on ≥b800 image with low ADC; no focal features, however, linear, triangular, or geographical features are allowed	2
	Intermediate appearances not in categories 1/2 or 4/5	3
	Focal area(s) of reduced ADC but iso-intense SI on high b-value images (≥b800)	4
	Focal area/mass of hyper SI on the high b-value images (≥b800) with reduced ADC	5
Dynamic contrast enhanced (DCE)-MRI	Type 1 enhancement curve	1
	Type 2 enhancement curve	2
	Type 3 enhancement curve	3
	For focal enhancing lesion with curve type 2–3	+1
	For asymmetric lesion or lesion at an unusual place with curve type 2–3	+1

Modified from [4]

Abbreviations: *ADC* apparent diffusion coefficient, *BPH* benign prostatic hyperplasia, *DCE* dynamic contrast enhanced, *DWI* diffusion weighted imaging, *PZ* peripheral zone, *SI* signal intensity, *TZ* transition zone

Fig. A.2 Schematic presentation of the location of prostatic zones

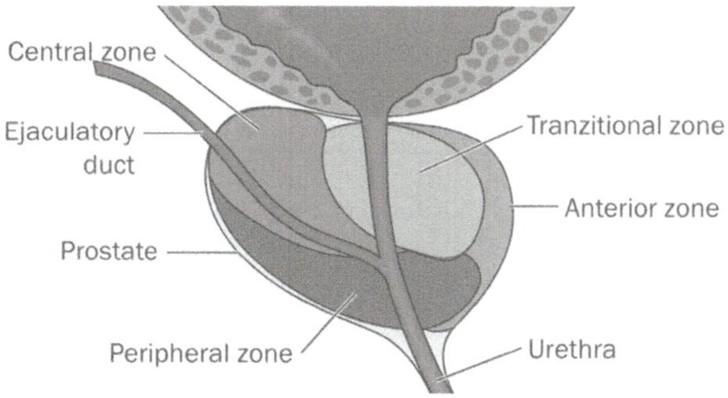

Table A.3 Scoring of extra-prostatic disease at MRI

Criteria	Findings	Score
Extracapsular extension	Abutment	1
	Irregularity	3
	Neurovascular bundle thickening	4
	Bulge, loss of capsule	4
	Measurable extracapsular disease	5
Seminal vesicles	Expansion	1
	Low T2 signal	2
	Filling in of angle	3
	Enhancement and impeded diffusion	4
Distal sphincter	Adjacent tumor	3
	Effacement of low signal sphincter muscle	3
	Abnormal enhancement extending into sphincter	4
Bladder nec	Adjacent tumor	2
	Loss of low T2 signal in bladder muscle	3
	Abnormal enhancement extending into bladder neck	4

References

1. Epstein JI, Allsbrook WC Jr, Amin MB, Egevad LL. ISUP Grading Committee. The 2005 International Society of Urological Pathology (ISUP) consensus conference on Gleason grading of prostatic carcinoma. Am J Surg Pathol. 2005;29:1228–42.
2. Barentsz JO, Richenberg J, Clements R, et al. ESUR prostate MR guidelines 2012. Eur Radiol. 2012;22:746–57.
3. Rosenkrantz AB, Kim S, Lim RP, et al. Prostate cancer localization using multiparametric MR imaging: comparison of Prostate Imaging Reporting and Data System (PI-RADS) and Likert scales. Radiology. 2013;269:482–92.
4. Röthke M, Blondin D, Schlemmer HP, Franiel T. PI-RADS-Klassifikation: Strukturiertes Befundungsschema für die MRT der Prostata [PI-RADS classification: structured reporting for MRI of the prostate]. Rofo. 2013;185:253–61.

GPSR Compliance

The European Union's (EU) General Product Safety Regulation (GPSR) is a set of rules that requires consumer products to be safe and our obligations to ensure this.

If you have any concerns about our products, you can contact us on ProductSafety@springernature.com

In case Publisher is established outside the EU, the EU authorized representative is:

Springer Nature Customer Service Center GmbH
Europaplatz 3
69115 Heidelberg, Germany

Batch number: 10732044

Printed by Printforce, the Netherlands